LABOUR OF LOVE

To my parents
Jean Strachan and Neville Strachan

LABOUR OF LOVE

The History of the Nurses' Association in Queensland, 1860–1950

GLENDA STRACHAN

ALLEN & UNWIN

Cover photographs: reproduction courtesy of (top and bottom left) Collection: John Oxley Library, Brisbane; (bottom right) Collection: John Oxley Library, Brisbane and Queensland Nurses' Union; badge courtesy of Queensland Nurses' Union.

Published with the assistance of the Queensland Nurses' Union

First published in 1996 by
Allen & Unwin Pty Ltd
9 Atchison Street, St Leonards, NSW 2065 Australia
Phone: (61 2) 9901 4088
Fax: (61 2) 9906 2218
E-mail: 100252.103@compuserve.com

National Library of Australia
Cataloguing-in-Publication entry:

Strachan, Glenda, 1951–
Labour of love: the history of the nurses' association in Queensland 1860–1950.

Bibliography.
Includes index.
ISBN 1 86448 053 X.

1. Australasian Trained Nurses' Association. Queensland Branch.
2. Nurses—Queensland—History. I. Queensland Nurses' Union of Employees. II. Title.

610.73060943

Set in 10.5/12 Goudy by DOCUPRO, Sydney
Printed by SRM Production Services Sdn Bhd, Malaysia

10 9 8 7 6 5 4 3 2 1

Contents

List of tables and illustrations

List of abbreviations

AANS	Australian Army Nursing Service
ACTU	Australian Council of Trade Unions
AIF	Australian Imperial Forces
ALP	Australian Labor Party
ANF	Australian Nursing Federation
ANJ	*Australasian Nurses' Journal*
ATNA	Australasian Trained Nurses' Association
BMA	British Medical Association
CAR	Commonwealth Arbitration Reports
CMCC	Central Medical Co-ordination Committee
HEF	Hospital Employees' Federation
MCC	Medical Co-ordination Committee
MJA	*Medical Journal of Australia*
NSWPD	*New South Wales Parliamentary Debates*
QGG	*Queensland Government Gazette*
QIC	Queensland Industrial Commission
QNA	Queensland Nurses' Association
QNRB	Queensland Nurses' Registration Board
QNU	Queensland Nurses' Union
QPD	*Queensland Parliamentary Debates*
QPOA	Queensland Professional Officers' Association
QPP	*Queensland Parliamentary Papers*
QSA	Queensland State Archives
QTU	Queensland Teachers' Union
RANF	Royal Australian Nursing Federation
RVTNA	Royal Victorian Trained Nurses' Association
TLC	Trades and Labour Council
VPP	*Victorian Parliamentary Papers*

List of abbreviations

VTNA Victorian Trained Nurses' Association
WEB Women's Employment Board

Currency conversion

Conversion from sterling to decimal currency occurred on 14 February 1966. Prior to this date 12 pence equalled one shilling, 20 shillings equalled one pound. A guinea equalled 21 shillings or one pound one shilling.

At conversion:
1 penny equalled 1 cent (1d = 1c)
6 pennies equalled 5 cents (6d = 5c)
1 shilling equalled 10 cents (1s or 1/- = 10c)
10 shillings equalled 1 dollar (10s or 10/- = $1)
1 pound equalled 2 dollars (1 = $2)

Acknowledgements

My initial inspiration and interest in labour history was kindled while an undergraduate at the University of Queensland by the late Dr Denis Murphy. His assistance and encouragement in my research led me to this topic, a choice I have never regretted as the subject of the nurses and their associations grew ever more fascinating as I investigated it. This book is based on my PhD thesis and I owe a great debt of gratitude to Dr Marion Diamond, my supervisor, for her continual guidance, advice and intellectual rigour and support for the project. It was a great privilege to work with her. While the process of academic research is generally lonely and isolated, I hope that my history of one part of women's working lives will reach those whose lives it is about. I also hope it does their story justice.

Researching and writing the thesis, and subsequently the book, have taken several years and there are many people and organisations who have helped me. The Queensland Nurses' Union have assisted with the publication of this book and I am most grateful for their support. I would like to thank Denis Jones and Gay Hawksworth for their support, as well as other officers of the union for their assistance. When I commenced research on this book the Queensland Branch of the Royal Australian Nursing Federation was the major nurses' union in Queensland and they were most helpful in giving me access to their records. Bartz Schultz, Dr Mary Dickenson and Shirley Donohue offered their friendship as well as help with information. I would like to thank the other branches of the nurses' associations which also allowed me to look at their records. Cecelia Brazil of the Royal Brisbane Hospital Graduate Nurses' Archive has assisted me greatly in the search for illustrations. My thanks are also due to the many librarians and archivists who have helped me along the way.

I would also like to thank the John Oxley Library; Fryer Library; University of Queensland Library; Royal Brisbane Hospital Graduate Nurses' Archive; Royal Brisbane Hospital Archives; Queensland Nurses' Union; Australian Nursing Federation, National Office and Victorian Branch; Department of Employment, Education and Training; Australian Consolidated Press; and Dr Ellen Jordan, for allowing me to reproduce illustrations. Every effort has been made to trace the copyright owners of the illustrations reproduced in this book. Should there be any omissions, the publisher would be grateful to be informed about them so that they may be rectified.

My thanks also go to the following people for their assistance in discussing topics and support in a myriad of ways: Anne Allingham, the late Margaret Cribb, Helen Gregory, Vivien Griffin, Dr Ellen Jordan, Chris Kynaston, Dr George Shaw, Maryanne Winter. Finally I would like to thank Jean Strachan, Neville Strachan, Rupert Owen and Sid Owen for the great support they have given me. This book is for them.

Introduction

Nurses' associations began in Australia in the 1890s as formally trained nurses looked towards the regulation of this occupation. In 1899 the Australasian Trained Nurses' Association (ATNA) was established in Sydney with its first branch formed in Queensland five years later. It served as the professional association for nurses and subsequently as their trade union.

The Queensland Branch maintained its links with the ATNA nationally, and from 1923 was part of a loose national federation of the branches, the Australian Nursing Federation (ANF). In 1955 the federation adopted the prefix 'Royal' and the Queensland Branch of the ATNA became known as the Queensland Branch of the Royal Australian Nursing Federation (RANF). By 1980, the majority of the association's work was carried on by the Royal Australian Nursing Federation, Queensland Branch, Union of Employees, which several years later became the Queensland Nurses Union (QNU). The QNU is today affiliated with the Australian Nursing Federation, the national organisation representing nurses' associations. This book examines the development of nursing in Australia from 1860 and analyses the influence of this on the ATNA in Queensland. It traces the development of this organisation, its aims and activities and emphasises its attitude towards involvement in industrial issues in the period to 1950.

During the second half of the nineteenth century the job of nursing was transformed from being the work of low status male and female servants to the work of educated women who received formal training. By the end of the century, the ideal of the nurse was an educated and trained woman who worked for the love of humanity and not the monetary rewards of the job. Although the reality frequently did not match the ideal, the ethos of the self-sacrificing nurse was a powerful influence on the beliefs and activities of the nursing associations.

Striving to raise the status of their occupation in the eyes of the community, the associations emphasised the ethos of service and sacrifice, with the result that concerns over poor working conditions were not seen as legitimate issues on which to take action.

Nursing associations in Australia, like those in Great Britain and the United States of America, sought to establish the new female occupation of trained nursing on a firm basis within the health-care system. They concentrated their efforts on the creation and regulation of training standards as they attempted to raise the status of nursing. In Australia they were set up to pursue a professional identity and raised status for trained nurses. Formed by influential doctors who frequently ran hospitals themselves, and recently trained nurses who were in charge of a new female hierarchy within these hospitals, the assocations aimed to establish a separate occupation of formally trained general nurses who would be capable of reliably carrying out the orders of the new medical profession. Their concerns centred on the standardisation of training and the gaining of State acceptance for this new profession through State registration, with the consequence that those who lacked the specified training were excluded from this unique group.

Far from wanting better wages and conditions for this new workforce within hospitals, these doctors and nurses were vitally interested in keeping the cost of running their hospitals as low as possible. The executives of the nursing organisations had little interest in regulating the wages and working conditions of the average nurse. Trainee nurses, for instance, who formed the bulk of the hospital workforce, were only granted the right to participate in the union's affairs in Queensland in 1933.[1] The desire of some women for a well-respected occupation and the needs of the community for relatively cheap labour in the changing system of health care coincided, for nursing as a women's occupation could fulfil both aims.

The ethos of nursing, one of serving humanity without thought of monetary reward, has played a critically important part in shaping the ideas of nurses themselves and the community in general, and consequently of the nurses' trade union. The council and executive of the union in Queensland saw nursing as different from other occupations, a view frequently shared by employers who thought that the promise of high wages would not attract the right sort of recruit.[2] The ATNA absorbed this view to an extraordinary degree with the result that it was unable to accept involvement in industrial activities as legitimate and was extremely loath to ask for increased wages and better conditions. The ATNA in Queensland was a very reluctant trade union, forced by outside circumstances to enter the industrial arena. In the period to 1950 it never fully acknowledged its additional industrial role. These attitudes, unusual for a trade union, mean that, until recently, the history of the nurses' union is quite different from that of other unions. The ethos of the occupation itself and its position within the health-care system have exerted the major determining influence on the beliefs and actions of the trade union, to a greater extent than has occurred in relation to other occupations and their trade unions. Because of this, the history of this union needs to be examined within the wider context of the changing occupation of nursing.

Although registered as a trade union in 1921, the operations of the ATNA in Queensland cannot be seen in terms of traditional union aims and objectives.[3] While akin in many of its activities to professional unions, the ATNA saw itself in the category of nurses' associations, with little in common with other groups of professional workers. The ideology of self-sacrifice and therefore difference from other workers, served to keep the association's vision focused solely on nursing. Flanders argues that trade unions are a mixture of movement and organisation, that is a community of purpose and an effective means for ensuring that its members comply with its decisions. He asserts that 'the members of a movement combine because, sharing in some measure the same sentiments and ideas, they want to achieve the same things'.[4] The community of purpose shared by formally trained nurses and doctors in the early years of the twentieth century was that of organising the training and regulation of nurses. Once established, the associations provided services related to this, as regulation ensured that there would be positions kept for trained nurses. But their goals were not 'the economic advancement of their members and . . . improvements in their terms and conditions of employment',[5] and involvement in industrial issues occurred as a result of overwhelming pressure at specific times from groups of members or the community at large.

The segregation of the labour market by gender and the different roles and opportunities offered women are crucial issues in an examination of the nurses' union. As Game and Pringle note, 'gender is fundamental to the way work is organised'.[6] This is a point which cannot be over-emphasised in the case of nursing. Apart from teaching, where women experienced distinct problems, the only socially acceptable work for middle and upper class women in the nineteenth century was that in which they did not compete with men and which mirrored women's caring functions within the family. Women's subordinate place in relation to husbands was replicated by nurses' subordinate position in relation to the male doctors. Thus nursing swiftly gained acceptability as suitable women's work. Conversely, this nurturing role was not seen as the province of men. Employed only until marriage, nurses led cloistered lives, reminiscent of the military and religious origins of the occupation. The development of general nursing as an exclusively female occupation had major ramifications for its role and status within the evolving hierarchical structure of the hospital and the delivery of health care generally, and determined its position in relation to medical practitioners and other health professionals. The fact that general nursing was solely women's work during the period to 1950 has determined many features of the development of its organisations.

Nursing had great difficulty in establishing its status as it was handicapped by its all-female membership, low levels of education and its position of subservience in relation to medicine. As a consequence of this, some nurses have looked to nursing history to assist their claims for professional identity and autonomy, urging that the history of nursing offers 'the promise of a sense of identity, a sense of continuity, and a sense of unity'.[7] Church argues that:

> this absence of a historical perspective could account for the current dilemma that relates to redefining nursing and determining its parameters of professional responsibility within the health care arena. A sense of history seems appropriate as a prerequisite to a professional mentality. For, ignorance of the past contributes to the inability to identify one's boundaries properly and retards the development of the essential autonomy that accompanies professional self-determination.[8]

Or, as Hardy and Rafferty say, history 'produces and sustains a professional image'.[9] In no other occupation do the practitioners seem to pursue this goal so vigorously.

In many ways nursing textbooks that deal with the history of nursing echo these views, although not as openly. In their discussions of nursing history 'from the earliest times' there is a desire to prove that nursing has always been an important and valued part of society. This desire for continuity, the idea of an unbroken line with each change making one more step towards progress, has been present in many nursing histories. These congratulatory histories paint a picture of an increasingly improving world, especially since the scientific advances of the nineteenth century and the changes in the twentieth century are regarded unquestionably as reforms for the better.

Many histories of nursing have adopted this global perspective. The four-volume *A History of Nursing* by the eminent American nurses Adelaide Nutting and Lavinia Dock, appeared from 1907 to 1912.[10] Commencing with chapters titled '"First Aid" Among Animals' and 'Care of the Sick of Primitive Man', it discussed nursing in Asia, the

Middle East, Greece and Rome before proceeding through the Middle Ages to the nineteenth century. The authors attempted to endow nursing 'with a past of active humane service going back to ancient civilizations'.[11] This approach has been replicated many times in nursing history texts and other recent nursing publications.[12]

All nursing texts emphasise the role of the individual in the development of nursing, particularly the role of Florence Nightingale. As James notes, 'an independent practitioner in the grand style is a powerful image in nursing, where very stressful vital services are performed with little individual recognition'. [13] Many recent textbooks have followed the path of Nutting and Dock and the early British work of Pavey.[14] This emphasis on the history of nursing from earliest times has persisted in Bullough and Bullough's *The Emergence of Modern Nursing* and Mellish's *A Basic History of Nursing*, published in a new edition in 1990.[15] Most histories of nursing, many of which have been designed primarily as textbooks for nurses, have relied solely on secondary sources and promoted what has gradually become a received wisdom. Nursing has not been seen within the context of work generally or the division of labour in society, as identified in the work of Gamarnikow[16] and Game and Pringle. Writers of these histories have seen their role as identifying the past in order to establish an identity of sacrifice and service for nurses today.

Many writers of texts on nursing history and articles in nursing journals stress that the history of nursing can assist in the struggle for professional status. Nutting and Dock's works, written at a time when trained nurses were trying hard to establish nursing as a separate profession, attempted to achieve this by examining and praising the movement for State registration, a movement that 'is new and of great significance'. This was of critical importance for Dock, especially as she was concerned with a perceived dilution of standards caused by 'faulty education' and the 'vast influx of young girls' into the occupation in the early part of the twentieth century.[17] Dock praised the work of the nursing organisations in Australia and the 'high uniform standard' in training that had been achieved.[18]

Nursing has usually been identified as something more than a mere job and this has been emphasised in nursing histories. Nutting and Dock believed that:

> the art of nursing, at once the oldest of the occupations of women and the youngest branch of medical science, must have been co-existent with the first mother who performed for her little ones all those services which made it possible for them to live and thrive . . . these

> maternal cares, as old as or even older than the human race, aid the foundation from which our profession of nursing has developed to its structure of to-day.[19]

Thus the first major history of nursing clearly identified nursing as woman's natural role.

Nursing has frequently been seen by nurses as different from other occupations. Lawler writes that 'what separates the (proper) nurse from those who are technically competent to perform nursing care is not *what* is done, but rather *how* it is done—that is, nursing is more a social entity than anything else'.[20] This echoes earlier writers like Isabel Stewart, noted American nurse educator, who believed that:

> the real essence of nursing, as of any fine art, lies not in the mechanical details of execution, nor yet in the dexterity of the performer, but in the creative imagination, the sensitive spirit, and the intelligent understanding lying back of these techniques and skills. Without these, nursing may become a highly skilled trade, but it cannot be a profession or a fine art.[21]

For 'the head, the heart, and the hands became truly united to provide the strong foundation for modern-day nursing'.[22] Emphasis is placed on the unique qualities of nursing and the element of devotion which supposedly makes nurses' work different from that of other mere workers:

> Lay nurses have the same right as do those in other vocations to be concerned about adequate income and working conditions, but it would be an unhappy outcome if nurses were to limit their outlook to these considerations. Society expects that nurses, like teachers, physicians, and clergymen, will be animated also by a desire to serve. If this spirit is maintained, nursing will continue to be a calling as well as a vocation; and the rewards of a calling transcend those of a trade.[23]

These values have produced nursing histories which eulogise the work of the nurse and emphasise self-sacrifice and have had the practical purpose of assisting the socialisation process of trainees. Yet the reality for most nurses was that they worked to earn a living. There was often a dichotomy between the needs of the ordinary nurse for an income and decent working conditions and the desires of nursing leaders, who emphasised the idea of selfless service to humanity in order to raise the status of the occupation in the eyes of the community.

In the last decade there has been an additional approach to nursing history by scholars who seek to place nurses' history within the wider social context of women's place in society. This approach has relied on researching original sources to detail the changes in nursing since the eighteenth century. In the early 1980s three collections of articles challenged the assumption of history as progress and did not aim to inculcate students of nursing with a wonderful faith in the profession and their unique position in society. As their titles implied (*Rewriting Nursing History*; *New Perspectives, New Possibilities*; *Nursing History: The State of the Art*), they were taking a different approach.[24] The subsequent works of Melosh and Reverby in America and Maggs in Britain placed nursing within the broader context of women's work and owed much to recent ideas about feminist history and the place of women in society. Melosh examined the culture of nursing and the experiences of ordinary nurses and questioned the view that nursing leaders necessarily represented the interests of the majority of nurses. Her work provided a new perspective on nursing history for, as she says, 'nursing offers an illuminating example of the ways in which gender informs work, and conversely, how work both reproduces and transforms existing relationships of power and inequality. Medical division of labor replicates a larger sexual division of labor'.[25]

Reverby drew on Melosh's work and looked at an earlier period in American history, examining the transition to trained nursing. She believes that 'nursing is a form of labor shaped by the obligation to care. But its history, and ultimately its identity, cannot be understood unless the bond that has wedded it to womanhood is also unravelled and revealed'.[26] In Britain, the work of Maggs added to the understanding of the changes that occurred in the occupation of nursing with his study of the nurses who completed formal training between 1881 and 1914. Once again, Maggs emphasised the group of nurses and not the nursing leaders.[27] Much recent work in Australia has not used these insights but has been purely descriptive and failed to place nursing within the wider context of events. It has accepted that the views of nursing leaders, including those in the nursing organisations, represented those of all nurses.[28]

The nature of nurses' work and the tasks which nurses performed are separate subjects to those dealt with in this book. They were dependent on the changes in medical and thus nursing practice and the 'demarcation' questions which could arise between nurses and other health practitioners. A large component of nurses' activities, particularly trainee and assistant nurses, related to cleaning and housework. For instance, trainee nurses performed the following tasks in the 1930s: scrubbing and re-papering lockers, boiling face washers and hanging them out to dry, cobwebbing, cleaning baths and toilets as well as pan rooms and their utensils, cleaning sterilisers, carbolising beds, sweeping floors, dusting, preparing and distributing morning and afternoon teas and suppers, washing up, cooking supper for night staff, serving and delivering patients' meals, collecting used dishes, and answering the telephone.[29] Severe shortages of nurses and domestic staff during the Second World War meant that these activities still formed a significant part of a nurse's work.

The issue of nurses doing 'non-nursing' duties has been discussed frequently as this was linked to 'battles' by nurses to divest themselves of much of this work. Yet other duties and the nursing treatment of diseases and injuries have not been so widely discussed. The period to 1950 predates the widespread use of antibiotics with sulphur drugs being used in 1940s. In the late nineteenth and early twentieth century the most common reasons for admission to the Brisbane Hospital were fractures, contusions, injuries and typhoid. These were followed by pulmonary tuberculosis, known as 'the white plague', which was the most common cause of death at the hospital.[30] Little surgery was performed in the nineteenth century apart from amputations and the Brisbane Hospital operating theatre was known as the Amputation Room.[31]

Many diseases were treated using intensive nursing care. This involved procedures such as the application of poultices and giving frequent cold baths in an effort to reduce the temperature of typhoid patients. Dr F.E. Hare, who developed a special system for this in the 1890s, noted that 'in private practice . . . if no specially-trained nurse is procurable, it will be necessary for the physician to supervise personally the first few baths, and to give detailed instructions concerning them; in fact, some time should be given at the beginning of the case to the careful training of the nurse'.[32] Hot foments and baths were a feature of the treatment of infantile paralysis.[33] Meticulous observation and charting of symptoms were a necessary part of these treatments and done by nurses. Nurses dressed wounds, prepared and fed special diets to patients, and performed 'household' tasks such as bedmaking. Cleanliness was stressed as a major feature of their work. In addition, trained nurses supervised other staff, such as trainees and the male orderlies who assisted in the fever wards.

In the early part of the twentieth century there was a move from antiseptic to aseptic surgery, the development of abdominal surgery, the introduction of pathology, bacteriology, radiology and blood transfusions. From 1900 to 1920 the Brisbane Hospital introduced medical specialities in gynaecology, radiology, pathology and dermatology, and an orthopaedic department was established in the 1920s.[34] But the nursing duties of students in the 1930s were similar to those of their predecessors: first year students sponged patients, gave out and collected bed pans, helped patients in and out of bed, measured patients' temperatures and applied poultices and foments. By second year students did small dressings, gave out extra fluids and sometimes escorted patients to and from the operating theatre. Third year students were responsible for dressings and other treatments which were supervised by a registered nurse. They were also responsible for the administration of medications, both orally and by injection. Fourth year nurses assisted the registered nurse in recording information in patients' charts and supervising the work of more junior nurses.[35]

This book examines the nurses' union in Queensland and emphasises the strong influence that the occupation of nursing had on the nature and activities of the union. The idea of nursing as sacrifice became the crux of the ethos of nursing and this had profound effects on the attitudes of the ATNA in Queensland, for nurses could not be seen to be sacrificing themselves and still receive good wages. Prestige for nurses often had to be gained through the ethic of self-sacrifice, and this belief was absorbed to a large degree by practitioners and was evident in practices such as starting work early and leaving late without asking for payment. Although nurses generally earned more than the female basic wage, their pay compared poorly to that of other female skilled workers and their hours of work were usually longer. Working within a rigid hierarchy of command in the hospital or beholden to the doctor in private practice, qualities of obedience, reminiscent of the military, were required of them. Nurses were reticent to ask for better conditions as working in adequate conditions for good pay would make it difficult to sustain the argument of selflessly serving humanity. These views were particularly important for nursing leaders (matrons and owners of private hospitals), who frequently saw longer hours as a benefit.

The voices of ordinary working nurses are not often heard, though at times their efforts to become involved in the ATNA provide some insight into their goals. On occasions nurses did break from the mould of unquestioning obedience and strive for better pay and conditions, even to the extent of threatening industrial action during the 1940s. At other times a picture of their lives can be gained through evidence given to Royal Commissions, (for example the 1892 Royal Commission on Charitable Institutions in Victoria) a government survey of hospital conditions in 1920 or occasional letters to the nursing journals. An indication of the working conditions of the ordinary nurse has been included in this book wherever possible.

During the last decade there has been some debate about whether nurses should be seen as feminists and part of the struggles for the franchise and women's rights.[36] It is difficult to see the history of nursing in this light. While a few nursing leaders in America were active in, for example, the campaign for the vote, most were not.[37] There is little evidence of such activity occurring in Australia. Spending long hours within the walls of the hospital or the private homes in which they worked, nurses had little time for activities outside the health sphere. The Melbourne campaign by Vida Goldstein for better conditions in 1904 or the Queensland campaign by women teachers for equal pay in the 1880s and 1890s did not have any impact on nurses. Historically their world was shaped by changes in the hospital and health care; their battles directed to establishing a respectable occupation for middle and upper class women. Successful in creating a women's occupation of high status, nursing remained the handmaiden of medicine.

The first chapter of this book traces the development of nursing in Australia from 1860 to 1900, taking account of the influences on the occupation which were occurring in Britain at this time. In Australia by the 1890s, the idea of female trained nurses was widely accepted, if not always implemented. Chapter 2 examines the beginnings of nursing organisations in Australia, especially the establishment of the Queensland Branch of the ATNA in 1904. Chapter 3 analyses the activities of the ATNA in Queensland from 1904 to 1912, emphasising the establishment of training standards for nurses. There were no heated debates about the merits of State registration of nurses as occurred in Britain and State registration was achieved in Queensland in 1912, in one of the first such Acts in the world. Registration set the seal on the efforts of the ATNA in its endeavour to establish trained nursing and chapter 4 examines the achievement of State regulation.

The ATNA started as a professional association and only later reluctantly accepted an industrial role. Trade unions, although numerous and well-developed in Australia by 1900, were not popular among many professional and white-collar workers who frequently preferred a professional association. Those that did exist, such as teachers' unions, eschewed industrial action and remained relatively conservative organisations industrially. So it is not surprising that nurses did not embrace unionism with enthusiasm, however the first steps in this direction came after World War I. Chapter 5 examines the working conditions of hospital nurses in Queensland in the 1920s and analyses the moves which propelled the ATNA into the industrial arena and registration as a trade union. The establishment of another nurses' association, the Queensland Nurses Association (QNA), which was viewed as a rival by the ATNA, provided the impetus for involvement in industrial issues. But operating as a trade union was certainly never considered by the founders and, during the period under study, the association was not comfortable with this role.

Longer working hours were received favourably by the decision makers in the ATNA in the 1930s and Chapter 6 examines these changes. Chapter 7 explores the working conditions of nurses in private practice, who formed the majority of trained nurses throughout the period studied, including the efforts of these nurses to gain increased remuneration and improved conditions through the ATNA. Chapters 8 and 9 deal with the 1940s and cover the effects of the Second World War on the nursing labour force. Shortages in nursing staff in this decade led to community demands for better conditions and the ATNA slowly achieved some changes through the Industrial Court. Settled in its role as a professional association, the ATNA in Queensland remained very uneasy with its industrial role. As the president stated in 1947,

> I have never liked Trade Unionism as applied to the profession of Nursing. The A.T.N.A. (Q) was forced . . . [to become] a union and over all these long years your Council had done its best, so far as possible, to keep that aspect in the background and yet improve Nurses' conditions and salaries.[38]

Nursing continued to be influenced by the conception of Florence Nightingale's work in the 1850s which was highly praised: 'her wondrous and truly heroic deeds—her pure "work and labour of love".'[39]

CHAPTER 1

Nursing in Australia in the nineteenth century

'. . . it is natural to every woman to be, to some extent, a nurse.'[1]

The ATNA was the product of a major movement to transform the work of caring for the sick from an unprestigious job performed by women and men with no formal training to a higher status occupation whose ranks were filled by educated women with a formal training in nursing. The aims of this movement became the central goals of the ATNA and these developments and the assumptions on which they were based set the scene for nursing in the twentieth century. These included a belief in the essentially female nature of the work. Female hierarchies were created within the hospitals to oversee nursing tasks, hierarchies which were divisive because of the strict ranking of grades of nurses and the unquestioning obedience to superiors that was required. This environment did not foster collective action. It was also an unquestioned assumption that this new female nursing was totally subordinate to the emerging male medical profession. Just as surely as women were excluded from this profession they were encouraged to join the nursing ranks where their place mirrored the subordinate position of women generally in Victorian society.

Between 1860 and 1900 the occupation of nursing was transformed and the public perception of what a nurse should be changed dramatically. Three overlapping phases are discernible in the transition from the form of nursing existing in 1800 to that which was common by 1900. Prior to the 1860s, formally untrained women and men worked as nurses in institutions in what was regarded as a lowly occupation. Following changes to the occupation in Britain, nursing in Australia changed in the three decades from 1860 to become almost exclusively an occupation for women of education. By the 1890s the predominant public view was that training was necessary for nurses. The supporters

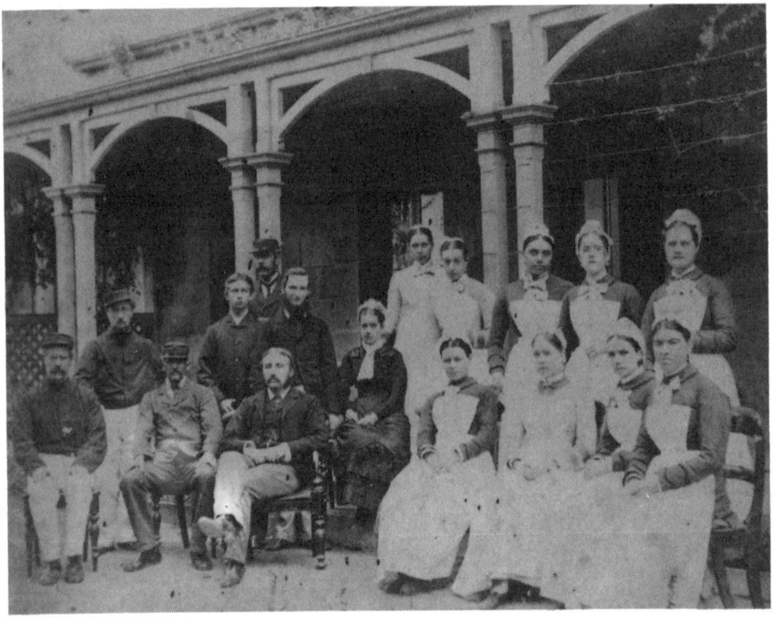

Staff of the Brisbane Hospital, about 1882, outside the Tower Block Building, one of the hospital's main buildings. Nurse training commenced at the hospital in 1886. (Photo courtesy of Royal Brisbane Hospital Archives.)

of female trained nursing were keen to consolidate their position and ensure that the status of the nurse and her living conditions within the hospital were such that they would continue to attract recruits from the educated classes.

There was concern that only those who had been trained should be able to call themselves nurses and the regulation of nursing as a profession for women within the bounds of specific training began. These aims were reflected in the late 1890s in the nursing organisations' concentration on professional goals which attempted to standardise and codify the training and raise the status of the occupation. The nurses and doctors who assumed positions of power in the new organisations were frequently the medical superintendents, matrons and senior medical and nursing personnel who ran the hospitals, indicating the groups for which the associations' goals were important. Such an attitude meant that professional, not industrial, goals were predominant in the nursing organisations.

Nurse as servant—pre-1860

Before about 1860, most nursing was carried out by women who looked after their family, relatives or neighbours in their homes. Women, usually older and often widowed, who needed to earn an income were paid for their services as private nurses in their own communities. Hospitals, which cared for the chronically ill and destitute, were staffed by nurses and wardsmen whose work 'amounted to little more than specialized charring'[2] and which society regarded as lowly and classified as the work of servants. Most hospital nursing was done by wardsmen, with female patients cared for by female nurses, the majority of whom in the 1820s were convicts or ex-convicts.[3] Standards of nursing varied from unsatisfactory to skilled as staff learnt their tasks by experience on the job. In the mid-nineteenth century the qualities of the nursing staff of the Melbourne Hospital were such that 'the typical nurse at the hospital was not a Dickensian vagrant; she was a moderately efficient maidservant'. This was perfectly reasonable as 'she was not expected to be anything else' until changes were made to nursing and publicity was given to Florence Nightingale's ideas.[4]

Nurses were regarded as servants and paid similar wages. In 1843 the average wage for a nurse in New South Wales was 12 pounds 10 shillings a year, comparable to that of a housemaid or a domestic servant, but slightly lower than ladies' maids and kitchen maids, while a governess' salary was 30 pounds.[5] However the position of matron, a job undertaken in female institutions and orphan schools, was different and 'provided employment for a limited number of free women of respectable background and credentials'.[6] Thus the nurse was placed firmly among the servant hierarchy while the matron was chosen for her managerial and supervisory skills, not for her training as a nurse.

For most of the nineteenth century hospitals were used by the chronically ill who had no alternative care. Those with relatives and friends, and those who could afford nursing help, were cared for in their own homes. In the new colony of Queensland there were more people without the support of home or family than in England or the more established colonies. As evidence to the 1866 Select Committee which enquired into the operations of Queensland hospitals showed, newly arrived immigrants, men working on the railways and stations, used the hospitals: 'a certain class of men, shepherds and others, who, from want of sufficient lodging accommodation, and proper attention when ill, prefer coming to the hospital and paying'.[7] The majority of patients however, could not pay. The Brisbane Hospital provided relief to the destitute who were usually women, new arrivals to the colony whose husbands were searching for work in country areas as well as some who were widows. The hospitals were partly funded by subscribers, who paid about one pound a year for the right to have one person admitted and some employers paid an amount per employee so that their workers could receive care when they needed it. Donations were also received but government funding remained a substantial and necessary part of the hospital's income.[8] Unlike Britain there were no pauper hospitals or workhouses and hospitals cared for the acutely ill, the chronic and long-term ill, the destitute, and provided outdoor relief to the destitute who had somewhere else to live.

Husband and wife teams were generally in charge of the domestic and nursing work in Queensland hospitals in 1866. The duties of the nursing staff and their experience for the work likened them to other servants. At Toowoomba Hospital the wardsman's wife acted as cook, laundress and general manager of the household and the nurse was also the cook for the dispenser. The wardsman at Rockhampton was married to the matron of the hospital. In this case the couple resided in the kitchen, with the assistant cook living in a small partitioned section of the kitchen. At Brisbane Hospital the head wardsman and his wife had their own room but other wardsmen and nurses slept in the wards.[9] There was thus little formal division between the public sphere of work and the private sphere of home and family when employed in a hospital.

Transition to female nurses, 1860–1890

Between 1860 and 1890 the community's perceptions of nursing changed, although the pace of this change was uneven. Nursing moved from a form of servant work available to either sex to a unique female occupation which aspired to professional status. By 1890, community preference was for female nurses as women were perceived as having a greater capacity for caring than men. Toward the end of the century the belief grew that this innate womanly ability had to be supplemented with formal training. At the same time nurses were needed to provide extensive hospital labour which gave them the experience that was always regarded as a vital part of training.

The transformation in the occupation of nursing in the Australian colonies followed the pattern in England where reformers, including the widely-publicised Florence Nightingale, had begun to make changes. News of her adventures and ideas spread rapidly to the Australian colonies. A committee was formed in Melbourne in 1856 to gather subscriptions to the British fund for the maintenance of women training to be nurses.[10] The 1866 Queensland Select Committee on the Hospitals of the Colony, concerned primarily about the funding of charitable relief in the colony, was well aware of the English innovation of trained female nurses, and they questioned hospital representatives about this. Dr Joseph Lansdowne, House Surgeon of the Brisbane Hospital, believed that it would be advantageous to appoint female nurses from Sydney or London where they had received proper training. Rev. Edward Griffith, a member of the Brisbane Hospital Committee, felt that there should be 'a superior excellent matron' and agreed with the Select Committee that a few trained nurses should be engaged from the 'Nightingale Institution' in London.[11] The Brisbane Hospital Committee discussed the importance of bringing trained nurses from England to work in the hospital in 1867. Despite the Premier's offer of assistance, the hospital committee felt that it was not feasible to attempt to import trained nurses from England because it could not guarantee the length of any engagement nor specify the salary. In 1868 Miss Lucy Osburn and five nurses trained at St Thomas' Hospital in London and selected by Florence Nightingale herself, came to work in the Sydney Infirmary. From there some of them moved to other jobs in the colonies[12] including Miss Annie Miller who worked briefly as matron at Brisbane Hospital but resigned over organisational difficulties.[13]

Pressures for changes in hospitals were exerted by the particular colonial conditions which increased their use by the community. Growing urbanisation exacerbated problems such as deserted families, illegitimate children and unemployment, which meant that more people were in need of care and assistance. As longevity increased there were more aged and infirm who needed care.[14] Crisis situations, such as the smallpox epidemic in Sydney in 1881, increased the government's role as supplier of medical services and the Depression of the 1890s added to the population who were forced to depend on hospitals and other charitable services.

In New South Wales between 1875 and 1900 the rate of hospital use grew twice as fast as the growth in population and 'the pressure for respectable hospitals meant increasingly that the respectable came to use them'.[15] Government funding for hospitals was significant and in New South Wales it exceeded other forms of funding in most years from 1858 to 1914.[16] From 1876 government subsidies accounted for 60 to 70 per cent of the total receipts of Brisbane Hospital[17] for 'in spite of the traditional frontier emphasis upon self-reliance and individualism, it was inevitable that the state would have to meet the growing need—no other source could supply it, and Australia had a history of wide government activity'.[18] In fact, 'a new generation of refined, prosperous colonists . . . turned to their governments to fund the new generation of general hospitals at a standard worthy of the middle class-dominated societies of colonial Australia. The governments—largely composed of such men—concurred'.[19]

As well as these pressures the changing nature of medical care meant that reliable nurses were needed to carry out doctor's orders. Innovations in cleanliness and the 'Listerian' practices of asepsis, better educated doctors and changes in nursing meant that 'hospital services were in the process of the most substantial revolution in standards they had ever experienced'.[20] From 1860 to 1890, significant changes occurred in the community's perception about what a nurse was and what she did.

Nursing was seen as an acceptable occupation for women because they did not compete with men but in fact carried out their orders in a way which was deemed suitable for women. As the popular English journal, *St Paul's Monthly Magazine* said in 1871,

> here is an opportunity for showing how a woman's work may complement man's in the true order of nature. Where does the character of the 'helpmeet' come out so strikingly as in the sick-room, where the quick eye, the soft hand, the light step, and the ready ear, second the wisdom of the physician, and execute his behests better than he himself could have imagined?[21]

This image replicated the relationship of husband and wife in the middle class home where the Victorian wife provided 'the proper environment of respectability. She became the guardian of morality, the citadel of respectability. "Helpmeet" to her husband required that she be righteous, gentle, sympathetic, and most of all submissive'.[22] This description could easily have been applied to the nurse, and it had ramifications when the new nursing organisations began at the turn of the century. The nurses, subordinate in society in general and in the hospital in particular, willingly let male medical practitioners play a leading role in the first decades of the organisations.

Nursing developed in its peculiar form in England, according to Abel-Smith, in order to meet the social need of providing a suitable occupation for daughters of the higher social classes. Demographic factors in Britain created a pool of single women who, denied marriage, the trades or learned professions, looked for another outlet for their energies. Performing charitable works was sanctioned by society and caring for the sick was an extension of this.[23] The supply of female labour in England did not exist in the Australian colonies. Until the late nineteenth century, males were the majority in the population and assisted immigration schemes encouraged young single women to come to the colonies.[24] There were 105 females to every 100 males in England and Wales in 1871, whereas there were fewer females to males in the Australian colonies, with Queensland having the lowest ratio of 67 females for every 100 males. By 1880 these figures had changed little, with almost 67.5 females to every 100 males.[25] Despite these demographic differences, the Australian colonies followed the British pattern of nursing changes.

By 1890 the overwhelming bulk of nursing work was done by women, at least in the larger hospitals in the cities. The 1891 census in Queensland recorded 128 people in the category of hospital or asylum nurse, only four of them men. There were also 390 midwives in the colony, all female, and 50 people in the category of 'Sick Nurse', only one of whom was male. The ages of these workers show the changes occurring in hospital staff, for the majority of female hospital nurses (73 per cent) were aged under 30, compared to the majority of midwives (96 per cent) who were older than 35.[26] Census data from Victoria shows the changing sexual division of labour in nursing. Until 1881 there were more wardsmen than female nurses in charitable institutions but by 1891 female nurses outnumbered wardsmen by approximately five to one, and by 1901 wardsmen had all but disappeared. In the three decades from 1871 to 1901 the number of female nurses working in charitable institutions increased from 128 to 783, while male numbers declined from 211 to 10.[27] Gradually wardsmen were restricted to areas where their strength was required for lifting patients.[28] Virtually all private nurses were women: 764 nurses worked outside charitable institutions in Victoria in 1871, increasing to 2469 in 1901.[29]

Assessment of the standard of nursing care varied. The 1866 Queensland Select Committee and the 1891 Victorian Royal Commission showed little dissatisfaction with the standard of nurses' work and a Victorian report in the 1860s stated that the inmates were 'cared for better than are many of the labouring classes in their own homes'.[30] In the 1880s the honorary medical officers at Melbourne Hospital reported that some of the nurses were 'intelligent, respectable women, thoroughly capable of doing their work, who had dedicated themselves to the care of the sick despite the absence of official encouragement'.[31] But the *Australian Medical Journal* in 1880 concluded that 'only a small percentage of hospital nursing staff remained to become skilful "in a haphazard sort of way" and that the majority of nurses "come and go aimlessly" '.[32] Although the work of these nurses was not criticised, the

Australian Medical Journal felt that women of a higher class would be better:

> considering the class from which they have been drawn, the head nurses in the Hospital have been remarkably efficient as far as regards their practical work, and many of them have picked up for themselves an amount of knowledge that is creditable to them in the highest degree. Still, none of them pretend to be gentlewomen, or to possess that sympathy and refinement which adds so much to the efficiency of a hospital sister in other places. It is not essential that all the nurses in the hospital should be ladies, but certainly some of them should be.[33]

Being able to do the job of nursing was not sufficient any more as refinement became a necessary quality. The *Australian Medical Journal* concluded that 'unless they are to be treated as ladies, however—that is to say, fairly paid, given a reasonable amount of leisure, a private room, and well-cooked, decently-served food—such a class will never be obtained, either as pupils or nurses'.[34]

By the 1880s, public discussion addressed the perceived need for formal education for nurses. There was much debate in the Melbourne press about nursing and a growing conviction that 'nursing was a sacred office, not a trade'.[35] The Melbourne Hospital, for instance, responded to public pressure to introduce training and a trained nurse was appointed as matron and a systematic training course introduced in 1890.

In 1885, Miss Mary Weedon, trained at the Charing Cross Hospital, was appointed Matron at the Brisbane Hospital. Her appointment marked the separation of nursing and housekeeping duties at the hospital, with the former matron becoming the housekeeper and Weedon supervising the nursing. She also instructed trainee nurses when a training scheme was started in 1886.[36] Shortly before this in early 1885 a six months' training course had been instituted at the Hospital for Sick Children in Brisbane. In 1884 the first qualified midwife, Mrs Doyle, was appointed Matron of the Lady Bowen Hospital, which dealt exclusively with maternity cases, and by 1890 she was assisted by one trained nurse and three pupil nurses.[37] There were few trained staff in the colonies until local hospitals instituted courses. In the 1880s there was a shortage of nurses in Brisbane and vacancies for nurses at the Brisbane Hospital were filled from the group of single women immigrants willing to work as domestic servants.[38]

In the transition from nurse as a general servant to the specially skilled nurse, the characteristics of the occupation and of its practition-

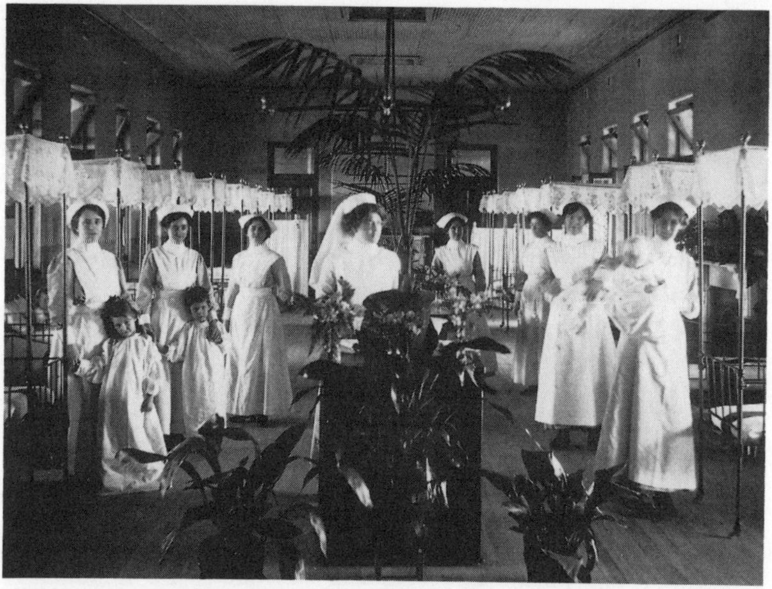

Sister L.A. Hardcastle and nurses and their young patients in the Raff Ward of the Hospital for Sick Children, Brisbane, in the 1890s. Training began at this hospital in 1885 with the first certificates issued the following year. (Collection: John Oxley Library, Brisbane and Royal Brisbane Graduate Nurses' Archive.)

ers changed. By 1890 in Australia, the ideal nurse was seen to be a woman of education and refinement who required a better standard of accommodation and living conditions at the hospital and who did not like the extensive cleaning that was involved in the work. Although public debate was raised in the press about educated women taking up nursing, poor working and living conditions were a great disincentive to these potential recruits. As Inglis has remarked, 'even young ladies who felt the greatest compassion toward the sick found all this hard to endure. They were trying to make nursing a profession, but they were treated still as domestic servants'.[39]

The move to female nursing gathered momentum and, although the question of training generally remained a matter of discussion rather than implementation, there would be no return to the acceptance of untrained nurses. The beginnings of the delineation of the nurse from other servants and hospital workers is seen in the discussions of the problems of accommodation for the nurse and the emphasis on separation from other classes of workers. In the years that followed, nurses' remuneration may not have been very different from that of the domestic staff of the hospital, but their position and uniqueness among hospital staff was.

Acceptance of trained nurses, 1890s

By 1890 there was wide community acceptance that nursing was exclusively a female occupation and most city hospitals had adopted this view. It was obvious that women were the preferred nurses, except for carrying out heavy jobs such as lifting and work in mental hospitals. The larger city hospitals, mirroring the changes in the larger voluntary hospitals in Britain, quickly instituted the employment of female nurses to the exclusion of males and many hospitals began some form of training.

The national picture is difficult to ascertain but the situation in the colony of Victoria is clear from the extensive evidence given to the 1891 Royal Commission on Charitable Institutions in Victoria. No other colony conducted such an enquiry in the 1890s but information about other capital city hospitals presents a similar picture of hospital nursing. Even though all but one of the small hospitals in the country regions of Victoria agreed that female nurses should be employed, many had not implemented this change.[40] Information about the pace of change in the small country hospitals of Queensland is not obtainable from other sources, but there are similarities between the hours and working conditions of the nurses in these small Victorian hospitals and the evidence of the 1921 enquiry into the staffing of Queensland hospitals,[41] so it is likely that the situation was similar.

Witnesses before the Victorian Royal Commission readily accepted the 'naturalness' of women being employed as nurses. Dr Walter Balls-Headley from the Medical Society of Victoria, elaborated why women were better nurses:

> they sit up better and endure better, and I think they are apt to be kinder. Their hands are more delicate; they understand the feeding of people better than men, and they do not, as a rule, drink . . . Then they do not go out and smoke, and loaf; they very often like their work. I think it is natural to every woman to be, to some extent, a nurse.[42]

His final comment reflects the belief that it was in every woman's nature to be a nurse, a belief that included the idea that women were superior to men in this work. Rev. Mervyn Whitton, a hospital

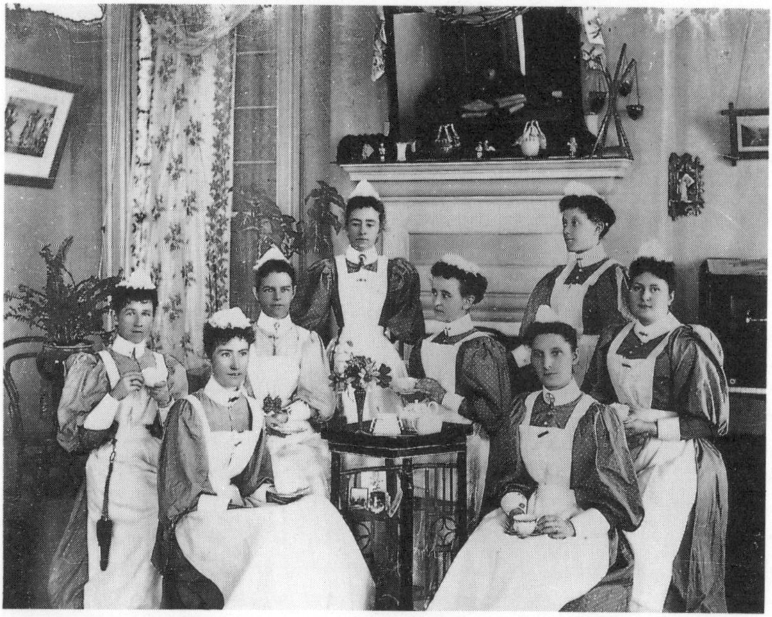

Nurses at the Hospital for Sick Children, Brisbane, 1899, taking tea in a sitting room which was probably adjacent to one of the wards. The transformation of nurses from formally untrained servants to educated ladies performing a unique job is clearly evident in this scene. (Collection: John Oxley Library, Brisbane.)

chaplain, endorsed female nursing, saying that 'females are more patient, enter more into details, are more sympathetic, and in nearly every way are better qualfied than men for sick nursing'.[43] Dr Robert Duncan, a surgeon working at Kyneton Hospital, believed that 'male nurses, except in very exceptional instances, are out of place as attendants on the sick, and it is astonishing how such a barbarous custom could have survived for the length of time it did'.[44]

The transformation to female nursing was associated with a change in the class of the applicants, at least in the minds of the hospital administrators, even if not always in reality. But this increased the cost of introducing female nurses, particularly the expense of new nurses' quarters, 'because nurses cannot be placed on the same footing as domestic servants, and proper arrangements must be made for their comfort'.[45] For country hospitals accommodation was not the only problem. The medical officer at Stawell Hospital saw another difficulty in that 'a trained nurse will not sit down and eat with the laundress, the cook, and the gardener'. Yet he felt that it was essential to have a woman in authority over the servants for 'there is no man living who can control more than one woman at a time. I cannot always be about the hospital, and I cannot always be hanging about to see that the girls are not gallivanting, as they always do when they get half a chance'.[46]

It was difficult to entice educated women to enter nursing while it contained such routine, hard domestic labour. The changes in nursing and hospital practice emphasised the necessity of cleanliness and meant that nurses were expected to know how to keep a room completely clean. For 'cleaning, domestic, or menial tasks were . . . performed because they were part of the science of nursing, asepsis and antisepsis, or were part of the characteristics of the new nurse'.[47] But the 'charring' was a discouragement to the middle class women whom hospitals were trying to attract as trainees and this work was transferred to other female servants, 'scrubbers' or ward maids. Although most trainees still did some domestic work, they did not have to do it routinely.[48] But the removal of this work from nurses at the Alfred Hospital in 1890 caused dissatisfaction among the ward servants, and several left.[49] There was controversy at Warrnambool Hospital over whether the nurse in the fever ward should do the scrubbing. The medical officer felt that:

> it depends a great deal on how many patients she has in. At the present moment there is only one patient in the ward, suffering from scarlet fever, and he is not very bad, so she can quite well do the scrubbing. If she had half-a-dozen patients to attend to she could not do the scrubbing. Speaking in the abstract I think it is a bad thing for a nurse to have to do the scrubbing.[50]

Theoretical arguments were clouded by the exigencies of staffing a small hospital with its fluctuations in patient numbers.

Although there was public pressure to introduce training, the question of what constituted training was a vexed one. By 1890, city and larger country hospitals had begun formal training courses involving lectures and examinations, but many country hospitals still saw training as experience gained on the job, with possibly some instruction from the doctor. Evidence from the 1891 Royal Commission shows that many hospitals were satisfied with this system. The medical officer at St Arnaud Hospital believed 'practice is better than any lectures you can give. You can read that in books. I do not believe in lectures'.[51]

Training in country hospitals might only have been intermittent instruction by the doctor. The surgeon at Hamilton Hospital preferred to train local women than to get 'strange nurses from Melbourne'. Then the training consisted of the irregular lectures he gave at the bedside:

'I train them to my own views of treating and nursing'.[52] At Daylesford Hospital the principal nurse was regarded by the surgeon as 'trained and experienced' as 'she is a widow who has brought up a large family, and has been accustomed to sickness a great deal'.[53] Thus this country hospital still maintained the traditions of previous decades. At Inglewood Hospital the female nurses were not trained but the president of the hospital committee reported that 'we know them by repute. They are generally appointed from the servants who get a good deal of training from being there'. He thought trained nurses would want a much larger salary and he feared that they would want someone to wait on them.[54]

The 1891 Royal Commission in Victoria was strongly in favour of trained female nurses, and carefully questioned and examined any witness who did not support this. It recommended courses of training and even the establishment of a register of trained nurses as this 'would tend to give a professional character to nursing as the handmaid of medicine'.[55] To the commissioners, nursing was not a form of domestic service but a separate function within the hospital, ancillary to the male domain of medicine.

By the 1890s, neither the Brisbane Hospital nor most of the larger hospitals in Victoria had any difficulty in recruiting trainees, despite the arduousness of the work. The spread of compulsory primary education created a larger pool of potential trainees and the 1890s Depression forced more single women to earn their living. However, this did not happen everywhere and benevolent asylums and small country hospitals had more trouble attracting staff.[56] Trainees were generally in their twenties when they began their hospital life. Brisbane Hospital trainees were aged between 19 and 30[57] and the average age at the Alfred Hospital was 25.[58] Miss Isabella Rathie, trained at the Edinburgh Royal Infirmary and Matron of the Melbourne Hospital from 1890, believed that:

> any one who contemplates the profession of nursing ought to be thoroughly healthy, young (not too young), well educated, of medium height, and of an even and sweet temper. The candidate must be prepared to take her life in her hand as it were, and for the coming two or three years as the case may be, make herself and her personal interests second to those of her patients and the hospital in which she is being trained.[59]

Proof of literacy and certificates of good moral character and physical health were usually obligatory.[60] The requirements were general and, as a contemporary nursing advice book stated, the intending probationer 'should be able to read and write clearly and have sufficient mental capacity for understanding the study of medical and surgical cases from the doctors' point of view, not that she might criticise, but intelligently receive his instructions and carry out his orders'.[61] The level of education required for trainees could not be too stringent as large numbers of recruits were needed to staff the hospitals.

By 1890 city and larger country hospitals had instituted formal training courses, although a large component of this training was gained through work in the wards. Modelled on the new training courses in England and America, many larger hospitals in the Australian colonies admitted two categories of trainees, lady probationers and ordinary probationers. This separation reflected the changed beliefs about the suitable class from which nurses should be drawn. Lady probationers paid for their maintenance at hospitals and underwent a shorter course, devoid of much cleaning and housework which was performed by the ordinary probationers. This group, always the numerically larger group, worked longer hours, generally undertook a longer training period and did not pay for their training and maintenance.

In Australia there was public pressure for a two-tiered system of training.[62] Although very few women could spend their whole lives without an income of their own, some could afford to spend a year or two without wages and even pay the hospital for the privilege of training. At the Alfred Hospital in Melbourne, Class A pupils paid a premium of 12 guineas for their twelve-month course, plus one guinea per month and an additional 2 guineas per month if they lived at the hospital. For this they were excused from household work, and worked the comparatively short day of ten hours with no weekend work. Class A candidates 'consisted of young women who expected to work for a living, but who had enough capital to buy freedom from the most onerous of the household chores'. Class B pupils received the same training, had to live in and performed the ordinary work of the wards. Their days were twelve to fourteen hours long, with one day off a week, and in return for their labours, their training and board were free. They received no wages and had to pay one guinea as a deposit which was returned on satisfactory completion of their training. At first there were very few Class A candidates but after the provision of better accommodation they represented about one in four of the trainees.[63] The hospital thus had not only the cheapest labour available but labour that paid the institution to work for it.

Brisbane Hospital implemented a system of two categories of trainees from 1891 with a difference in daily hours and payments. The training period for the ordinary probationers was six months longer than the two-year course for the other group.[64] The system of training provided hospitals with a labour force that was guaranteed to stay for a set time, as long as three years in some cases, at little or no wages. This need for a reliable workforce remained after more systematic training was introduced, and the training needs were often subordinate to the work to be done.

In England, lady probationers were separated from the other probationers by their class origin and their social superiority and 'class snobbery remained explicitly a part of recruitment'.[65] In accordance with the views of Nightingale, the matrons put faith in women of their own class to become nursing leaders in the future and everything was done to encourage them to take on this role. These ladies were supposed to qualify for the superior positions in the new nursing hierarchy.[66] This may have occurred frequently in England but in the colonies it was so difficult to employ a woman who had received any formal training as a matron, that the financial terms of their training were probably of little relevance.

In England as well as in the Australian colonies, the special class of probationer remained a numerically smaller group than the regular probationers. Maggs has characterised the first generation of trained general nurses in England as 'women who turned to nursing as a choice of work, paid work, rather than one of the many other occupations then available to women'.[67] This view was mirrored by the surgeon at Bendigo District Hospital when he was asked at the 1891 Royal Commission: 'Are there any of your nurses who take up the work from the enthusiasm of the work, apart from the pay?' He replied that he thought that 'all the young ladies who have come there to learn nursing have come with the intention of making a livelihood by nursing. I do not know of one who has come without that intention'.[68] This practical reality was not often popularly portrayed or incorporated into the mystique of the self-sacrificing nurse. Most nurses had to earn a living, but this was generally forgotten in the image of total dedication that could be created by nurses working long hours under difficult conditions for little remuneration.

In most hospitals in Victoria the class origins of the trainees were mixed.[69] The social stratum from which nurses came to the Alfred Hospital was typical with the majority coming 'from the lower middle class or that of the superior domestic servant'.[70] At Bendigo Hospital Miss Dorothy Smith, one of the nurses, told the 1891 commission that the majority of nurses were from 'the class of domestic servants' and were 'simply there in order to gain a livelihood'. She did not think that it was 'from the love of nursing that the majority go there'. She added that they took it up 'as a profession; but there is a great advantage to them because they have shorter hours than they would have in domestic service, from which most of them come, and there is a better position'.[71] Miss Catherine Caffyn, a private nurse who had trained at St Thomas' Hospital, felt that there were 'a good many' applicants for nurses' jobs from the housemaid class, 'who are not common women, but they are not quite ladies, and they want to raise their position by becoming nurses'. She would not debar these women from training,

> certainly not if they have a real vocation, or go into it from a better motive than earning a livelihood. I think they will never make as trustworthy nurses as women of education, because women of education like the work from a scientific point of view, whereas it often becomes a drudgery to people of the other class.[72]

Yet the ideal remained, even though it was contradicted by reality. One member of the British Medical Association (BMA) thought that 'the higher they are educated the more gentle they are, and kinder, and better to the patients'.[73] Miss Alice Martelli, a nurse who had trained at the Alfred Hospital, told the Victorian Royal Commission: 'I think the educated brain will do better at any work, especially as women of this class take it up with the view of perfecting themselves in the art. The domestic servant class take it up, as it would any domestic service, to make wages'. Later in her evidence Martelli stated that nurses were underpaid and if nurses were paid more the services would be 'performed by a better class, and therefore more efficiently performed'.[74]

Nurses worked long hours. The evidence of the 1891 Victorian Royal Commission shows daily shifts of ten to fifteen hours, with time off each week varying from half a day to one and a half days.[75] In 1890, the Brisbane Hospital reduced nurses' hours from fourteen to twelve a day.[76] Nurses in small country hospitals often worked long and irregular hours as fluctuating patient numbers demanded. Miss Margaret Watson, trained at the Alfred Hospital, was the sole nurse in charge of the female part of the Horsham Hospital and in her month at the hospital, she claimed, she had not had a whole night in bed. She felt that her work was no harder than at the Melbourne Hospital, for with only five patients she had very little to do, but 'it is hard in this way that I am on duty all the time, night and day. Any night I may expect to be called up by some of the patients'.[77] Other workers such as shop assistants toiled long hours, also often working from early morning until 9 pm on weekdays and until 10 pm or 11 pm on Saturdays.[78] Pupil-teachers, the majority of whom were women, also led a gruelling life characterised by large, unruly classes and long hours which led to charges of sweated labour being made in Parliament.[79]

Although there was some expectation in the community that women should not work longer than 48 hours a week, this was not the general view in relation to nurses. For instance, neither the resident surgeon nor Miss Dorothy Smith, a nurse at the Bendigo District Hospital for four years, felt that the nurses' twelve-hour days (with one afternoon off each week and alternate Sundays free) was excessive. The hours were shorter than in domestic service, Smith argued, for they were free after 6 pm, whereas in service they could be called on to do anything until 10 pm or 11 pm.[80] Others thought the hours were too long and 'cruelty'.[81] Ten hours were long enough, for the nurses looked tired and exhausted and often complained.[82] Some even thought that eight hours was sufficient and Dr Thomas Rowan of the Victorian Branch of the BMA believed this should be the maximum or nurses soon became ill. He added that 'I do not see why the law should make women work longer than men; I have always thought it a hardship'.[83]

The hospital matrons generally considered that shorter hours should be worked but they were loath to implement this because of the extra expense it would entail. Miss Henrietta Strong, Matron of the Alfred Hospital, believed that eight hours per day should be worked but this would be difficult to do in a charitable institution because of the added expense of extra staff and their accommodation.[84] However Isabella Rathie, Matron of Melbourne Hospital, felt that a maximum of eleven or twelve hours was acceptable, with nurses on duty from 7 am to 9 pm.[85] The matrons were thus firmly part of the hospital management and efficient mouthpieces of hospital committees. Yet according to Miss Alice Martelli, 'nine hours is quite sufficient for any woman to work at anything, more especially at the task of nursing the sick, with the responsibility attached to it, and the cool nerve, light hand, and even temper she has to keep'. She added that 'you will not get more than nine hours' good work out of any women, and the patients suffer'.[86]

By the 1890s there was some regulation of working hours of women and children in Australia. For instance, in Victoria legislation prevented women and children from working more than 48 hours a week without express permission, although such permission seems to have been easy to obtain.[87] Such industrial legislation never included nurses. In 1896, an amendment to the Factories and Shops Legislation[88] proposed that no woman or boy under sixteen years of age should work as a nurse for longer than 52 hours a week but the amendment was lost because the charities persuaded the opposition that these nine-hour shifts would be unworkable and that the government was meddling in the private affairs of autonomous institutions. Although one proponent of the clause could class nurses amongst the most sweated workers in the community, others felt that certificated nurses did not want to be classed with factory workers.

W.H. Embling, Legislative Council member and chairman of the Alfred Hospital's medical staff agreed that nurses worked long hours but they 'were so imbued with a love for the work, so self-denying, and so thoroughly womanly, that they could scarcely be prevented from working too hard'. Trained hospital nurses 'were ladies—some of them ladies of birth, and all of them ladies of education'.[89] Queensland's *Factories and Shops Act of 1896* likewise did not cover the work of nurses and although the subsequent Act in 1900 stipulated the amount of overtime worked by women in factories and shops, it, too, left nurses' conditions unregulated.[90]

Similar debates regarding nurses and labour legislation occurred in the USA early in the twentieth century, but by 1920 California was the only state to include student nurses in laws governing women's working hours. In fact, in 1913 the California State Nurses Association joined with the hospitals to oppose a Bill to restrict the hours of women workers, including student nurses, because 'it did not want nursing classed as a trade and nurses as workers. As the association argued, "Real nursing, self-sacrificing service, cannot be timed by the clock. It never has been, and it never will be" '.[91] On the other hand the hospital association—

> willingly classed nursing as a profession, albeit a womanly one, to justify exclusion from the law. Nursing stands, they asserted, 'in the same relation to the sick of the world as the medical profession. The work of nurses can no more be regulated by a hard-and-fast law than the work of doctors or mothers'.[92]

A similar ethos prevailed in Queensland. There was, consequently, no attempt to bring nurses under labour legislation during the nineteenth century. Not until 1921, with the first nurses' award, were the hours of some hospital nurses in Queensland finally regulated.

Although by the 1890s nurses were increasingly differentiated from servants because of their specialisation and training, their salaries remained close to those of domestic servants, as they had 30 years earlier. This was even the case for formally qualified nurses. At the Brisbane Hospital probationers earned 12 pounds a year rising to 65 pounds for experienced charge nurses.[93] Figures for Victoria in the 1890s suggest that a recently certificated nurse could expect to earn 30 pounds a year, rising eventually to a maximum of 60 pounds. For most of her working life she would earn less than 50 pounds. Trainees often were not paid for all[94] or part of their training, making them the ultimate in cheap labour. Some trainees even had to pay a premium to the hospital.[95] The Women's Hospital in Brisbane charged trainees a premium of 10 guineas in 1892, increasing to 25 guineas in 1920.[96] Work without payment occurred in other areas as well, and apprentices in the clothing trades normally received no payment for up to twelve months. In an attempt to curtail the abuses of the apprenticeship system the *Factories and Shops Act 1900* (Qld) established a minimum wage for minors of 2 shillings 6 pence per week after one month's probation.[97]

A significant feature of the life of the hospital nurse was that she lived at her place of work. The antecedents of this practice lay in Victorian England where the new classes of nurses needed to be guarded from unwholesome influences. Living-in was generally thought desirable as nurses were seen to need supervision even in their off-duty hours. Its purpose was control of the staff and this belief was clearly stated by the resident surgeon at the Bendigo District Hospital who opposed the idea of nurses living outside the hospital on the grounds that 'it would have to be a home in which they were under careful supervision'.[98]

Yet accommodation was an added expense for hospitals and there were constant complaints about its standard. Quite frequently nurses shared a bedroom, had an inadequate sitting room and poorly cooked and served food.[99] At Warrnambool Hospital the accommodation was bad with nurses sleeping in wards and two nurses had left because of this. The medical officer felt that 'as long as the place is like it is now there will be a difficulty in getting nurses who have been used to better things. You might get a woman who is not a lady, but a good and efficient nurse, who would be willing to go there, but nurses with any pretensions to being ladies do not like it'.[100]

The nurses' quarters at the Brisbane Hospital were inadequate until a new building was commenced in 1896 and Dr E.S. Jackson, the senior medical officer, commented in 1893 that 'apart from the disciplinary need of suitable accommodation for nurses, it is anomalous that those whose lives are spent in ministering to the comfort of others should themselves lack comfortable provision'.[101]

Miss Isabella Rathie, Matron at Melbourne Hospital, had strong ideas on what the nurses' accommodation should be, although this was not reflected in the actual conditions at the hospital in 1890. She thought that head nurses ought to have a bedroom to themselves with other nurses no more than two in a room. Head nurses and junior nurses ought to have a sitting room each, 'where they can see their friends, when off duty, brightly furnished, with piano'. These conditions signal the new type of desired recruit, one who was presumably educated enough to play the piano. She believed that:

> the housing and feeding of hospital nurses is a matter of much importance. Their home ought to be comfortable and cheerful, their food well cooked, and, if possible, even dainty. One can easily imagine how a badly-cooked dinner and a gloomy uninviting room would not be helpful to a tired or foot-sore nurse.

Yet although this was the ideal, Matron Rathie felt that suffering should be accepted:

> It must always be borne in mind by us nurses, that let our surroundings be what they may, we must live independently of them, and that in no way shall our patients or our work suffer through the neglect of those in authority toward us. A nurse, during her training time especially, is to all intents and purposes a soldier (a good soldier, I hope, in most instances), and must do quietly and without question just as she is bid.[102]

Yet she readily accepted that the accommodation at Melbourne Hospital was inadequate. Sleeping up to three in not very large bedrooms which were cold in winter and hot in summer, they had a dining room but no sitting room and no piano.[103] Nurses called their home 'Ratland' and in 1910 the matron agreed with them. It was not until the hospital was rebuilt in 1915 that she was satisfied with the accommodation.[104]

Details of the daily life of the nurse have not often been recorded, however, given the long hours, the discipline, heavy back-breaking work such as that in the fever tents and often the lack of training for the tasks which had to be performed, the routine was undoubtedly hard. Information from disaffected nurses, or those who did not survive their training, is scarce, but the Victorian Royal Commission did take evidence from one such nurse. Miss Marie Magill commenced training at the Alfred Hospital and lasted three months. She was sent to the fever tents and her experience sounds like that of a nurse at war. Rising at 5.30 am from her bed alongside eight to ten other nurses in a tent five feet from the ones where she worked, and starting work a half hour later, the day was punctuated by the regular sponging of the patients, sweeping wards and carrying heavy loads. Her duties in the tents ended at 6.30 pm or 8.30 pm on alternate days, but she sometimes remained on duty as late as 11.15 pm. At the end of the day 'I then carry to the laundry, sort out, and put in tubs of hot or cold water all the soiled linen from the tents for the day. I then betake my aching wearied limbs to my sleeping tent. To take a bath means a walk to the hospital, an ascent of three flights of stairs, and a probable long wait'. There were only three baths, one for the matron, one for the nurses and one for the housemaids.

The sleeping tent too had some problems as an open drain from the fever tents 'runs so near to where I lay that I could put out my hands and touch the contents: and five feet from me on the other side is the only deposit of all that is most offensive and loathsome'. (The drains contained slops and excreta which ran into the street.) She complained about the food at the Alfred Hospital, saying it was 'coarsely and roughly cooked and served, so much so that I have very frequently been unable to touch it until sharp hunger has compelled me'.

The one day off a week could not always be enjoyed. Miss Magill said that the nurse might be 'deprived' of her day off 'if you have had any ailment and been obliged to lay up. Nurses usually, those in training especially, use this day to lay up. Lying on flat of the back to regain strength to do next day's duty takes the place of fresh air and recreation'.

> At no time during any day had I any rest or cessation from work more than . . . for my hasty meals, neither was I privileged to be present when doctors were examining patients, as should have been allowed. I became ill from exhaustion and blood poisoning. I was told that the hours would be quite as long, in addition to scrubbing wards, when the tents were removed . . . I also knew that I should have to be in my ward at 5 a.m. I knew it was impossible to recover my lost strength, I therefore resigned. What hope had I of recovery when my fellow-nurses were often called to duty at 4 a.m. on scrubbing days, remaining until 8 p.m. For them compensation was arranged in the form of meat for tea, but only for them. It is now said that scrubbing is removed from the nurses' duties, but an hour longer is added, viz., until 9 p.m.

She felt that 'not many women of strong sympathies and keen perceptions have muscle to do the menial work. They are, therefore, debarred from becoming nurses'. She reported that of the twelve nurses whom she knew to sleep in the tent near the fever tent, six developed typhoid symptoms, four of them seriously and one died.[105] Miss Magill left following an attack by one of the patients in which she was injured. At the Brisbane Hospital the nurses were 'frequently assailed by epidemics of contagious diseases . . . The hospital committee became so concerned by the number of nurses who contracted typhoid from patients that it conducted a full scale enquiry into ways of reducing hazards to the health of the nurses'.[106]

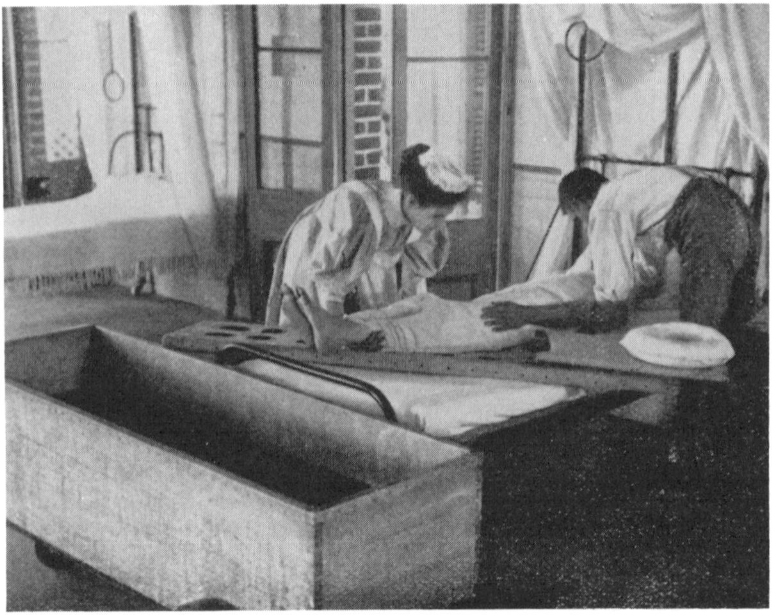

Nurse and male attendant lifting a patient suffering from typhoid fever into a bath of cold water, Brisbane Hospital, about 1898. The cold bath treatment used by Dr F.E. Hare at this hospital involved regular baths to lower the patient's temperature. The wooden bathtubs, lined with galvanised iron and mounted on wheels, were particularly heavy when filled with 75 gallons of water. The nurses' backbreaking work in the fever wards was fraught with the risk of infection. (F.E. Hare, The Cold-bath Treatment of Typhoid Fever, *Macmillan, London, 1898.* Courtesy of the University of Queensland Library.)

Development of nursing as a unique occupation

As nursing tasks became more complex and ward administration more standardised, hierarchies were developed within hospitals so that the transmission line for orders was clear. At the Brisbane Hospital the 1886 by-laws created a distinct hierarchy, from medical superintendent to newest nurse. The ward nurses were 'required to supervise the instruction of assistant nurses and . . . to "control" them'.[107] Structures like this gave way to a rigid hierarchy within the nursing service, from matron to probationer. This was established and perpetuated in order to mould the new category of trained nurse out of the raw recruits who came from a variety of backgrounds. The hospital world became 'a strict hierarchy of responsibility and duty between doctors and nurses and between trained and untrained nurses. Any attempts on the part of the trainee to question or reject that order had to be immediately given up'.[108]

Codes of nursing behaviour, hospital discipline and etiquette were extensive and included basic rules such as standing up in the presence of doctors and senior nurses, not speaking to a senior unless spoken to first, using specific staircases only if you were a probationer and appearing before superiors in a clean apron.[109] Rules such as taking orders from nurses only three weeks senior still remained in place at the Brisbane Hospital during the Second World War.[110] The military images used to describe nurses ('nursing is warfare, and the nurses are soldiers')[111] were not incongrous in the new disciplined hospital setting. Yet administrators also hoped to create a family-like atmosphere, as much of the discussion in the Victorian Royal Commission over accommodation and comforts for the nurse showed. Vicinus has concluded that most sisters,

> tired and overworked . . . used discipline to cover mistakes and to enforce order. Moreover, even the most adroit might have had trouble juggling the dual role of army officer and sympathetic mother. If she took her duties seriously, a sister could not risk intimacy with those under her. The sister was, after all, controlled by her 'general,' the matron.[112]

The discipline and hierarchical structure had a practical purpose when students were used to do most of the work of the hospital, for they were often placed in situations before they had the knowledge and maturity to handle the work asked of them.[113] The ideology of nursing and the practical purpose of cheap hospital labour coalesced.

Much of the training was directed towards the moral and character development of the nurses, rather than specific technical knowledge. The art of nursing 'addressed itself to the specific personal qualities of the entrant, rather than her ability to take in the formal education'.[114] These qualities included sobriety, honesty, punctuality, truthfulness and patience, as spelt out for Nightingale probationers at St Thomas' Hospital in London. Matrons strove to inculcate these qualities into their trainees.

The independence and power of nursing within the hospital setting had been Nightingale's goal, but, in numerous battles with doctors and hospital committees, nurses' power within the hospital was reduced. What was left was a hierarchy of nurses alone, with those at the top rigidly exercising power over those below them. Vicinus has characterised this situation saying that 'as arguments for the nurses' autonomy failed, nursing leaders tightened their hold upon those they trained; a woman's world ruled by a few at the top became the goal'.[115] The nursing hierarchy was separate from and subordinate to the male medical hierarchy and the male hospital administration. For nurses the result was—

> not a family . . . but rather a rigid ordering of women that masquer-aded as a family while mimicking the medical hierarchy under which the nurses labored. The constant rotation of probationers from ward to ward, the class divisions in the training home, and the exploitative work all acted to inhibit a sense of community among women nurses.[116]

In addition, 'given the stress on separating the nursing student from contact with the hospital's other workers, trained nursing began with an elitist ideology that precluded alliances across occupational boundaries'.[117]

These views were to have ramifications for the beliefs and activities of the nursing organisations. Not only was the newly founded nursing profession divided horizontally through the hospital hierarchy, it was divided vertically between hospital and private nursing, and it was cut off from collaboration with other workers. Its aspirations to be seen as equal but different to medicine were not achieved and 'separate became unequal and less important'.[118] Links with other groups of women workers or other groups of hospital workers were not likely because the efforts of the aspiring nursing profession to establish itself rested on proving its uniqueness. This militated against nurses seeing themselves as part of a wider group of women workers or hospital workers. It would take until the second half of the twentieth century for the nursing organisations in Australia to feel they were similar to and had ties with other workers and therefore other trade unions.

The hierarchical organisation of the hospital nursing structure and the diverse class origins of the recruits led to little community of interest among the different classes of women. Their views mirrored those of middle and upper class women towards their servants in their home even though, a generation earlier, nurses had themselves been akin to domestic servants. There was no universal sisterhood that crossed class boundaries. Hewitt has stated the case generally, saying that:

> no such universal sisterhood existed, and in fact . . . the develop-ment of a sense of community among various classes of women served as a barrier to an all-embracing bond of womanhood . . . it is now clear that privileged women were willing to wield their sex-specific influence in ways that, intentionally or unintentionally, exploited other women.[119]

In order to make nursing a respectable occupation for middle and upper class women it had to be shifted away from the domestic classes even if many of its recruits still came from there. Reverby concludes that 'nursing's history provides us with a specific example of a group of women so divided by class that their common oppression based on gender could not unite them'.[120] The Victorian Royal Commission evidence shows the class divisions with which hospital administrators, doctors and nurses all identified. While the tradition of social egalitarianism was of enormous importance in Australia it was a matter of manners only.[121]

Marriage was the ultimate destiny of most women. Although by the 1890s young women worked longer and married later in life than their mothers had, 'the majority still looked to marriage as their prime goal and to the home as their natural and proper sphere'.[122] It was clear that 'social pressures . . . set marriage as the prime female goal; and a majority of women accepted that only widowed or deserted married women should work'.[123] Most female teachers, for example, resigned when they married and few 'considered it necessary to have a career and those who did soon gave teaching away for marriage or other employment opportunities'.[124] Mr James Stewart, Rockhampton North Member of the Legislative Assembly, believed that:

> the great majority of young women who took up teaching as a profession . . . knew that the chief end of woman was man. Young ladies did not take up the profession of teaching with the view of going on with it all the days of their lives, and finally subsiding into old maidenhood. Their purpose was to devote a few years to teaching, at the end of which time they hoped to be taken under the wing of some man who would be their companion during the remainder of their lives.[125]

Without marriage, for the 'new' nurses remained unmarried, status in the community could only be gained from the higher status of their reformed occupation.

The idea that cultured, educated ladies undertook the work of nursing was very important in transforming the occupation from one likened to the work of servants to one appropriate and attractive to educated women of the middle classes. Yet the mixed origins and expectations of recruits could be an element of division amongst nurses. Although the majority of the women who entered nursing needed to earn a living, the distinction was frequently made between those for whom this was a necessity and those for whom it was not. As a totally female occupation in which high educational attainments were not required of recruits, and in which the training was at best like that of an apprentice tradesperson, nursing had to prove its status by other means. Its recruits, if not ladies when they came to the hospital, had to be trained to be indistinguishable from them. As Maggs has said:

> most nurse commentators knew the occupation to be at least 'mixed as to rank', if not absolutely composed of women from the 'lower orders'; however, even when admitting this, the nurses did not speak of women from the working-class in general, but women from an 'earnest class'; it would seem that such women could be found in all walks of life, working- and middle-class, and indeed their earnestness was what wiped out the social distinctions of class of which contemporaries were acutely aware . . . the standard form of instruction and the standardisation of the training programme itself would wipe out any vestiges of 'class', and turn all women into trained nurses and thus members of the earnest class.[126]

Their reward was the unique designation of being a nurse, but this had to be created in the public mind, for there was to be no great monetary reward. In fact, financial reward was counterproductive to the image of self-sacrifice that nursing needed to guarantee its uniqueness.

By the 1890s nurses were no longer seen as servants. John Taylor, Secretary of the Manchester Unity Independent Order of Oddfellows, believed that:

> females who have qualified themselves to become trained nurses and passed an examination must necessarily have devoted a considerable time to reading and educational attainments that would entitle them to a social status higher than a person who is engaged in scrubbing floors. I take it that would be by giving them a status something like the non-commissioned officers in the army and navy, and that they might be addressed by a title a little above those who wash dishes and scrub floors. I think from what is expected from women who go into that work there should be a social status given besides emolument.[127]

David Bennett, Melbourne Trades Hall Council secretary, felt that female nurses should be treated with more respect than menial servants for 'in respect of their training and superior education, they are entitled to every consideration. They are not taken from the most ignorant classes of the community' and 'should be treated a little better than kitchen maids'.[128] Mrs Edith Morris, honorary secretary of the Nurses' Home in Melbourne, drew the distinction between trained and untrained nurses:

> Not many years ago the nursing and tending of the sick was thought to be a work for which any one was fitted; success in it seemed open even to those who had failed in all other attempts to earn a livelihood . . . Slowly but steadily this state of things is passing away, and in Europe and America women of high position and education are constantly coming forward and devoting their lives to the work of nursing, thereby raising the tone of the profession. Nurses who have been properly trained are now recognised as holding a distinct position, and one that is highly and generally respected. To belong to a profession which has included in its ranks such women as Florence Nightingale, Agnes Jones, and Sister Dora, not to mention others, is surely a position of which any woman should be proud.

In her delineation of the formally trained from the untrained nurse, she foreshadowed the role of the early nursing organisations:

> That position should be jealously guarded, and it should not be permitted that women without proper training and a right to the name should call themselves trained nurses. This abuse should be especially guarded against in this country, where the public is only learning what a trained nurse means, and where no opportunity seems to be lost to speak slightingly of the nursing profession, when in many cases some individual is to blame who has been sailing under false colours . . . All that is possible should be done to raise the status of the nursing profession in Victoria and to encourage women of good education and position to join its ranks.[129]

Within several decades there had been a transition from the belief that every woman was a born nurse by virtue of her sex, to the belief that every woman had the potential to become a trained nurse, by virtue of her sex. For 'genteel "good" women were to become disciplined soldiers in the war against disease and disorder, self-sacrificing mothers to the patients, efficient housekeepers for the hospitals, loyal and subordinate assistants to the physicians, and firm supervisors of the hospital's other workers'.[130] Nevertheless, the ideal of the nurse had not changed since it was described by the Sydney Infirmary's report in 1869:

> There cannot be a doubt that the best and most efficient nursing is that which simply and faithfully carries out the instructions of the Medical Officers, attends cheerfully to the domestic comforts of the patients, manages the wards with the strictest economy, method, and cleanliness, and meets every emergency with unflinching self-sacrifice.[131]

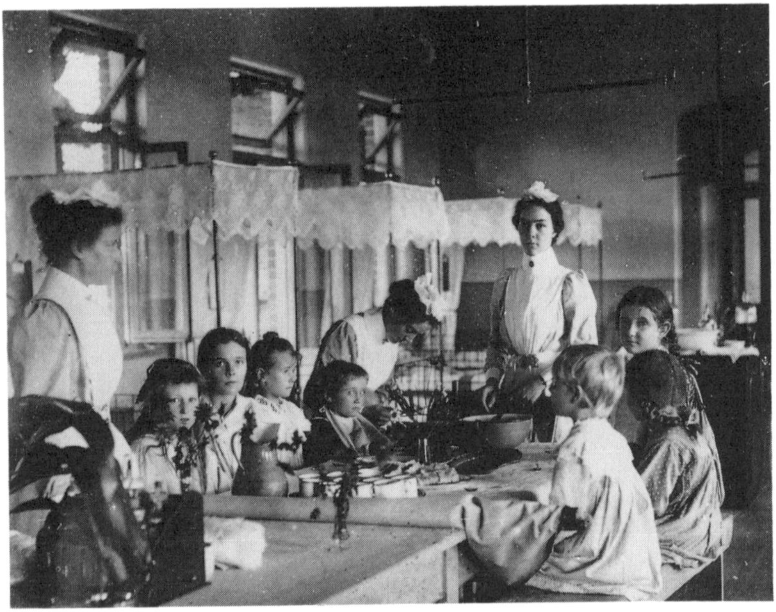

Nurses serving a meal to young patients in the Hospital for Sick Children, Brisbane, in the 1890s. The table and benches in the centre of the ward were a typical arrangement. Photographs of nurses performing their everyday duties like this are rare. (Collection: John Oxley Library, Brisbane.)

Instead of earning a large salary as other mere mortals did, the nurse's reward for long hours of work and training at little or no cost to the hospital was to be a 'ministering angel',[132] a member of 'one of woman's noblest professions'.[133]

By the last decade of the nineteenth century the occupation of nursing was characterised not only by its totally female nature, but by its long hours, low or non-existent pay during training, and by the cloistered life that hospital nurses led. Within 50 years nursing had been transformed from work done by servants to a paid living for women from many different classes. It was an occupation that was characterised in the public mind by selfless sacrifice, a belief that its members absorbed to a large degree. As a consequence they were loath to complain about problems and they lacked a community of interest with other women workers, who were not part of their select band. Yet the female hierarchy of the hospital had many divisions rather than being united.

The importance given to the ideal that nurses did not work merely for money but for the sheer love of the job had as its obverse the fiction that income and working conditions were unimportant. Nurses were trapped into poor working conditions by the success of their own rhetoric. In this debate their selflessness accorded them status but this very characteristic locked them into long hours of work. Nurses were also trapped because they provided indispensable labour for hospitals. This labour had to be cheap, since the institutions were charitable ones, although this argument never applied to medical practitioners.

These characteristics were to have profound ramifications for the goals and methods of operation of the nursing organisations when they emerged in Australia at the turn of the century. The main aim for these organisations was to transform the infant profession into a publicly-accepted one in which all members were trained and certificated. The trained nurses wanted to protect their hold on their newly-gained skills and wanted a way of raising their public profile. Their aim was to establish a monopoly in nursing through the promotion of public acceptance of trained nurses as the only nurses that the community should have. Their concerns, therefore, were not those of the diverse group of nurses, trained and untrained, young and old, in city or country hospitals, newest probationer, private practitioner, matron of a hospital or proprietor of a nurses' home.

The establishment and organisation of the profession of nursing were thus the goals of the nursing organisations which were founded in Australia at the end of the nineteenth century. Questions of wages and working conditions played no part in the aims or activities of these organisations. Yet their members, the newly-trained nurses, were overwhelmingly in need of earning a sufficient income to support themselves.

CHAPTER 2

The beginnings of nursing organisations in Australia

'. . . *in no mere spirit of trades unionism.*'[1]

At the turn of the century in Australia, trained female nurses worked alongside those who had not received a formal nursing education. As in England and America, Australian trained nurses sought to delineate their services from those of others who called themselves nurses, thereby gaining a more secure market for themselves and, they believed, giving the public a reliable standard of service. The major way they did this was by creating their own organisations to promote their specialised interests. The nursing organisations set out to regulate training and obtain recognition for the profession by the public and the State, and within a decade of their establishment they had travelled a long way towards achieving this. The activities of the associations created a trained elite of respectable female nurses who were widely employed in the larger towns. In contrast, the working conditions of nurses were of little or no concern to the newly emerging nursing organisations.

In Australia, the first on-going nursing organisation was established in 1899 and within a few years several states had associations which looked after the interests of trained nurses. There had been some unsuccessful attempts to form associations throughout the 1890s. A short-lived nurses' association began in Sydney in 1892 but 'nothing was accomplished then owing to a diversity of opinion as to what constituted a trained nurse'.[2] However, on Friday 26 May 1899, nurses and medical practitioners met in the Royal Society's Rooms, Elizabeth Street, Sydney, to make plans for a nurses' association.[3] At a subsequent meeting on 21 June, Dr Graham suggested specific objectives for the organisation and these were adopted:

1. To promote the interests of trained nurses in all matters affecting their work as a class.

2. To establish a system of registration for trained nurses.
3. To afford opportunities for discussing subjects bearing on the work of nursing.
4. To initiate and control schemes that will afford to nurses a means of providing an allowance during incapacity for work caused by sickness, accident, age or other necessitous circumstances.[4]

These objectives were to remain substantially the same for the next 50 years and guided the work of the association.

The ATNA began chiefly in the larger training hospitals in Sydney at the instigation of prominent medical practitioners and nurses who held the most senior positions within the nursing community. The influence of the medical profession and its place of regard in the eyes of the nursing profession is seen in the positions that doctors assumed on the association's council. Until the first annual meeting the only member of the nursing profession represented among the executive officers was Miss Susan McGahey, Lady Superintendent of Prince Alfred Hospital, Sydney, who acted as joint honorary secretary. The remainder of the executive positions were held by male medical practitioners. Dr Manning, Inspector-General for the Insane in New South Wales from 1879 and a trustee of Prince Alfred Hospital, was president. On his death in 1903 one nursing journal declared that he had been 'the originator, the trusted councillor, the life and soul of the movement that raised the nursing profession of New South Wales to its present enviable position'.[5] Other members of the executive were Dr Goode, vice-president, Mr J. Oswald Fairfax, treasurer, and Dr Mills, honorary physician at the Prince Alfred Hospital as joint honorary secretary.[6] The initial rules of the ATNA in New South Wales established an annually elected council of seventeen members, exclusive of executive officers, (with three representatives of midwifery nurses added in 1904). Of these seventeen, five had to be qualified medical practitioners, five matrons or superintendents of nurses, five sisters and nurses, and two might be honorary members.[7] This formally set the seal on who were to be influential in the decision-making process of the organisation, with at least ten out of the seventeen council members being those at the pinnacle of the medical and nursing professions.

From the earliest meetings the daily running of the ATNA and the overwhelming majority of its policies were decided at council meetings, which had to be held at least quarterly. Ordinary members would have the opportunity to influence the running of the association through the annual general meeting, any general meeting called by the council, and the election of councillors. Special meetings could be called on the written request of ten or more members.[8] Although contentious questions were sometimes put to general meetings, only metropolitan members were able to attend and voice their opinions. Nurses in country areas had very little chance to take part in ATNA affairs, and the structure of the association did not encourage their involvement. The council became the guardian of the standards and training of the nursing profession and there was very little contact with the lower echelons of the nursing hierarchy. This was to be the pattern for years to come, with few specific problems of members being handled.

Those who formed the ATNA wanted to standardise the nurse's training and raise her public status. The nurses' association, called the Australasian Trained Nurses' Association from December 1899, can be classified as a professional association, whose primary functions are the organisation of a specific group of trained workers; the implementation of standard qualifications which have to be met before membership is granted; the inclusion of activities which further the study of the subject and the communication of subsequent findings; the maintenance of a register of competent professionals; the promotion and preservation of a high standard of professional conduct.[9] These functions can all be identified in the early activities of the ATNA as it established educational standards, set up a register of nurses who met the organisation's criteria of trained nurse and published its own journal.

The ATNA acted as a qualifying association,[10] a particular type of professional association, and aimed to examine and qualify individuals in the specific occupation of nursing, to control entry to the profession and to protect the profession and the public through the knowledge that all members of the association met the organisation's qualification standards. Since the express purpose of the ATNA was the delineation of a trained nurse, it set out requirements for formal training and examination. By establishing minimum qualifications for membership the ATNA limited the numbers in the category of trained nurse, thereby reducing competition from those with work experience only. It aimed to publicise the relatively new distinction between formally trained and informally trained nurses with the professed goal of providing the public with a choice of nurse. The ATNA thus created a fence around the occupation and aimed to control the gateway through which others could enter. The instigators were those most concerned with the training and qualification of nurses: nurses and medical practitioners in senior positions. This match of goals and personnel reinforced the aims of the ATNA as a professional organisation little concerned with the everyday needs of the ordinary nurse.

These moves were not unique. In Britain and the USA too, similar steps were being taken by trained nurses trying to achieve professional identity and raised status. Nursing leaders 'committed themselves to the assumptions and strategies of professionalization. They used professional ideology to defend nursing as paid work, distinguishing it from the diffuse category of women's domestic duty'.[11] The aspirations of the ATNA also reflected the moves for standardisation and professionalisation that were occurring in other occupations. In the final decades of the nineteenth century, groups trying to do this in England included teachers, chemists, dentists, midwives, veterinary surgeons, health inspectors, surveyors and journalists, as well as nurses.[12]

As the major purpose of the ATNA was to delineate the trained nurse and separate her from the untrained, it was crucial to set the criteria for membership of the association. Not surprisingly, this was one of the first points debated at length with the aim of setting a high standard of working ability, yet not debarring those nurses who had gained their position through experience but with little or no formal training. Stringent qualifications were laid down: a nurse had to prove that she had been engaged for three years in a general hospital containing not less than a daily average of 40 occupied beds, four years in a hospital with at least 20 beds, or five years in a hospital with no less than ten occupied beds. In all cases the hospital had to be recognised as a training school for nurses by the ATNA Council and in hospitals with fewer than 40 beds, the matron had to possess a certificate from an approved training school. All candidates had to provide references as to their moral character, certificates of competency from their hospital, and to account for any interruptions in their nursing career.[13]

A concessional clause was introduced enabling experienced nurses who did not comply with these conditions to register. Training of a shorter duration was allowed in certain circumstances. In addition, the concessional rule meant that a nurse was eligible for registration if she could show that she had been engaged for not less than three years 'in the bona fide work of medical and surgical nursing, either in Hospitals or in private nursing, and can produce certificates of competency and good conduct satisfactory to the Council, from at least three reputable Medical Practitioners as to her attainments and repute'. The nurse qualified under these concessional rules was to have 'Admitted by the Council under the provisions of Rule xxi' after her name in the association's register.[14]

The ATNA thus allowed wide entry to the association when it was formed, while remaining conscious of its role in restricting entry to the occupation in the future. The concessional clause was adopted by a general meeting of members 'in order to give all respectable nurses in the Colony the opportunity of becoming members'. In a speech to the

International Congress of Nurses, Miss Susan McGahey reported that 'the Council realised that a grave injustice was being done by excluding from membership a certain section of the Nursing profession who were not fortunate enough to receive their training when a three years' course was compulsory'.[15]

The organisation quickly extended training standards to cover midwifery nurses by establishing a Midwifery Nurses' Auxiliary Branch. A six-month course in a recognised maternity hospital, participation in not less than 20 cases of labour, an examination, and a certificate of good moral character entitled the practitioner to registration with the ATNA. General nurses with midwifery qualifications could be registered as both.[16] There were moves to form a register for massage nurses but though a sub-committee was formed to consider this proposal, no such register was established by the association.[17]

The earliest method used by the association to differentiate trained from untrained practitioners was publication of a register of members. It was designed to ensure that the former were easily recognised by the public, a significant goal when the majority of nurses worked in private practice. The first register, published in mid-1900, listed 327 nurses, 60 medical practitioners and eight honorary members. This number included eighteen Queensland nurses, nine of whom had been admitted under the concessional rule xxi.[18] Fears were held in the community that proficient nurses might miss out on being registered with the result that they would eventually lose their livelihood. It was emphasised that much care had to be taken in compiling the register as 'this register will be accepted by the public as a standard book of reference, and the time will come when very few nurses will be employed whose names do not appear in the list of those who bear the hall-mark of competency'.[19]

Within four years of its formation the ATNA in New South Wales had made great strides towards the standardisation of nursing training by setting training criteria in general nursing and midwifery and qualifications for membership of the association. Moves were made to promote the organisation as the professional association for nurses and gain recognition for its standards from medical and nursing practitioners, hospitals and government. The ATNA began activities to implement its objective of discussing nursing subjects and in 1901 commenced regular lectures for members, usually given by medical practitioners on clinical topics, though these were only held in Sydney. The formation of a benevolent fund for destitute nurses put objective (4) of the ATNA into practice which aimed to provide for nurses when out of work, infirm or aged.[20]

The interests of trained nurses were further promoted by the publication of an association journal. On 24 March 1903, 1400 copies of the first issue of the *Australasian Nurses' Journal* (*ANJ*) were printed and distributed free to members.[21] The journal carried association news and reports of meetings, lectures given to the association, articles of a clinical nature or other aspects of nursing. In its first editorial the *ANJ* proudly related the achievements of the association saying that the register of trained nurses contained almost all qualified nurses in New South Wales as well as many from other states, New Zealand and Fiji. Minimum educational standards had been accepted by training schools and the New South Wales Government recognised the association's standards by appointing only matrons and nurses who held a certificate from an approved hospital training school to positions in hospitals which received government subsidies.

The editorial felt that the ATNA still had important work to do such as discouraging the employment of trainee nurses in the smaller hospitals where, it believed, a nurse could not receive adequate training. As well as this, the association needed to organise a central examination board which would examine all nurses at the end of their training, instead of leaving this to the hospital doctors and matrons. However the association felt that:

> most of the work it has already done, as well as of that which it is still called on to undertake, is work which might more fitly have been carried out by the Government; and perhaps a bill providing for the examination and registration of Nurses, as well as to define their status and accord to them certain privileges, may be submitted to Parliament in the near future.

The editorial added that the ATNA was:

> entitled to claim that it has so far carried out its work in no mere spirit of trades unionism and merely for the benefit of its members. In raising the standard of education among Nurses, and in publishing the Register, it has conferred benefits on the public both by providing for it Nurses better qualified to carry out the important duties of their calling, and by enabling the public with but little trouble to distinguish between those Nurses who are qualified by training and experience to undertake those duties, and those Nurses (so-called) who possess neither the training nor experience to render their employment safe or expedient.[22]

Thus the ATNA commenced its life with a firm hand over the training and certification of nurses, setting standards that were to apply in all training hospitals. In doing so it saw itself as performing a service for the public.

Although the ATNA was controlled by an elite within the nursing and medical professions, its membership was broad. Concessional clauses, extended over some years, meant that nurses who had not received a formal training could become members, although they were barred from some positions such as matrons of training hospitals. Training was standardised sooner and more completely across training schools and, once there was a final examination held by the ATNA, all training ostensibly became equal. The ATNA was not concerned primarily with the immediate problems of working nurses in the period until 1950 as it concentrated on the professional issues which had been the reason for its formation.

The establishment of nursing organisations in other states

Several years after the formation of the ATNA councillors considered expanding the influence of the association in other states. Copies of the constitution were sent to hospitals throughout the country, 'nurses of standing' were contacted, and in January 1901 a letter was sent to the heads of different hospitals and to 'leading medical men and nurse members' throughout Australia.[23] Branches were formed in Queensland in 1904, South Australia in 1905, Western Australia in 1907 and Tasmania in 1908.[24] The pattern of nursing associations was similar throughout Australia. For instance, the impetus for the formation of the nurses' association in Victoria, the Victorian Trained Nurses' Assocation (VTNA),[25] came from the ATNA in Sydney when the council wrote to Dr W.A. Wood of Melbourne asking him to stimulate interest in the formation of such an association.

The VTNA commenced in June 1901 with 'almost all the organising work . . . done by a handful of doctors'. In fact, Dr Wood was 'convinced that unless it is supported by the medical profession it will not succeed'. One of the first councillors of the association endorsed this saying 'women were not the promoters. However if we cannot lead, we can follow'. Most of the nurses were matrons or proprietors of Nurses' Homes and once again male medical practitioners dominated the council of this nurses' organisation. Although only five out of fifteen on the council were male doctors, the 'men affectively dominated the executive positions' with the only nurse to hold an executive position being Miss Glover as joint honorary secretary. Like the New South Wales and Queensland associations, this was not seen as a cause for concern but was accepted by the nurses as normal with the 'automatic assumption that the paternalistic rule of doctors was in nurses' best interests'.[26]

The formation of the ATNA and the Victorian association show the unanimity of purpose between the nursing and medical professions. There was no apparent dissent and the nurses certainly posed no threat to the doctors, with the former's place clearly defined as subordinate to that of the doctor.

Formation of ATNA branch in Queensland

The first branch of the ATNA was formed in Queensland in 1904. This occurred during a period of general activity in nursing throughout the country, but local factors also played a part, for there was dissatisfaction with some nursing practices in the state. Mr A.M. Payne, Secretary of Brisbane Hospital, wrote that:

> the effect of the Australasian Trained Nurses' Association in limiting the practice of nursing to qualified persons does not appear to be felt here in Brisbane as it should. It is represented that there are instances in recognised Nurses' Homes where trained nurses have to wait their turn after unqualified nurses.[27]

The nurses behind the move to establish the branch had been trained at the Brisbane Hospital and Payne pointed out that he was 'really the spokesman for a few of our old nurses, headed by Miss Beatrice L. Macnish', to whom he referred the correspondence from the ATNA secretary.[28] This group believed that the influence of the ATNA could be felt more directly if a Queensland Branch, with headquarters in Brisbane, could be established.[29] A 'very well attended' public meeting of those interested in forming an association was held at the Technical College, Brisbane, on the afternoon of 25 February 1904. Dr Ernest Sandford Jackson presided, while those present included thirteen other medical practitioners, Nurse Marks, the Matron of Brisbane General Hospital, Mr Payne and numerous nurses. Dr Jackson read a letter from Dr Sinclair Gillies, secretary of the ATNA in Sydney, expressing pleasure at the proposed Queensland Branch. The meeting agreed to form a Queensland Branch of the ATNA and Lady Chermside, the wife of the Governor, was invited to be its patroness.[30]

A formal request to establish a Queensland Branch, signed by 22 medical practitioners and 71 nurses, was sent to the parent organisation in Sydney.[31] The draft rules submitted by the New South Wales body were adopted at a general meeting held in Brisbane on 27 April 1904. The council sent application forms to all who sent in ballot papers for the election of the council, asking them to forward copies of certificates, testimonials and subscription fees to the secretaries.[32] Unlike the parent association, midwifery nurses were admitted immediately as part of the branch as a whole, and not merely to an auxiliary branch as in New South Wales.[33] The concessional rule xxi was to be extended to 31 March 1905 in the case of Queensland nurses.[34]

The membership of the Queensland Branch expanded and by April 1922 it was over one thousand.[35] Like its parent association, the potential decision-making roles were centralised in the people on the council and in the capital city, with the result that members not living in Brisbane had virtually no chance to participate in the organisation's affairs. The council held monthly meetings with sub-committee meetings when necessary but usually held only one general meeting a year, the annual general meeting. The branch dealt with members' individual problems and gave advice or offered monetary assistance for legal fees if, for instance, a nurse had to take steps to recover fees owing to her. There were intermittent calls on the benevolent fund and small amounts paid to nurses.[36] As more tasks were undertaken the council found it necessary to appoint a paid secretary and Mr Henry Bolton began work early in 1907.[37] But the prime concern of the ATNA in its first sixteen years was to have the trained nurse recognised as such with training of a uniform and sufficiently high standard. In this it succeeded; State registration set the seal on its efforts in 1912.

An outward manifestation of the superiority of male medical practitioners within the health services can be seen in the allocation of the executive positions, all of which were to be held by medical practitioners except for one of the vice-presidents and one of the secretaries, who were to be nurses. As well as these key executive posts, almost half of the executive and council positions, eleven out of 27, were to go to medical practitioners.[38] Such an allocation of positions, strongly weighted towards male doctors, powerfully illustrates the superior authority assumed by them within the health services. In the absence of any contrary evidence, it must be assumed that nurses acquiesced in these arrangements which replicated the hierarchy within the hospital and the power relationship between nurses and doctors in private practice; if nurses objected to such an assumption of male power, they have left no record of those objections.

The Queensland Branch mirrored the characteristics of its parent organisation. Male medical practitioners were prominent in its formation and continuing operations. Matrons and proprietors of private

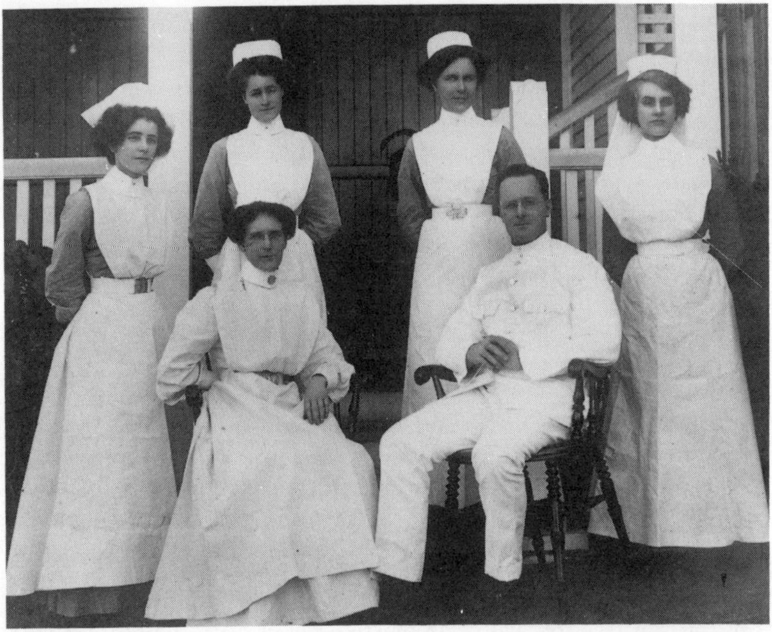

Medical practitioners and nurses from the Brisbane Hospital were prominent in the formation of the Queensland Branch of the ATNA. When this photograph was taken about 1908, both Miss Emily Hunter, *Matron of the Brisbane Hospital from 1906 to 1914, and Dr John Barr McLean, Medical Superintendent from 1904 to 1931, (seated) were secretaries of the ATNA.* Miss Hunter *served as secretary from 1907 to 1914 and Dr McLean served as secretary from 1904 to 1912, president from 1912 to 1923 and vice-president from 1924 to 1926.* (Collection: John Oxley Library, Brisbane.)

hospitals were dominant among the nurses on the council and this governing body made the majority of decisions concerning the policy and operations of the association.

Dr Ernest Sandford Jackson, the branch's inaugural president, had formerly been Medical Superintendent of the Brisbane Hospital and was instrumental in establishing nursing training there.[39] In 1904 he was a surgeon in private practice and owner of St Helen's Hospital. Dr John Barr McLean, Medical Superintendent of the Brisbane Hospital and known as 'Father' to the nursing staff of that hospital,[40] was joint secretary along with Miss Appleton. Dr Arthur Halford and Miss Mary Weedon, Matron of the Brisbane Hospital from 1885 to 1890, were the vice-presidents and Dr Page was treasurer.[41] It was not until 1912 that the Queensland Branch rules were changed to allow two nurses to act as honorary secretaries. This motion, sponsored by Dr McLean, came about because he had decided to resign from this position and felt that there might be some difficulty in getting a medical practitioner to replace him.[42] Not until 1943 did a nurse take over the role of president from male medical practitioners. The superior profession and more powerful sex had numerical superiority on the executive and strength on the council. The coalition of interests between the male medical practitioners and nurses in Australia is clearly seen in comments made during a lecture given to the Queensland Branch in October 1904 by Dr Jackson. He stated that:

> one supposes that no intelligent person would doubt that anything which will be to the best interests of trained Nurses will be also to the interests of the medical men with whom they work, and, what is more important than all perhaps, in the best interests of the patients whom they are caring for.[43]

The nurses and doctors who served on the Queensland Council of the ATNA overwhelmingly were not rank and file nurses in hospitals, for this job was done by students or untrained nurses who could not be members of the association. Nor were there many nurses in private practice on the council. When private nurses started to agitate for increases in fees, their pleas were taken up reluctantly by the council. Neither fees, nor working conditions, nor hours of work were the predominant concerns of the council. It is difficult therefore, to agree with Trembath and Hellier when they say that 'like the councils of the A.T.N.A., the Victorian council might have been dominated by doctors and matrons, but their aims were those of the ordinary nurse'.[44] There is no evidence to suggest that this was so, or that the opposite was the case, as so little is ever heard from 'the ordinary nurse' or those who commenced training but failed to reach the destination of trained nurse. It is highly unlikely that the councils did represent the concerns of the average nurse and this is borne out by the struggles of the private nurses within the ATNA to increase their earnings.

Nursing organisations in the United States have been characterised as being out-of-touch with nurses' everyday needs, for 'as nursing organizations focused on state registration laws and educational reforms in the schools, they became isolated from the majority of working nurses, whose concerns were different'.[45] Like them, the ATNA certainly did not voice concerns about trainee nurses and the cheap labour that they provided to keep the hospitals running. Indeed, at one meeting of the ATNA in New South Wales it was declared that 'it has come to the ears of the members of the Council that some of our Nurses feel that they would be better pleased if the Council contained some representatives who are not the heads of hospitals and kindred bodies, but, so to speak, members of the rank and file'. At this time each one of the ten nursing members on this council was head of a large or small hospital or nursing home. The editorial stated that any nurse could nominate and be elected to the council, however it continued: 'Our critics reply that unless the representation is so arranged that some members of the rank and file must be elected, it is impossible to secure the return of such against the better-known heads of institutions'.[46] If they had concerned themselves with questions of the wages and working conditions of nurses this would have been difficult to reconcile with their positions as administrators and keepers of the hospital purses.

An *ANJ* editorial spoke of the difficulty of obtaining staff for country hospitals because 'the remuneration is absurdly inadequate to the services rendered'.[47] Although the council occasionally answered queries from hospital committees about nurses' wages by stating a minimum salary, no effort was made to have these wage scales more widely known or accepted. Certainly no steps were taken to have any salary scales brought into effect legally via the industrial system.

There was a minor discussion of the hours nurses had to work and a 1909 conference of ATNA branches discussed an eight-hour day for hospital nurses. Dr McLean, secretary of the Queensland Branch and Medical Superintendent of the Brisbane Hospital, felt that from the hospital's point of view there would be great difficulty implementing this because of the increased expenditure, with Brisbane Hospital probably facing an additional expense of £800 a year. Dr Blackburn of New South Wales believed that the average nurse's hours were too long but thought that it was 'going rather far to make a limit of fifty-six hours a week, as a Nurse's work was not continuously hard, some of it, indeed, being comparatively light'. He added that it was not the function of the ATNA conference to fix the working hours of hospital nurses. The conference unanimously resolved that the 'hours on duty per week should be reduced'.[48]

Although an *ANJ* editorial remarked on the benefits to a hospital from having a nursing staff that were not tired and worn out, the introduction of an eight-hour day for nurses would have upset the hospital system so it was suggested that the nurses' total hours of work per week should be shortened by allowing them 36 consecutive hours off duty each week, that is, two nights and a day. It concluded: 'It is

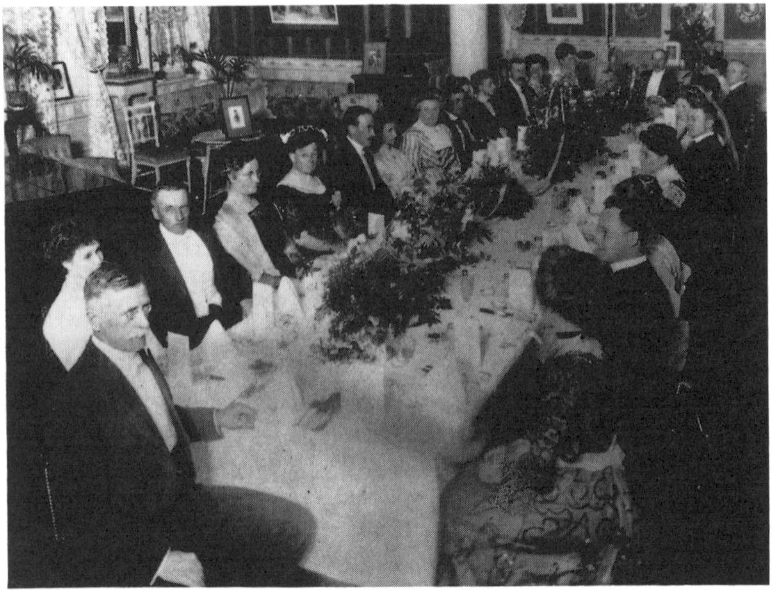

ATNA Conference of Delegates, Sydney, 9 July 1909. Participants are (left side of table, foreground to rear of table): Mrs Chennell, SA; Dr Brenney; Miss Creal; Miss K. Davies; Dr Cumpston, WA; Mrs Davidson; Miss Ryan, WA; Dr Dansey; Miss Newell; Miss Godson; Dr Wilson, SA; M.Watson; Miss Hunter, Qld; Dr Gillies, vice-president; Dr Fiaschi (at the head of the table); (right side of table, foreground to rear of table): Miss McGahey; Dr McLean, Qld; Miss Thomas; Miss McMaster; Dr Blackburn; Miss Wayne, Tas; Miss Garron; Miss Sanders; Mrs Scott, WA; Dr Ramsay; Mrs Thompson. Councillors represented New South Wales unless otherwise identified. (Courtesy of Queensland Nurses' Union.)

to be hoped that in the near future the large general hospitals in the various States will of themselves adopt some means of shortening the hours on duty of their Nurses, and not wait till an outburst of public opinion renders such imperative'.[49] Yet the ATNA did not apply any pressure to hospitals to comply with this recommendation. There was never any agitation for there was always the consideration that the introduction of an eight-hour day would mean that more nurses would need to be employed, thus adding to hospital expenditure.

The ATNA's objectives and activities were concerned with other issues. As Dr Jackson, president of the Queensland Branch, commented, it was the ATNA's objective that every nurse should have received proper training:

> The foremost duty of a Nurse to her patient is . . . that she shall take pains to know her work. With a good knowledge of her work she must bring a determination to let nothing she can do for the welfare of her patient be left undone. To know her work she must, of course, have been in the way of a proper training. Her determination to do all she can is for her own character, and may be influenced but not controlled by the Association.[50]

The aims and activities of the ATNA embodied the goals of those who had risen through the ranks of nurses to reach positions of power and who wished to entrench the place of the trained nurse.

CHAPTER 3

The education and training of nurses, 1904 to 1912

' . . . eager, enthusiastic, and highly-trained women, and yet women of refinement and "all womanliness" .'[1]

When the ATNA began in Queensland its main aim was the establishment and regulation of a standardised system of nurse training and this remained its major focus until 1920. There was little debate about the style of training because once this work became the province of women, different forms of education were not an option. Apprenticeship-style training with a few theoretical lectures supplementing the long hours of work in the hospital wards was universally accepted. The type of recruit and the form of training of the nurse were invariably linked to the idea of what a nurse should be. This relied on beliefs about the supposedly innate virtues of women and reflected the view of women in society as subordinate to men and as submissive, pliant individuals. The ideal nurse was a woman who would sacrifice herself for the work and was not concerned with the level of remuneration or working conditions. The reward was the work itself.

By 1900 however, it was not enough to possess womanly virtues to be a nurse, for it was accepted widely that nurses needed to undergo training which would give them specific practical and scientific knowledge. Thus the image of the nurse that was constructed and replicated was that of an altruistic, educated woman unconcerned with payment for her work.

The Queensland Council of the ATNA was involved in the supervision of nurse training in order to produce well-qualified trained nurse members. This covered checking the level of education of nursing recruits; recognising and registering hospital training schools and continually supervising their standards; setting training standards by outlining a schedule of lectures for each year of training; and conducting examinations for nursing trainees. The emphasis was on a training that was essentially practical rather than theoretical and combined the demands of training with the needs of the hospital for large amounts of reliable labour.

The association carefully considered the question of the minimum standards for entry as a trainee nurse. As the ATNA recognised, 'the education of girls is extraordinarily unequal and . . . with the exception of the State Schools there is nothing like the uniformity of standard maintained in schools for girls that there is in those for boys'.[2] The low qualification level for entry was directly related to the low standard of education generally for girls and meant that any discussion of an alternative to hospital-based training, such as university education, was effectively meaningless. The 1906 Circular to Training Schools specified that the minimum educational standard for trainee nurses was the sixth form of primary school[3] but the minimum standard finally adopted was the fifth form,[4] the general school leaving standard for girls. An editorial in the *ANJ* commented that 'though many think it errs on the low side, it is on the whole probably the best that could be at present devised'.[5] The entry standard remained essentially the same in Queensland (completion of primary school) until 1968 when the standard was raised to the Junior Examination (equivalent of grade 10), fifteen years after this had occurred in New South Wales.[6]

At the turn of the century in Queensland, schooling was compulsory for children aged six to eleven years old. It was usual for twelve and thirteen year olds to be in the fourth and fifth classes with an extremely small percentage completing the sixth class.[7] Most girls in Queensland did not reach sixth class and few proceeded to secondary education, which was 'still narrowly conceived as the education of . . . "the brightest of the bright", in academic courses leading to the university'.[8]

Education beyond primary school was rare as 'the ability of parents to extend their children's schooling depended very much on whether the family unit could forgo the income those children could earn if they left school and entered the workforce'. Girls who were not in paid work themselves were 'very likely to be at home attending to domestic duties and minding children while their mother worked'.[9] The 1911 census showed that 92 per cent of twelve year olds were receiving an education compared with 78 per cent of thirteen year olds. By the age of fourteen less than half the population (42 per cent) were receiving an education, with only 20 per cent in education at the age of fifteen.[10] From this system 'the great majority emerged as they reached their teens . . . with a rudimentary capacity for reading, writing and arithmetic'.[11] Girls who 'persisted with their secondary education in the state high school, like those in the private sector, had to have financial support, parental encouragement and high personal ambition'.[12]

In Queensland, secondary schooling leading to university entrance was only available through private, protestant denominational schools or grammar schools until 1912 when the first state high schools were opened. The charges at the private and grammar schools meant that they were prohibitively expensive for most parents. Although a few scholarships were offered to secondary schools in Queensland, even fewer country children could actually go to the city schools to utilise them.[13]

As well as lack of opportunity to pursue secondary education, the purpose of education was different for girls and boys. About the turn of the century, a greater differentiation between the subjects taught to boys and to girls was advocated. Whereas boys were thought to need a wide variety of schooling so that they could undertake many different occupations in the paid workforce, girls were seen to need 'a common education for their single role as wives and mothers'.[14] This reflected late nineteenth and early twentieth century changes in the skills needed to care for a home and family and 'it was argued that instincts were not enough for the modern world: household management and cookery must become part of the school curriculum for girls'.[15] 'Housewifery' came to be 'the common denominator' in the emphasis of much of girls' education and 'according to the proponents of the domestic ideal, education for their total development was to be firmly rooted in the environment of home and family'.[16]

Having completed school before the age of fourteen, what would a young woman do until she could begin nurse training at the age of 20 in some country hospitals or even 23 at some of the city hospitals? Dr Robert Scott, surgeon at Ballarat Hospital from 1886 to 1911[17] felt that 'experience shows that the best nurses are those who have had some preliminary training, not specially as a nurse, but such as will tend to refine her character, make her more companionable to her patients, and prevent her profession from having any hardening tendency'. How was this training in character to be achieved? Scott felt that:

> after having formed an ideal, she should go through a course of introspection. Let her examine her own character; seek out relentlessly her failings. Is she easily put out of temper? Correct this by playing tennis or croquet or even bridge with a bad partner, and when she is congratulated on being a 'good loser,' let her consider she has conquered this defect.[18]

Scott obviously believed that only women of middle class backgrounds entered nursing and the potential trainee could fill her days with leisure pursuits. But what was the young woman without independent means to do? Women who had to earn a living upon leaving school were presumably lost to nursing as they entered other occupations in which they remained. Some country hospitals solved their own staffing problems by obtaining probationers from the long waiting lists of the metropolitan hospitals.[19] The editor of the Royal Victorian Trained Nurses' Association (RVTNA) magazine *Una* felt that working as a probationer in a private hospital, which often accepted a woman a few years younger than the public hospitals, was not useful as 'the arduous work must of necessity sap the girl's powers, both nervous and physical. She therefore later starts her actual training with her initial store of force materially lessened'.[20]

Girls wishing to become probationers were directed by the ATNA to apply to the matron of the hospital of their choice with three personal references and a certificate of health. After 1 June 1906 (January 1907 for prospective midwifery trainees) all applicants were referred to the newly constituted Educational Committee of the ATNA in each state.[21] This committee of three was elected annually by each branch council and had the duty of deciding if an applicant had sufficient educational qualifications. In Queensland the Board of Examiners consisted of matrons in active work and medical practitioners; Misses Jane Bell (Matron of the Brisbane Hospital from 1904 to 1906) and Edith Annie Best (Lady Superintendent of the Hospital for Sick Children, Brisbane, 1898 to 1906) and doctors Hopkins, Turner and J. McLean (Medical Superintendent, Brisbane Hospital, 1904 to 1931) were appointed as the first committee.[22]

As most nurses entered private nursing on completion of their training, there had to be a constant stream of probationers to staff the hospitals cheaply. By setting entry qualifications at the level of primary school completion, hospitals were assured of a sufficient number of trainees. A higher standard would have meant that very few girls would have been eligible for entry. For those who did not possess these qualifications provision was made for an examination in general education, conducted under the supervision of the education committee. The examination included reading aloud, a composition or essay written on a simple subject and arithmetic. Once they were accepted at a hospital, the students embarked on three months probation, at the end of which, with a satisfactory report from the matron, they could continue with their training.[23]

The prominent feature of nurse training was the apprenticeship-style, on-the-job training with some theoretical lectures to complement this. As the work of the trained nurse was seen as 'essentially practical' it was 'obviously of first importance that the practical part of her training should receive the greatest attention'.[24] Registration of hospitals as training schools was the primary means by which the ATNA sought to supervise the standard of nurse education. Ten years after the establishment of the ATNA in New South Wales, 97 hospitals throughout Queensland, New South Wales, Tasmania, South Australia, Western Australia and Fiji were recognised as training schools. There was reciprocal recognition for hospitals registered with the RVTNA and in New Zealand by arrangement with the Hospitals Department.[25]

The length of training recommended by the ATNA differed according to the size of hospital, with three years in a hospital with a daily average number of occupied beds of over 40, four years in a hospital of 20 to 40 beds and five years in a hospital of ten to 20 beds.[26] Prior to the formation of the Queensland Branch in 1904 there were thirteen hospitals registered in this state as training schools.[27] By 1909 there were seven hospitals in Queensland with a daily average of more than 40 beds which were registered as three-year training schools with the ATNA. These were the Brisbane Hospital and Brisbane Children's Hospital, and the hospitals in Charters Towers, Ipswich, Rockhampton, Toowoomba and Townsville. Ten hospitals in Queensland were registered as four-year training schools and four were registered with a five-year course.[28] This lower limit helped small regional hospitals gain cheap staff as otherwise the town would have faced the expense of having to employ trained nurses.[29]

There was some disquiet about the non-recognition of even smaller hospitals but the ATNA Council felt that advances in medical and surgical techniques meant that a nurse in a small hospital could not get a 'sufficiently varied and up-to-date experience to entitle her to be registered as fully trained'.[30] The concern with costs was the chief reason small hospitals wanted to be registered as training hospitals with the ATNA. As an *ANJ* editorial argued,

> most country hospitals employ probationers, and the aim of most probationers is to qualify for membership of the Australasian Trained Nurses' Association. Hence those hospitals which are not recognised have considerable difficulty in obtaining probationers, and are so driven to the expense of employing fully trained Nurses—an expense which they say they can ill afford.[31]

The councils of the ATNA and RVTNA argued about the recognition of private hospitals as training schools, with the ATNA recognising them and the RVTNA not doing so. The RVTNA felt that accepting these training schools was unfair to trained nurses as it deprived them of 'a large amount of legitimate practice' and

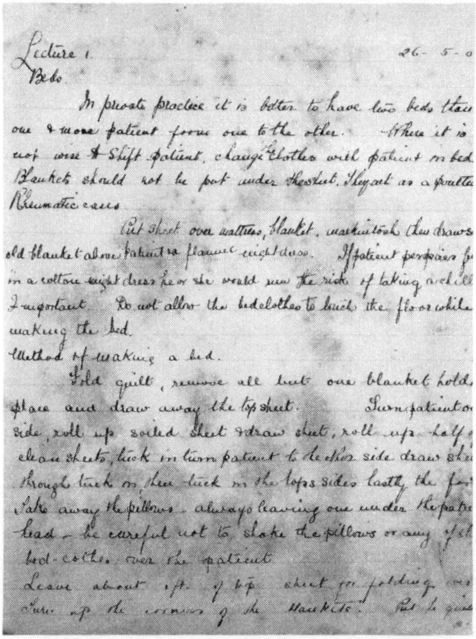

Lecture 1. 26-5-0

Beds.

In private practice it is better to have two beds than one & move patient from one to the other. Where it is not wise to shift patient, change clothes with patient in bed. Blankets should not be put under the sheet. They act as a poultice [illegible] Rheumatic cases

Put sheet over mattress, blanket, mackintosh then draws [illegible] old blanket above patient in flannel nightdress. If patient perspires [illegible] in a cotton nightdress he or she would run the risk of taking a chill. Important. Do not allow the bedclothes to touch the floor while making the bed.

Method of making a bed.

Fold quilt, remove all but one blanket hold [illegible] place and draw away the top sheet. Turn patient on side, roll up soiled sheet & draw sheet, roll up half [illegible] clean sheets, tuck in turn patient to the other side draw sheet through tuck in, then tuck in the tops sides lastly the [illegible] Take away the pillows always leaving one under the patient's head – be careful not to shake the pillows or any of the bed-clothes over the patient.

Leave about 1 ft. of top sheet for folding over. Turn up the corners of the blankets. [illegible]

Notes on bedmaking taken by Miss Eunice Paten on 26 May 1905 at her first lecture given by Matron Jane Bell when she commenced training at the Brisbane Hospital. Eunice Paten graduated in 1908 and was an active member of the ATNA for many years. She became a councillor in 1919, a position she held until she became vice-president (1933–1934, 1939–1943) and subsequently the first nurse president in 1943, a position she held until 1948. (Courtesy of Queensland Nurses' Union.)

was unfair to the public who 'pay for and expect to get trained nursing',[32] while the ATNA believed that private hospital fees 'would have to be raised to such an extent that many of the patients now admitted to them would be driven into the public hospitals'. The average patient was most concerned with keeping the cost of hospital care as low as possible and 'trusts to his doctor to see to it that he is efficiently cared for, without concerning himself with the various diplomas held by each individual concerned in the nursing'.[33] The *ANJ* concluded that training in private hospitals was satisfactory, the system was 'convenient and advantageous to the public and the medical profession'. But as well as this the system was 'a means of livelihood for those who have invested their savings in these institutions'.[34] The collision of the needs of the hospitals for labour and of the nurse for education clearly existed but was not an issue for the ATNA. The prominent role of private hospital owners and matrons in the organisation and their influence in shaping its views were attested to in the editorial's comments:

> We should, therefore, surely be diffident about following the example of so many industrial unions, and using the strength our unity has given us in endeavouring to abolish the apprenticeship system . . . and thus seriously hampering this form of private enterprise . . .

> It would be well to remember also that many of the matrons of those private hospitals have taken a very prominent part in establishing this Association.[35]

Hospitals were required to meet extensive conditions to be recognised as training schools by the ATNA. The matron had to be on the general register of the association and hold a certificate from a recognised training school for nurses; the nurses had to receive practical instruction in the hospital wards from a trained and registered matron or sister; a systematic course of lectures had to be delivered by 'duly qualified and registered medical men'; and the curriculum had to be at least equal to that set out by the ATNA. Each hospital was required to conduct annual examinations in the practical and theoretical subjects nurses had studied. A final examination in general nursing, conducted by the lecturers or other examiners specially appointed by the council of the hospital, was necessary. Nurses who passed received a certificate in the form set by the ATNA and were then eligible to become members of the association. When the ATNA instituted its own final examinations, these were substituted for those given by the hospital itself.[36]

As a means of enforcing these regulations the ATNA required the hospitals to report annually to the association with information on the daily average number of occupied beds during the previous year; the names of the teaching staff; the subjects taught and the number of lectures given; the names of the nurses attending lectures; the dates they commenced their study; and evidence that they had attended at least four-fifths of the lectures in each subject.[37]

As early as 1903, the association in New South Wales was dissatisfied with many of the hospital reports. Out of 57 hospitals it had received reports from only 39 and of these only seventeen had been satisfactory. Of the remainder the lectures were in most cases unsatisfactory or insufficient and in three cases the average number of occupied beds had fallen below the minimum of ten.[38] If the hospital did not comply satisfactorily with any of these requirements, the ATNA could withhold, suspend or withdraw recognition and registration of the hospital as a training school.[39] Recognition was withdrawn from Gladstone Hospital in 1904 because the average daily occupied beds had fallen to 7.9 and a nurse, trained only four years at the hospital, had been appointed matron. At Hughenden Hospital the average daily occupancy rate fell to six, for nine months there was no matron and the one probationer was also head nurse and acting matron. Recognition was withdrawn.[40] ATNA membership by matrons of registered training schools was enforced and the Committee of the Hospital for Sick Children in Brisbane was reminded that the acting matron should be an ATNA member.[41]

In the years following the issue of the 1906 Circular to Training Schools there was very little change in the pattern of training. The Queensland Branch answered queries from training schools and dealt with minor matters of policy, submitting some queries to the New South Wales Branch. The question arose, for instance, as to whether a nurse could change training schools or had to complete her training in one hospital.[42] The ATNA decided that her training should be carried out entirely in one hospital, for

> knowledge that she will have her probationers with her during their entire apprenticeships enables the Matron to more easily map out their period of training so as to ensure their having a suitable proportion of medical, surgical and special work. This also applies to the important question of responsibility, for it is difficult under other circumstances to test the ability of the steadily maturing Nurse by placing increasing responsibility upon her shoulders.[43]

This remained a strict rule unless there was hardship such as ill-health preventing the return of a trainee to the hospital, or if the hospital was deregistered due to a fall in the number of average daily occupied beds. The Queensland Council later approved the principle of graduation from a small to a large hospital 'provided the Council is satisfied that the training carried out is equivalent to that carried out in a single Hospital'.[44]

Trying to control the standard of training given by the various hospitals was difficult when the only means of checking what was done was through the hospitals' own annual reports.[45] The lack of a central examination meant that in 1904 New Zealand refused to recognise the ATNA certificate.[46] Victoria instituted a system of bi-annual central examinations and the larger hospitals in that state had 'quite fallen in with the scheme'.[47] Although discussions proceeded for several years it was not until 1905 that any scheme for holding central examinations was instituted by the New South Wales Council. Regulations were compiled and after June 1906 no nurse trained at a training school under the control of the ATNA was admitted to membership of the ATNA until she had passed the final examination of the association. Examinations were conducted in regional centres and an entrance fee of one guinea was charged for the final examination which entitled the successful candidate to membership of the ATNA for one year,[48] thus ensuring a captive membership. Until 1912 the ATNA in Queensland

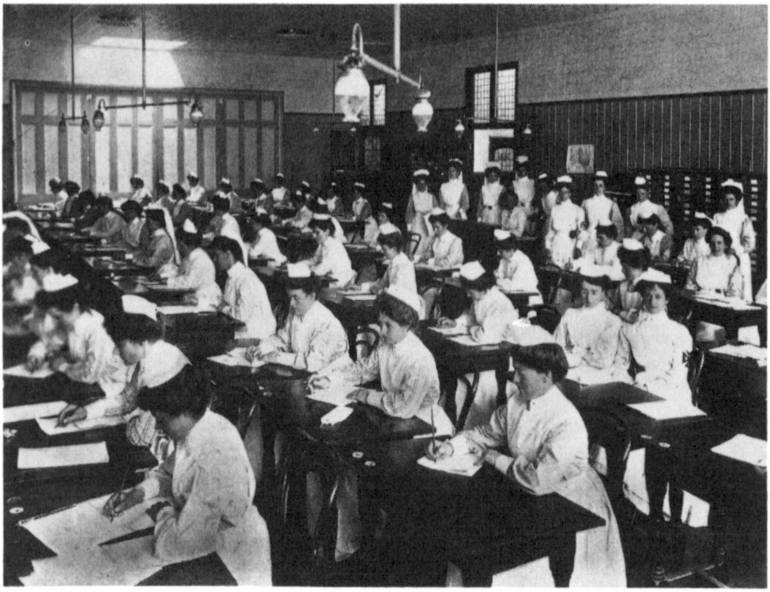

Nurses in Victoria, about 1908, sitting for their final examination conducted by the Royal Victorian Trained Nurses' Association. A pass would entitle them to become members of the RVTNA and give them recognition as trained nurses. Both the ATNA and RVTNA conducted their own examinations until State registration boards took over this function. (Una, Jan. 1909. Courtesy of Australian Nursing Federation.)

was the sole organisation which conducted final examinations for nurses, with successful candidates accepted for registration with the ATNA.[49] Following State registration of nurses this role was taken over by the state board.

The other major difficulty was the unsatisfactory quality or insufficient number of lectures given by many of the hospitals. In the Register of Members published by the association in 1904 a 'Schedule of Study to be accepted as Minimum Course for Registration by the ATNA' was set out. It advised that the matron should give practical instruction with the resident and honorary staff delivering lectures. In her first year the nurse received twelve lectures in anatomy and physiology and twelve in general nursing, including 'Distinction between the Doctor's work and that of the Nurse, Hospital etiquette'. Also included under the heading of the 'Nurse's general work' were bedmaking, hygiene of the sick room, baths, cleansing and padding splints, and prevention of infection.

In the second year there were twelve lectures in medical nursing and twelve in surgical nursing with demonstrations. In the third year, students had six practical lectures in invalid cookery and lectures in urine testing and housekeeping. It was stressed that this course 'is to be accepted as a Minimum Course, but all teachers [are] to be urged to make such Course as complete as possible'.[50] Before being eligible for the final examination, candidates had to pass an examination in anatomy and physiology at their training school and an examination in invalid cookery was necessary unless the nurse had successfully completed an approved course.[51] Within a few years some alterations to the study schedule were made, including the addition of six lectures in hygiene. This was considered vital because of 'the important part played by a Nurse as a public instructor in the prevention of disease'.[52]

The subjects for the final examination were general nursing, medical nursing, surgical nursing, hygiene and invalid cookery, unless previously passed. The papers were set by the Central Examining Board who were appointed by the ATNA and initially consisted of one nurse and one doctor, with the practical examination being conducted by the local board of examiners, who determined if the candidate possessed a sound knowledge of practical nursing.[53]

In the subject of housekeeping, instruction was given in keeping house for patients, nursing staff and men employed; the superintendence of the work of servants; the price and relative values of all food stuffs, household requisites, linen; and keeping accounts of moneys received in connection with housekeeping. It was suggested that, where possible, pupils should, for a time, personally carry out the repairs to linen, receive stores as they were bought or issued, give them out day by day as required, and be responsible for their preservation in good order. Instruction should also be given in the drawing up of official reports for the hospital committee relating to these matters.[54] Mundane cleaning and housework functions were part of the work of hospital wards and the importance of housekeeping reflected the role hygiene and cleanliness had played in reforming nursing and medicine in the nineteenth century. It also reflected the growing importance of the domestic science movement which attempted to extend scientific principles to the household[55] and its increasing place in the school curriculum for girls in the first decades of the twentieth century.

Direct comparisons are easily made between this work in the home and that in the hospital. In one lecture on housekeeping given to nurses in 1904 Miss Glennon stated that:

> the highest aim of the good housewife is to make the real man so comfortable and happy as to supply him with that unfailing energy

> which is productive of sound thought and true life. What the engineer is to the machine, that and more the true woman is to the household . . . She must see that in the home there is no obstacle to prevent man from doing the best possible work.

Of course, ladies did not actually have to do all this work: 'Although the lady of the house is not expected to do the work of the housemaid or cook, still she should have a practical knowledge of how such work is to be done, in order that she may properly appreciate those who do it'.[56]

The work of the nurse came to mirror this division within the upper class household. The scrubbing and menial chores obviously had to be performed in hospitals and in the nineteenth century nurses had usually done these tasks. Gradually, as nurses saw their work as more skilled, many wished to divest themselves of these duties and they were handed over to other poorly paid female workers, effectively passing these chores from one group of female workers to another who were classified as servants. But it was always done by women. However, for decades nursing trainees actually did cleaning and scrubbing, so that they knew how to do it and could supervise this work in the future, in the same fashion as was required of upper class wives. For 'until one has actually done a particular piece of work, one cannot claim credit for competency to perform it, still less to instruct others in its performance; the mere fact of having watched the doing of a thing a score of times is no guarantee of ability to do it'.[57] Or, as Miss E. Glover, a member of the RVTNA Council, believed,

> surely the sweeping and dusting of hospital wards, together with the small amount of indifferent cookery done in the ward pantries, will not pass for training in domestic work. After many years' experience amongst many hundreds of nurses, in hospital and out, I have met very few who could by any stretch of imagination be called domesticated women. If we accept the statement that most of us come from the middle and lower classes, this is no guarantee that we know how to do housework properly.[58]

In the first decade of the twentieth century at the Brisbane Hospital the matron, Miss Bell, asked the hospital committee to employ wardsmaids so that trainee nurses did not have to do cleaning. But she regarded this work as important and taught scrubbing herself to the trainees. Student nurses also had to stir the straw in the heavy mattresses, carbolize the beds each week and scrub the lead around the hand basins until it shone like silver. In fact, Miss Eunice Paten, first nurse president of the Queensland Branch of the ATNA, 'remembered feeling very proud when Miss Bell told her she had become a "good scrubber".'[59]

Womanly virtues and scientific education

Discussions about the nursing recruit and the details of training frequently referred to the qualities that were seen as necessary for the ideal nurse. Women who wanted to be nurses had to possess certain qualities which would be enhanced by the training they received. In developing standards for this training, those who assumed the leadership of the professional organisations worked within the framework of the beliefs about the attributes one needed to be a good nurse. Developments in the nineteenth century resulted in the model for trained nursing which 'stressed discipline, self-sacrifice, order, and a separate sphere for nursing within the hospital structure'.[60]

In the Australian nursing journals of the early twentieth century some confusion in thinking is evident, as writers attempted to link the idea that a nurse had to possess special innate womanly qualities with the idea that a nurse needed specific training. This debate emerges explicitly in the pages of the journal of the RVTNA but the ideas are borne out in the sentiments and actions of the ATNA in Queensland. Even the name of the RVTNA journal exemplified the main strand of the debate. The name *Una* was chosen because she was 'the "lovely lady" of the Red Cross Knight of the Faery Queen' who brought St George to a hospital where he was nursed back to strength. She was thus seen by the journal editor as 'the embodiment of gentle and devoted womanhood'.[61]

In the exploration of what constituted an ideal nurse and therefore what sort of person should become a nurse emphasis was placed on innate womanly or mothering attributes. In a lecture on the preliminary training of nurses, Dr Robert Scott felt that 'a nurse must, like a poet, be "born, not made." She must be wholesouled and devoted to her calling, and train herself to cheerfully give up many pleasures and make many self denials to endeavour to live up to a high ideal'.[62] In fact, he believed that 'in no profession more than that of a nurse is a high ideal of such importance' and quoted Ruskin to support his views: 'She must be enduringly . . . wise—wise, not for self improvement, but for self renunciation: wise, not with the narrowness of insolent and loveless pride, but with the passionate gentleness of an infinitely variable . . . modesty of service—the true changefulness of woman'.[63]

The nurses and doctors active in the ATNA faced a dilemma regarding the educational standard of nurses. On the one hand they stated that formal, even scientific, education was necessary to become a trained nurse, while on the other hand they believed that nursing was linked to womanly virtues. The emphasis on innate qualities was exemplified in a 1904 newspaper comment that 'all the training in the world will not . . . necessarily make a good nurse. She is born, not made, and she must add to her technical knowledge sympathy, tact, and common sense'.[64] Or, as an editorial in the Victorian nursing journal put it:

> a very large, if not the largest, usefulness of the nurse will, of course, always lie in those womanly feelings of sympathy and devotion which urged Florence Nightingale to that great initiative, which is the starting point of the present profession. But the feelings must be directed by the intellect, and upon her intellectual acquirements will inevitably depend very much of the success or failure which attends the nurse's efforts.[65]

Other writers painted the nurse as saint-like: 'In the ideal nurse we look for an infinite patience, and sympathy born of understanding, for a breadth of heart and mind that is unfortunately too rare, for perfect sincerity, loyalty, and refinement'.[66]

Nurses were seen to belong to 'the noblest and most self-sacrificing profession open to women'.[67] One nurse felt that 'nursing must mean to some extent self-renunciation'.[68] For one correspondent at least these refinements could not be found in the lower classes, a view which echoed the nursing reformers of the nineteenth century. These qualities were:

> more likely to be found among women whose homes are the abode of refinement and culture, whose parents are educated and refined, and whose minds have been trained and developed in their youth by study and discipline. The woman who is not sufficiently cultured to care to read anything but the most ephemeral trash, misses the broadening and educative influence of good literature and its consequent effect on character. The woman whose mind is bounded by her technical training, who can only talk hospital and cases, who has no knowledge of literature and art, who knows little and cares less about events outside her own sphere, who is touched not at all by the currents of thought that stir humanity, how is she to supply a convalescent's need of companionship as well as nursing, or to raise and uplift a mind disordered and depressed by physical suffering?[69]

This writer felt that a high educational entry standard would result in nursing gaining 'more cultured and refined' women.[70] Dr Robert

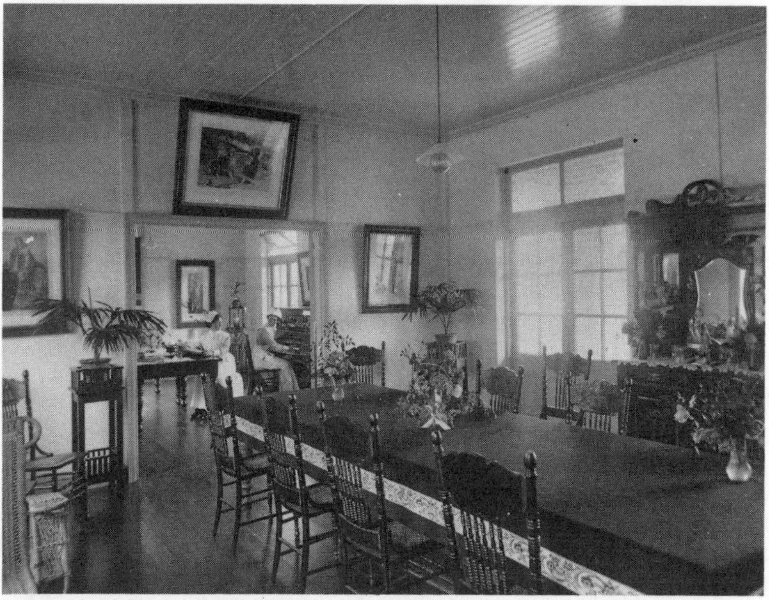

Nurses' dining and sitting room in St Mary's Home, Mater Misericordiae Hospital, Brisbane, 1914. These rooms were typical of those in city hospitals. This new nurses' home included a piano, a feature that was seen as essential for the enjoyment of nurses and was frequently mentioned in the debates over suitable nurse accommodation in the nineteenth century. (Collection: John Oxley Library, Brisbane.)

Scott felt that nursing needed to fill its ranks with 'eager, enthusiastic, and highly-trained women, and yet women of refinement and "all womanliness" '.[71]

Nursing was still linked with the idea of being a lady. A *Una* editorial maintained that:

> the evolution of the nurse has progressed, and will continue to progress, on lines that appeal to intelligent and high-minded women. And so we feel assured that all right-thinking men and women will accord the nurse . . . that position in the social scale which is due to her womanly worth and her high calling.[72]

The editorial concluded with the words:

> the greatest nurse that ever was—Florence Nightingale—had no higher honour bestowed on her than the title of 'Lady-in-Chief,' and the more closely the nurse can mould her life on the lines of her

> noblest exemplar, the more justly can she claim, and the more certainly will she attain to, her true social position.[73]

However a few years, later an *ANJ* editorial chided a matron who did not want to accept a young woman as a trainee because her parents were illiterate and of 'humble occupation' even though she had passed the ATNA's educational test. It urged 'those in charge of training schools to satisfy themselves that candidates . . . are educated, of high moral character and likely to be a credit to the nursing profession, and, if confident that they possess these qualifications, to pay no attention to their family trees'.[74]

Entry standards remained a serious concern for, as an editorial in *Una* said, nursing called for:

> the noblest qualities in woman, and raised as it now is to the rank of a science, the portals of the nursing profession should be wide enough to permit the entrance of all whom Nature has endowed with a sympathetic disposition, and whose physical and mental capacities are equal to the demands made upon them.[75]

Besides possessing 'sound health' the prospective entrant to 'this noble profession' had to have 'a natural inclination'. This meant that 'she must be sympathetic, self-sacrificing, and patient, and she must be so constituted as to realize to the full the helplessness of those whom she has to serve, and the responsibility which that service places upon her'. These qualities could be judged by the matron during probation. The nurse needed 'a special mental equipment' to cope with the study now involved in her training:

> For her own sake, for the sake of her patients, and for the advancement of her profession, she must be equal not only to the educational requirements of the curriculum, but also to the intelligent observation, recording, and interpretation of the innumerable phases of disease which she will be called upon to nurse, which more often than not necessitates educational acquirements considerably above the average.[76]

A major characteristic of the nurse's role was that it had to be subordinate to the superior males in their environment, the doctors. It was seen as:

> essential that she recognise that the doctor, before all others, is the commander-in-chief, that her first duty is to loyally carry out his orders, and that in the execution of that duty she should not alone do nothing [*sic*] to disturb the patient's confidence, but rather strive, by every legitimate means, to impress her charge with the value of his

> services. With this spirit underlying her work, she should bring to the performance of her important task all the skill of which she is mistress, all the thoroughness and attention to detail that she can command, all the sympathy and tact that she has inherited or acquired.[77]

It would be many decades before nurses could accept an identity independent of doctors, while still carrying out their orders as part of their work and would take until the second half of the twentieth century for the independent role of the nurse to be widely accepted.

Working conditions

If the work of a nurse involved self-sacrifice there needed to be extraordinary conditions in which she could give of herself. This was found in the harsh working conditions. The work was characterised as drudgery and the nurse had to be 'a strong, capable, practical, sweet-tempered woman, whose work can never be comfortably rounded into eight hours, but more often runs into 18'.[78] The training was 'long and arduous' and her work once she had qualified was 'frequently more arduous still'.[79]

Working conditions were discussed in a way that was akin to the trials of faith demanded of those with a religious vocation. Dr Scott said that nurses should impress on prospective trainees—

> the very highest traditions of nursing as a profession—let her see that what she wishes to become can only be done by hard work, combined with true love for her work; put before her, truthfully, the hardships she will have to put up with; the selfishness and ingratitude, and ofttimes the deliberate, and it may be malignant, misconstructions from those to whom one's best service has been given; above all, do not allow her to go into the profession for the glamour of novelty, which will be destroyed, like the gloss on new paint, after very little wear and tear.[80]

The nurse had to be a woman of virtue with unfailing patience, physically very strong and intelligent enough to absorb theoretical training. Nurses were clearly marked as different from other workers, even other women workers. As an occupation, trained nursing was in a peculiar position with 'an ambiguous and uncertain status. Although wage labor, it was seen as akin to a woman's devotional acts on behalf of her family. As women's work in a field dominated by male physicians, it was subordinate labor. As woman's labor, it demanded self-sacrifice and self-abnegation'.[81]

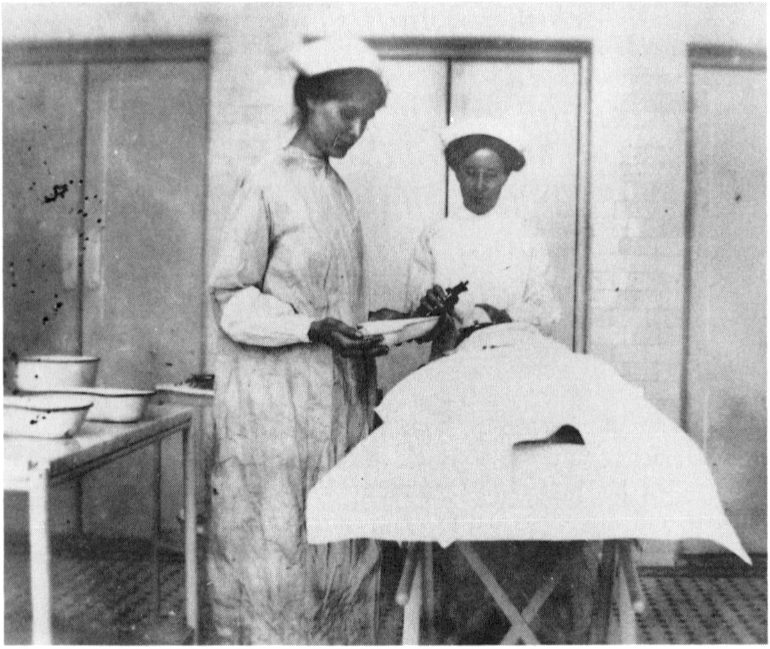

Nurse Freeman administers anaesthetic at the Hospital for Sick Children, Brisbane, 10 November 1914. (Collection: Royal Brisbane Hospital Graduate Nurses' Archive and John Oxley Library, Brisbane.)

Nurses were expected to have a vocation and a moral development that was not required of other workers. No wonder nurses had great difficulty in coming to grips with the belief that they could expect decent working conditions like other workers. These views which singled out nursing's special characteristics of sacrifice and service had the very practical consequence that nursing organisations showed little concern for, and rarely took action on, the working conditions of their members. The dilemma was that self-sacrifice gave nurses status but meant that the regulation of working conditions was not seen as a proper sphere of action. Miss MacLean, Matron of the Women's Hospital in Melbourne, felt that:

> our work, in its very nature, needs a spirit of self-sacrifice, quite outside all question of recompense. We cannot measure our work and charge so much per hour; we must throw ourselves into it and work while there is need, and because we wish to do all that is possible, and not merely all that is absolutely necessary.[82]

Defined hours and regulated working conditions were often seen as the hallmarks of a trade, something that the nursing leaders were trying to move away from. If nurses worked a set number of hours it would be 'at the greatest sacrifice of the dignity of our profession, bringing it down to the level of a trade'.[83] Also 'the eight hour system' was considered impractical because of the expense of the extra staff that would be required.[84] Miss Glover stated firmly that:

> we are not of trade, and therefore the eight hours question does not, and I hope never will, apply to nursing. We are professional women, and work for the benefit of mankind—not for twelve hours, but twenty-four if necessity arises. A nurse who is willing to leave her patient at a critical moment, on the stroke of the clock, is not worth being called a nurse . . . A nurse's life is hard, and full of self-sacrifice. Anyone going into the profession must go in fully prepared to sacrifice a great deal for the sake of her work. We must not measure our hours of labour, but rather regret that we cannot do more.[85]

These views were widespread. One hospital association in the USA in 1917 asserted that 'the work of nurses can no more be regulated by a hard-and-fast law than the work of doctors or mothers'.[86] Miss Glover thought an eight-hour day was possible for nurses 'if sufficient pressure be brought to bear', but that it would be of 'doubtful benefit to nurses'. Hospitals and private patients could not afford to pay the costs that this arrangement would entail and, after all, 'a good nurse can never be fully compensated by money. She must be paid, as she undoubtedly is, a fair remuneration, but her work must be something better, something higher, and I may add purer and holier than the ordinary commerce of to-day'.[87]

In 1904 ,the Brisbane Hospital reduced the working hours of nurses to nine and a half hours a day, six and a half days a week.[88] Six years later at the annual general meeting of the ATNA in Queensland it was resolved that 'the hours for Hospital nurses are excessive, and that the number of hours on duty per week should be reduced',[89] but steps were not taken actively to pursue this goal. In England, Maggs records that the eight-hour day was not discussed by nurses themselves until 1921 at the earliest.[90]

Agitation over industrial issues was rare, although some groups of nurses in the USA in the second decade of the century took strike action because of harsh conditions, bad food and overwork. These strikes were 'mainly the ephemeral and desperate actions of women angered by overwork and the abuse of power'.[91] In the end,

> for most nursing students the moral dilemma of leaving ill patients, the professional dilemma of classing oneself with workers, and the psychological dilemma of openly thwarting authority were overwhelming. Instead they sought survival through more subtle tactics on a day-to-day basis, or simply quit.[92]

The ATNA in Queensland was vehemently against nurses taking strike action, or any manner of industrial action. At a time of considerable industrial activity and protracted strikes throughout Australia[93] an editorial in the *ANJ* in 1911 clearly showed the ATNA's anti-strike stance:

> We view with regret that the unrest at present existing among industrial workers should have invaded the nursing profession. The right of protesting to the proper authorities against oppression and injustice, real or imaginary, is one all will admit, but to threaten a strike of the nursing staff—most of whom are trainees—of a large public hospital must be deplored from every point of view.[94]

The ideal of the nurse was used in justifying this position: 'It is certainly a retrograde step in a profession whose present high traditions have been built up by the unselfish and loyal devotion to work of its members'. An almost military discipline had to be accepted: 'When a probationer enters a hospital she must accept the discipline necessary for the protection and welfare of patients, and also for her own proper training'.[95]

These were the predominant views expressed through the ATNA and RVTNA journals and only rarely is a dissenting voice heard. Unlike women teachers,[96] for instance, the ATNA was not concerned with wider political issues or questions of women's suffrage. The only mention comes from the Victorian journal in connection with the efforts of Vida Goldstein, prominent suffragist,[97] who urged nurses to support women's suffrage 'for the sake, if need be, of their own self-protection, and of reaching the causes of the evils that drive thousands of people into our hospitals'.[98] She dared to open a debate in the press, saying that many nurses and their parents had told her that they were 'broken down' after their training and that the food for nurses was very poor.[99] 'Until I have satisfactory evidence that the rank and file of the hospital nurses disapprove of my action', she wrote, 'I shall take every favourable opportunity to speak and work on their behalf'.[100] A number of letters disagreed with her views. 'A Wellwisher' felt that any grievances about food or conditions should be taken up with the RVTNA.[101] Another correspondent, saying that she represented the opinions of 'a large section of the profession', vehemently stated that:

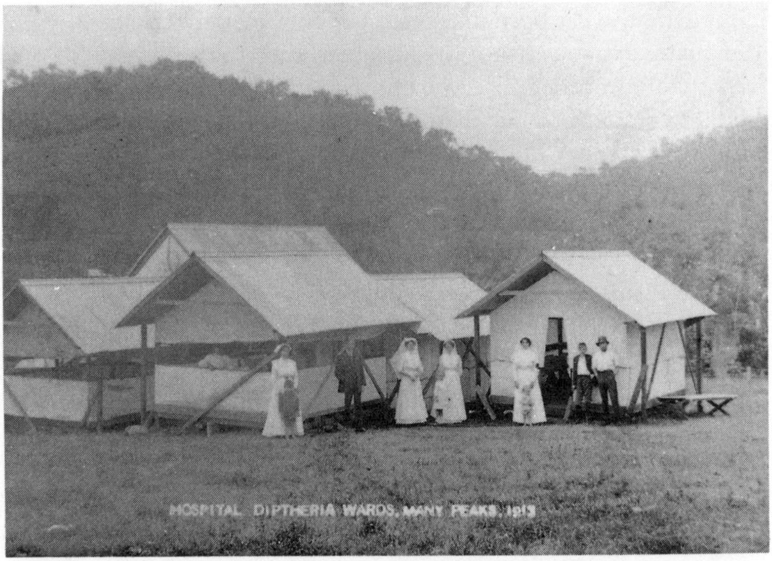

Nursing conditions were harsh in many country districts where nurses lacked the amenities of large city hospitals. This 1913 photograph shows nurses standing outside the diphtheria wards at Many Peaks Hospital, a town with a population of 1200 in the centre of a mining district, 93 kilometres south-west of Gladstone in central Queensland. Isolation in special wards, often tents, was common for infectious diseases such as diphtheria which was a major cause of death in this period. (Collection: John Oxley Library, Brisbane and Queensland Nurses Union.)

> trained nurses do not need any political influence used on their behalf, simply because the long hours and hard work inseparable from private nursing is their willing and cheerful contribution to the cause of suffering humanity, and is not in any sense exacted from them. The Trades Hall spirit of measuring out so many hours and so much exertion to each day, regardless of the public need, has so far found no favour among our nurses, and it will be an evil day for profession and public when it does so.[102]

However, 'Trained Nurse' disagreed:

> The fact that the hospitals are insufficiently supported is not an adequate reason why one section of the community should be oppressed to benefit another section. There is more sweating done in the name of charity than people have any idea of. An inspection of the salaries paid to employees in charitable institutions, in conjunction with the hours of duty, would convince any inquiring person of this fact.

She felt that, with hospital nurses working 60 or 70 hours a week, often with extra overtime in an emergency, nurses were 'shorter lived than any other . . . women of their class'. They also looked older and more worn out than their age and frequently took several months sick leave during their training. This writer stated that nurses were 'full of readiness to sacrifice themselves for their patients in any case of necessity, often in cases where no real necessity exists, but this does not give the community any right to sacrifice them to its poor'. But she did not blame the hospital authorities for this state of affairs. She concluded that:

> nurses, as a class, will never use their vote for their own aggrandisement—they are a much nobler-spirited class of women than that—but they should understand that if their strength is worn out, and their lives shortened needlessly, they have less service to give to humanity, and on this higher ground they should demand better food than is often supplied, and more reasonable hours of duty.[103]

Thus conditions could be improved if nurses' service to humanity was threatened. This would be the reason for asking for better wages and conditions: without higher pay nurses could not save enough money to exist in their old age or without better conditions nurses would become ill and therefore could not serve their patients well. This was the justification that the Queensland Branch of the ATNA used when it was forced to deal with these industrial issues. While tied to the reality of providing cheap labour in hospitals, nurses were socialised into behaviour which always put others' needs before their own.

The possibility of a nurse's training taking place within a university and thus removing this supply of labour was canvassed only briefly. An editorial in the *ANJ* in 1912 stated:

> in this age of progressive higher education, when universities all over the world are opening their doors to students of the many commercial and utilitarian sciences and arts of today, should not the profession of nursing—the hand-maiden of medicine—be considered worthy of recognition by the Universities of the States? There are Faculties of Veterinary, Agricultural, Dental, and Pharmaceutical sciences. Are these of greater value to the citizens of the State than a Faculty of Nursing, where women and men would receive the highest teaching in the nursing and the care of the young and sick?

The ultimate prize would be that:

> a Faculty of Nursing at the Sydney University would assure the future teaching and training of the Nurses in this State being placed on the highest level of efficiency, and the nursing profession given a status recognised by the highest seat of learning, to which it has every right by reason of its many high and noble traditions of the past.[104]

This cry was taken up after the First World War at an annual meeting of the New South Wales Branch by Miss Isla Blomfield, who argued for the establishment of a College of Nursing where nurses would attend lectures and pass examinations for twelve months and then move into the hospitals. She felt that:

> during this war so many untrained women have been made use of to do the work of nurses, that it is especially necessary that the standard of the trained nurse should be raised. With this end in view, the educational standard should be higher and a Nursing College be established. What the University training has done to improve the status of the masseuses a College of Nursing would do for the nurse.[105]

'Interested' was also in favour of a College of Nursing, as 'the present system of training imposes too severe a tax on the health of trainees. In some hospitals nurses are required to do 12 hours hard physical labour and attend lectures at the end of the day'. It was 'in the hands of the nurses themselves to raise or lower the profession. The good work of nursing is worthy of the best training obtainable, and I feel sure a College of Nursing would help the work along'.[106]

However, university or tertiary college training for nurses never progressed any further than the discussion stages and was not implemented until the 1970s and 1980s. One issue that would have hampered any moves in this direction was the low level of education accepted as sufficient for entrance to the training schools. Although other ways of training nurses were discussed on rare occasions, none were seriously entertained, nor would this have been realistic. Given that large numbers of new recruits to nurse training were needed each year, a primary school education was the only achievable level that could be set. Besides this, university education was only beginning to be accessible to women, and the University of Queensland did not begin offering courses until 1911. University education was seen as serving a different purpose for women than it did for men. As Summers has stated, there was:

> the notion that a woman's academic qualifications were to be measured in terms of her maternal, which then amounted to her marital, status. The educated woman who, perhaps after a short period of pursuing a career, renounced all to become a wife and mother was

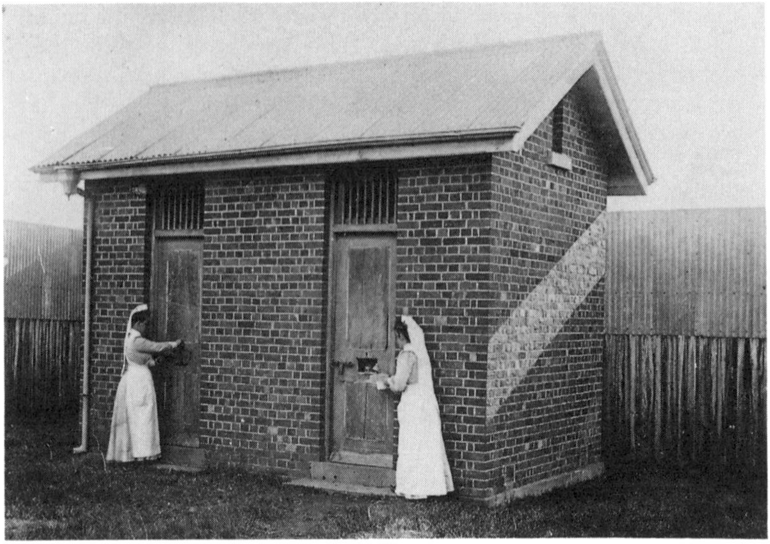

Nurses tending to patients with pneumonic plague in Maryborough, Queensland, in 1905. Pneumonic plague, one of the deadliest of diseases, is a droplet infection spread by sneezing, coughing or speaking, with death occurring within a few days. Eight people died in the only outbreak of this form of plague in Australia. Nurses Cecelia Bauer and Rose Wiles, staff nurses at the Maryborough Hospital, nursed infected patients before a diagnosis of plague was made. They contracted the plague and died in June 1905 at the ages of 22 and 28 respectively. Their sacrifice is commemorated by a fountain in Maryborough and the Bauer-Wiles Bursary for nurses. (P. Curson & K. McCracken, Plague in Sydney: The Anatomy of an Epidemic, *New South Wales University Press, Sydney, 1989, pp. 66–67.* Collection: John Oxley Library, Brisbane.)

> deemed to have successfully carried out her 'highest' vocation, but the woman who chose to follow her profession and did not marry was regarded as not being a 'real' woman.[107]

This dichotomy of choice was, of course, never an imperative for men whose accepted world lay at work.

Nurses never came in for the opprobrium reserved for other educated, unmarried women workers, for they bore the stamp of altruism and dedication to humanity which was seen as a suitable role for women and an acceptable alternative to the individual humanitarian role of caring for husband and children. Or, as Archbishop Duhig announced at a graduation ceremony for nurses in 1945, 'next to Motherhood, Nursing is the most important career for a girl'.[108] In this public acceptance of their vocation they stood apart from other women and became 'the third sex'. Maggs has used this term, coined in a 1913 book titled *The Night Nurse*, because 'their training as new nurses made them have such a view of the world, and of sex and gender in particular, as to make "their inherent femininity recede into the background" '.[109]

This can be clearly seen in the novel *A Bride for St Thomas*, about an Australian woman who applies to St Thomas' Hospital in London to train as a nurse in the 1930s. While waiting to be interviewed by the matron she realises that she is wearing a frivolous hat and cannot approach the senior nurse in this. The woman sitting next to her wore 'a grey felt hat with a brim, a formless object that served to keep her hair tidy and effectually protect her from any side-long glance of male admiration'. For Mary Bates 'it was the most desirable object in the world'. She borrows it for the interview and comments that 'once it was resting on my ears I had a chance of being mistaken for a girl whose only interest was a mission in life'.[110] The result was that 'nurses became . . . not pseudo-men, semi-doctors or especially-feminine women; they became, if they stayed in nursing, members of the "third sex" and were thus exploited twice over'.[111] They were the survivors of the arduous hospital training who had chosen to remain in the profession and not marry. In the words of a poem published in *The Hospital* in 1896 they were those who could say:

> And so in spite of all that's hard, in spite of tired feet,
> There's something in this busy life, a something that is sweet;
> And if I had my choice again I still would be a nurse,
> And take the cap and apron—for better or for worse.[112]

The ideas and beliefs about a woman's place in the world and what constituted the ideal nurse exerted a powerful influence over the concerns and activities of the ATNA. Their occupation was seen as a suitable one for women and, as the overwhelming majority remained unmarried, one that presented probably the only acceptable occupational alternative to marriage which did not impugn a woman's maternal role. That maternal role had been firmly established in the public mind with the images of Florence Nightingale and her lamp making her way among the soldiers at Scutari. It was an image of self-sacrifice and service to humanity, an image of a woman who would do this work and not ask for reward, for the reward was the work itself. They were unlike other women workers who needed to be married to be seen as whole. They were not like other workers who might bargain for their wages and form trade unions. They were indeed different, they were 'the third sex'.

CHAPTER 4

State registration of nurses in Queensland, 1912

'The only guarantee which can be offered that the standard of medical and nursing attendance is as efficient as modern teaching admits of.'[1]

State registration of nurses marked the ultimate acceptance of nursing as an occupation requiring standardised training. In August 1911, the Queensland Government became the first in Australia and one of the first in the world to pass this legislation. Other Australian states did not introduce similar legislation until the 1920s.[2] The system for organising the training of nurses had been the prime function of the ATNA in Queensland for nearly a decade; by 1911 it was almost totally accepted by the government under the legal requirements for registration. Anxieties about the state of health of the population and low birthrates led to wide-ranging health legislation being passed in Queensland and elsewhere. The regulation of private hospitals and the State registration of nurses was introduced as part of these moves. The regulation of midwives had been introduced in Britain in 1902 and New Zealand in 1904.

Registration effectively acknowledged the occupational viability of one group, the trained, and kept out another group, the formally untrained. Willis has characterised this licensing as 'a form of legal protection for the occupational territories of various health occupations from competitors. The state . . . provides those occupations with statutory registration . . . as a means of self-defence against encroachment upon their means of livelihood'.[3] State registration of nurses meant that public acceptance of this group of health workers was complete.

Reasons for registration

At the end of the nineteenth century, nursing leaders in Australia, Britain and the United States chose registration as the way to proceed and develop a relatively exclusive occupation for women. Nurse registration was avidly discussed in Britain and the United States, and New Zealand introduced such legislation in 1901. The ATNA had established standards of entry and training which assisted these moves for regulation and laid the basis for the legislation. Lavinia Dock, noted American nursing spokeswoman and honorary secretary of the International Council of Nurses, observed that Australia was 'doing excellent and energetic work on lines of general education, and preparing for State registration by a voluntary system'. She felt that 'their most excellent and practical provision' was that the head of an approved training school had to be a fully trained nurse. In her address to the New York Nurses' Association in October 1905, reprinted in the Victorian journal *Una*, she characterised the registration movement as 'part of the movement toward betterment of general education; it is a part of the movement to elevate women by fitting them for the better performance of their duties. It is a part of the effort to develop the human race and bring it to a nobler type'.[4]

According to Melosh, these women, 'like members of many struggling occupations, have long sought to identify themselves with the prestige and the privileges of the professions'.[5] Professional aspirations 'empowered nurses, pushing them beyond the confines of domestic ideology into the new possibilities of the labor market . . . In identifying themselves with professionals, they tried to act as men's equals in the world of paid work. They refused the limiting conventions of gender in their own lives and in their goals for nursing as an occupation'. But professionalisation as an ideology divided nurses[6] because, by

> adopting the exclusionary tactics of professionalization, leaders sought to secure the privileges of a few at the expense of many . . . To the extent that the leaders endorsed a professional hierarchy based on expertise, they participated in maintaining their own subordination. Within the logic of professionalization, doctors had an unshakeable claim to the controlling position in the medical division of labor: they could be unseated only by a direct challenge to the values of professional ideology.[7]

She speculates that other occupational strategies such as trade unionism might have proved more effective. In Australia, the culture of the women who trained as nurses in the early years of the century made them see themselves as different from trade unionists. Even though other white-collar workers such as teachers had formed associations which included industrial functions, nurses and the ATNA looked to the registration model of doctors.

Nurse registration had always been one of the ATNA's major objectives, with the association preferring a federal Act or 'precisely similar' state legislation so that there were uniform provisions thoughout Australia.[8] The ATNA had 'only established the system of voluntary registration as a makeshift to serve till the time was ripe and the public sufficiently enlightened to be entrusted with the task of passing a sufficiently comprehensive Act'.[9] As early as 1903, the ATNA Council in New South Wales felt that it should be prepared with suggestions for any proposed Bill on this subject and a sub-committee drafted an outline of one.[10] A year or so after this, an informal meeting was held in Sydney to discuss State registration for Australasia[11] which would 'set the seal of efficiency on the well-trained Nurse'.[12] From its inception the ATNA had endeavoured to gain recognition for trained nurses, both as a means of protecting the public against the possible malpractice of untrained women and of ensuring the employment of trained over untrained nurses:

> The public has a right while paying for a trained Nurse to some guarantee that it receives what it pays for, and there can be no question that the surest way to obtain this guarantee is for the State to require all those wishing to practice as Nurses to give proof of a minimum of training, and, further, to test their knowledge by examination . . . The system, while protecting the people, at the same time protects the trained Nurse by preventing anyone whose name is not upon the Register from receiving fees for nursing.[13]

Neither the ATNA nor the RVTNA favoured the separate registration of midwives as they believed it would create an occupation of midwifery which was separate and independent of nursing.[14] In some districts, particularly country areas, midwives competed directly with doctors for cases and thus posed a direct threat to the livelihood of some doctors. As general nursing developed it also came into competition with midwifery when it tried to incorporate childbirth within its occupational core. Although midwives 'resisted being incorporated into nursing with the subordination that entailed',[15] they could not succeed in retaining their separate identity against the combined opposition of the established medical profession and general nursing. Both doctors and nurses agreed on this, 'nurses because it extended their occupational territory to include the tasks associated with childbirth, doctors because the incorporation of midwifery into nursing ensured its subordination'.[16] The ATNA felt that it was better for a person dealing with childbirth to be trained as a general nurse first and then to do six months' specific training in midwifery. It reluctantly accepted six months' training in midwifery, without training as a general nurse, because, it believed,

> Sydney was overrun by unqualified, dirty old women, to the detriment of the poorer public. They agreed that the fully-trained nurse with an obstetric certificate was the ideal if she could be got to take obstetric cases. If perfection could not be obtained, it was desirable to do the best possible to get rid of the old 'Sarah Gamp'.[17]

By the time consideration was given to the question of maternal and infant health in the 1900s and the regulation of the practice of midwives, the issue overlapped with the regulation of nurses generally.

The international debate about nurse registration coincided with widespread concern over public health issues in Australia, including the lack of population growth and the health of mothers and infants because, with fewer babies born, it was felt that they should be provided with a better standard of care. These concerns led to the New South Wales Royal Commission on the Decline of the Birth-Rate in 1904, which concluded that there should be more public maternity hospitals available to 'allow better training of obstetric nurses, closer control of puerperal fever and the earlier hospitalisation of women experiencing complicated pregnancies'. It recommended that the state government regulate and inspect all private hospitals and maternity homes and proposed that each of these establishments should have a trained obstetric nurse in charge.[18]

Dr Charles Kinnaird Mackellar, who had chaired the 1904 Royal Commission, introduced a Bill for a Private Hospitals Act into the New South Wales Parliament in 1906. The Act aimed to institute government supervision of private hospitals, particularly those where it was believed that 'the murder of unborn children is callously committed almost daily'.[19] It also aimed at gaining jurisdiction over 'the class of untrained women who call themselves Nurses for the purposes of gain, taking in lying-in cases and treating them in a way little short of murder', and included a system of judging the qualifications of nurses in charge of these hospitals.[20]

The *Private Hospitals Act of 1908* (NSW) specified that managers of private hospitals had to be qualified nurses or qualified medical practitioners. A qualified nurse was one who had worked in a recognised medical and surgical hospital for at least three years and had passed an examination approved of by the Board of Health, while a 'midwifery nurse' had to have at least one year's training.[21] The ATNA concluded that:

> the Act will do much good, and though we should have liked to see a better definition of a Hospital Nurse, we fail to see how anything much better could have been decided upon until a Nurses' Registration Act comes into force. It is rather a case of putting the cart before the horse to legislate about what a Nurse may do before we have decided what a Nurse is.[22]

Although the Act was not one which was primarily concerned with State recognition of trained nurses, it strongly indicated State and community acceptance for nurse registration. The days of having untrained nurses in positions of responsibility or acting under their own direction were plainly over, except in remote country areas.

In 1909, Dr Mackellar introduced a specific nurse registration Bill in New South Wales, based on one which had been introduced into the British Parliament. It provided for the registration of general nurses, mental nurses and midwifery nurses, and proposed a specific Nurses' Registration Board whose membership included medical practitioners and matrons (in later amendments a representative of the ATNA was included),[23] to organise examinations, appoint examiners and issue registration certificates. Dr Mackellar stated that 'modern science demands not only that medical men shall be proficient in the science they practice, but that the nurses who carry out their orders shall be so educated that they may do their duty in a scientific way'.[24] A meeting of delegates from all ATNA branches, 'fully representative' of trained nurses in these states, decided that it was an excellent Bill[25] and the ATNA presented a petition to Parliament in favour of it.[26] The Nurse Registration Bill proposed in New South Wales overcame the fears of the ATNA council about being the recipients of an unsatisfactory Act. They had wanted a separate Act for the registration of nurses which provided a minimum standard of training acceptable to the association. It was important to the ATNA that nurses were represented on the registering body as 'no body upon which the Nurses are not directly represented is qualified to justly appreciate their interests'.[27] Or, as an editorial put it,

> the only safety for us lies in our pointing out that we have a right to be treated in exactly the same way as the medical and dental professions, and to have a special Board appointed upon which we are properly represented by members of our profession conversant with the needs of modern nursing, and assisted by medical men in active practice.[28]

The ATNA believed that the nurses' nominees on this board should be able to exert 'a reasonable weight in the voting upon vital questions'.[29] However, the council had been afraid this might not happen as Dr Mackellar 'had repeatedly stated that he would not consent to move any bill to register Nurses unless they were to be registered by the Board of Health. He . . . refused to be a party to the appointment of any Board which had Nurses on it. He did not consider that any Board with women on it would work satisfactorily'.[30]

The New South Wales Bill did not seek to stop anyone practising as a nurse, but proposed that a person could not state or imply that she was a registered nurse unless she was registered under the Act. Also included in the Bill was a clause which entitled a registered nurse to wear a distinctive badge.[31] As one parliamentarian said,

> if it is a wise thing to protect people with regard to medical practitioners, chemists, and dentists, I think it is still wiser to protect them with regard to nurses. A man has, perhaps, weeks to consider what dentist he will go to; he may have a very considerable time to consider what doctor he will call in . . . But with regard to nursing, in ninety-nine cases out of a hundred a nurse is called in when people have no expectation, perhaps the day before, that a nurse would be required.[32]

There was little opposition to the idea of registering nurses though Mr B. O'Conor wondered why three years training was necessary to become a nurse. He compared this with the five years it took to become a medical practitioner and could not understand why,

> if a girl shows aptitude, and gives evidence of it by examination . . . she cannot go for her certificate without going through the formality of serving three years. After all, an examination is merely a test of knowledge, and it seems to me that three years is a long time in a woman's life to train for a nurse.[33]

Dr Nash, however, felt that three years was the minimum time needed 'unless she is prepared to work abnormally hard; and you are not going to ask women to work their finger nails off and their brains dry'. A medical student, by contrast, had to be 'an educated man before he starts'. As well, he had to study for at least twelve hours each day and, Nash avowed, 'surely the hon. member would not ask a woman to do that?'[34] The necessity for hospital labour was not raised.

One member of Parliament was concerned about the hours nurses worked. Mr F. Flowers felt that the legislature should regulate the hours of labour of 'the grandest body of women in the community'. Hospitals in country areas 'could be termed nothing else but sweating dens' and he thought that the Bill would be of very little consequence to nurses

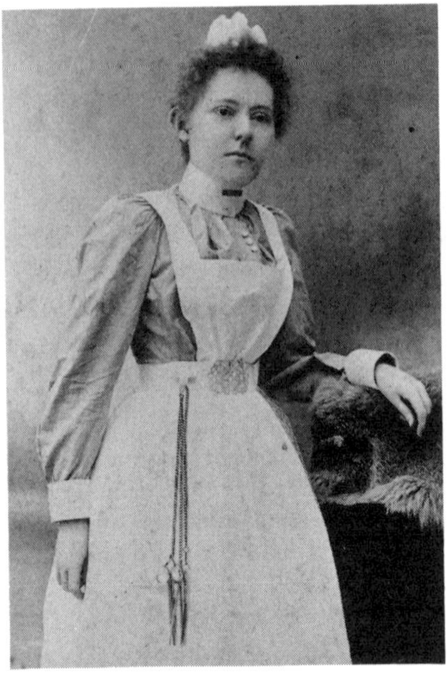

Elizabeth Harrison, nee Beames, trained as a nurse in Townsville Hospital from 1900 to 1903. She married and worked as a private nurse in Ravenswood in north Queensland until 1914, when, widowed with three children, she went to Brisbane and trained for six months at the Lady Bowen Hospital to become a qualified midwifery nurse. At this time she became a member of the ATNA. She returned to north Queensland and ran a private hospital, Mt Alma Park, in Charters Towers. (Courtesy of E. Jordan.)

unless it could prevent the working of these long hours.[35] He moved an unsuccessful amendment that would have given the government board power to regulate the working hours of nurses in both public and private hospitals.[36] But as another member noted, it was not the Bill's intention to 'interfere with the management of any hospital'.[37] The Bill was widely supported in Parliament with the major concerns being that women who practiced nursing for years, especially in country areas, might be deprived of their living.[38] However, it had an uneasy passage through Parliament, lapsed, and was re-introduced unsuccessfully in 1910 and 1913.[39] The First World War and Mackellar's advancing years[40] meant that the matter was not pursued. It was finally enacted in 1924, the same year as similar legislation in Victoria.

State registration of nurses in Queensland

Registration in Queensland was introduced in 1911 without the least pressure from nurses in this state. The *ANJ* reported that 'State Registration came as a great surprise. They had always regarded it as something to aim at in the future, but a matter in which they would follow New South Wales'.[41] Thus, as in other areas of activity and achievement, the Queensland Branch had not taken the initiative but had decided to follow the lead of the parent organisation. The honorary secretaries, Dr McLean and Miss Hunter, admitted that 'the whole is a Government measure, and there seems to be no reason why it should not be carried through in its present form'.[42] Nurse registration was included in the 1911 amendments to the Health Act along with clauses relating to the control of private hospitals similar to those in the *Private Hospitals Act* (NSW).[43]

The Health Act Amendment Bill had reached the committee stage before the ATNA became aware that it included provisions for the State registration of nurses. When the news reached the ATNA a special council meeting was hastily called and a sub-committee of Drs Halford and McLean, Misses Hunter and Chatfield was appointed to consider the Bill.[44]

The Queensland Branch of the ATNA felt that it had a right to be consulted about the provisions of any Act so crucial to the well-being of its membership of over 500 nurses.[45] The original Bill provided for the registration of nurses under the Queensland Medical Board.[46] The ATNA suggested amendments to cover midwives and mental nurses, changes concerning the length of training of nurses (the Bill specified three years, irrespective of the size of the hospital), and the representation of nurses on the board. The ATNA wanted the Bill to include a provision for general nurses to gain a certificate of training in midwifery in six months while persons without previous training should serve twelve months in a maternity hospital before obtaining a certificate.[47] The final Queensland Act registered nurses in the three categories of general nurses, midwifery nurses and mental nurses and followed the ATNA suggestions on length of training for midwifery nurses.[48]

Like their counterpart in New South Wales, the Queensland Council felt it was very important to have nurses well represented on their own registration board and wanted two representatives appointed by the Queensland Council of the ATNA on a five-person board. The Act included provision for nurse representatives on the board, but they were not nominated by the ATNA. Two medical practitioners or qualified nurses nominated by the registered nurses would join three medical practitioners on the registration board.[49] An ATNA council meeting in January 1912 felt that as the Act

> depends entirely upon the rules and regulations that are to be framed, and as it is very probable that the two members of the Board nominated by the Medical Board, together with the member of the

> Board who represents the mental Nurses, will draw up the rules and regulations, it is of the utmost importance that the A.T.N.A. should endeavour to induce the Medical Board to nominate two medical men who have the interests of nursing at heart and who are thoroughly acquainted with the rules and regulations of such an Association as the A.T.N.A.[50]

Despite these difficulties the ATNA was satisfied with the Bill and an *ANJ* editorial congratulated Queensland on its achievement, saying it was 'a Bill concise and to the point, and above all one which institutes a Board thoroughly representative to control and adjust its workings'.[51]

With the establishment of the Queensland Nurses' Registration Board (QNRB) problems associated with the nomination of a member of the board by registered nurses were overcome in the first instance by using all members of the Queensland Branch of the ATNA as the electorate. The joint honorary secretaries of the Queensland Branch, Misses Emily Hunter (Matron of the Brisbane General Hospital) and Florence Chatfield (Superintendent of the Diamentina Hospital), were nominated by the council as the representatives of the nursing profession. Their nomination was 'heartily commended' to every branch member[52] and they were elected. The other members of the board in February 1912 were Drs A.C.F. Halford, J.B. McLean, president and secretary of the ATNA, and H. Byam Ellerton, Inspector General of the Insane.

The Labor Opposition ironically pointed out that in their opinion the registration of nurses would mean that the government was giving preference to unionists. Mr John Mann commented that, 'under this amendment it was possible that the Australasian Trained Nurses' Association would boss the whole show'. Mr William Murphy of Croydon stated that he knew that 'the members of the Trained Nurses' Association were just putting themselves in the same position as members of other unions, and he did not blame them, but they wanted to make it as difficult as possible for other persons to become trained nurses'. However Mr Robert Philp from Townsville felt that it was a good thing to have two women on the board as the representatives of nurses, as 'surely the nurses had a right to be represented on the board, and to examine members of their own sex'.[53]

There was little opposition in Parliament to the clauses of the Health Act Amendment Bill which dealt with the nursing profession. The main concern of the opposition Australian Labor Party (ALP) was that country districts should be sufficiently served by nurses. Mr Vincent

Lesina, the Labor member for Clermont in western Queensland, expressed a common concern when he said that:

> it was impossible, in a sparsely populated country like Queensland, to apply the rigorous conditions which might be applied in a country like Great Britain, where people were in close touch with medical assistance. In Queensland, where people had to do pioneering work, necessarily a great deal of nursing had to be done by amateurs, and some of the most successful nurses in the back country were women who could barely write their names.[54]

Members of the ALP were not the only ones concerned about the rural population. Mr Godfrey Morgan, conservative party member for Murilla, was worried that women practising satisfactorily as midwives in remote districts would not be able to pass the examination required by the Bill and 'it would be inflicting a serious hardship on the people in these districts if these women were prevented from practising'.[55] Mr James O'Sullivan, the member for Kennedy in the far north of the state, said that there were 'scores of women who were well versed in midwifery who had never been in a private hospital'. In his district there were women 'who were as capable nurses as any to be found in the city of Brisbane . . . they knew that these women in the bush, who had got no diplomas, did far better work than the qualified nurse did here'.[56]

There was partial acceptance that nursing was an occupation which required a lengthy and standardised training. Murphy felt that:

> those who lived in the backblocks for a number of years must realise how necessary it was, especially in sparsely populated places, that the motherly women should be allowed to act as midwives. They did not want any women of the 'Sairey Gamp' variety, but there were plenty of women who carried on nursing in the far out places who were just as competent to do that work as those who receive their training in a lying-in hospital.[57]

He also believed that:

> the girls working in the outside hospitals were entitled to as much consideration as the nurses. In many outside places the doctors found it difficult to get nurses, and they had to get girls who were born in the places to do the work, sometimes for very small pay; and in passing a Bill of this nature they should see that those girls were given a fair deal.[58]

The fears of these parliamentarians were relieved by the amendment which provided that the Governor-in-Council could advise that the

Act should be brought into operation only in certain districts, and by this means sparsely settled areas of the state could be excluded from the operation of the Act. Similar concerns were expressed in relation to midwives and Mr J.G. Appel, Home Secretary, felt that this change would 'prevent an injustice being done to the women carrying on the profession of midwifery'. Nor would the Act—

> affect those women who went round and attended in private houses to the different women whom they assisted in giving birth to children. It did not affect them in the least, but if they had a private lying-in hospital, the Bill provided that the matron or nurse in charge must be registered, and that any nurse assisting in that private hospital must be registered.[59]

Appel said that the government's 'sole intention' was to have 'the most perfect and up-to-date legislation possible, which, while protecting the public, and affording it the best possible services, would inflict no injustice on nurses'.[60]

The Act that registered nurses in Queensland embodied most of the points the ATNA requested. After its commencement in 1912, registration was granted to 'every person who has attained the age of twenty-one years, and is certified as having had three years' training as a general nurse in such hospital, together with systematic instruction in theoretical and practical nursing from the medical officer and the matron . . . and who passes the prescribed examination'. Provision was made for nurses already practising in the community. A general nurse could be registered if, prior to 1 January 1912, she had a certificate of three years training as a nurse in a hospital recognised by the board, with proof 'to the satisfaction of the Board that during her training she received systematic instruction in theoretical and practical nursing from the medical officer and matron'. If the nurse wished she could sit for the prescribed examination. A further sub-clause stated that nurses who, prior to 1 January 1912, 'have obtained certificates issued by any such hospital, or who have had not less than three years' experience as general nurses' could be registered. 'Grandfather' or 'grandmother' clauses, which allowed for the registration of those currently practising but who did not comply with the new educational requirements, had been included in other Acts registering health professionals.[61] This would have given most women who had worked as a nurse for at least three years, whether or not they had received any formal training, the chance to gain registration until 31 December 1912. Moreover, the minister could dispense with any of these provisions.

The terms for registration of midwifery nurses were similar. Those who held a certificate of midwifery prior to the implementation of the Act were entitled to registration. The length of training was six months if registered as a general nurse and twelve months in all other cases, as recommended by the ATNA, plus a pass in the prescribed examination. The length of training specified for registration as a mental nurse was three years.[62]

Registration of nurses was supported by the BMA:

> The only guarantee which can be offered that the standard of medical and nursing attendance is as efficient as modern teaching admits of is to place the two professions under the control of a special board, which shall have the power of publishing the lists of persons registered, and of removing names from the lists when evidence is produced that the persons concerned are either incompetent or of bad repute. The principle involved, if carried to its logical conclusion, would include an absolute prohibition of all practice by unregistered persons. Sooner or later, the demands of the medical profession and of the nursing profession in this respect must be recognized, and the care of the sick will then be placed exclusively in the hands of doctors and nurses who have been found to possess knowledge and skill necessary to render their services safe and beneficial.[63]

The attitude of the BMA, and the members it represented, had thus changed dramatically from the days of Miss Lucy Osburn and the first Nightingale trained nurses who faced resistance from doctors in Sydney in the 1860s.[64]

In no way had the Act been initiated or influenced in its early stages by the Queensland Branch, however, in 1911 the branch was the surprised recipient of an Act that provided for nurses' registration. Thus a major point in the ATNA's policy was first enacted in Queensland, a mere twelve years after it had been included in the association's policies. In the first year of its operation 1401 nurses were registered, including 79 by ministerial direction.[65] The QNRB held its first examinations in December 1913 and only nurses trained at recognised training hospitals were eligible to sit.[66]

The process of registering nurses

After the introduction of registration in 1912, the employment of registered nurses increasingly became the accepted standard. There was nothing in the health Acts, however, that prevented a woman from practising as an unregistered nurse,[67] and in 1926 the QNRB was still

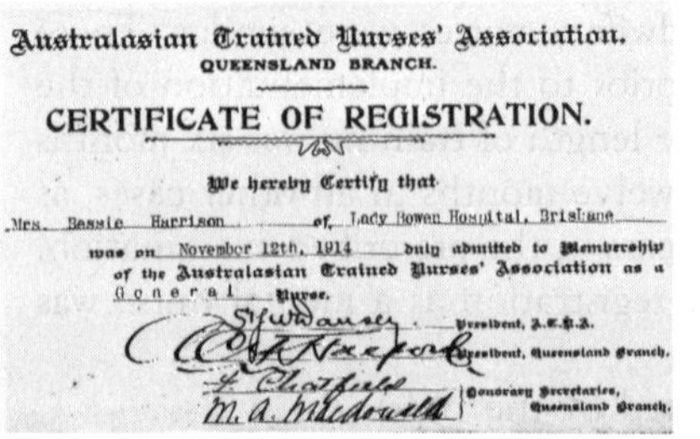

Australasian Trained Nurses' Association.
QUEENSLAND BRANCH.

CERTIFICATE OF REGISTRATION.

We hereby Certify that

Mrs. Bessie Harrison of Lady Bowen Hospital, Brisbane

was on November 12th, 1914 duly admitted to Membership of the Australasian Trained Nurses' Association as a General Nurse.

President, A.T.N.A.

President, Queensland Branch.

F. Chatfield

M. A. Macdonald

Honorary Secretaries, Queensland Branch.

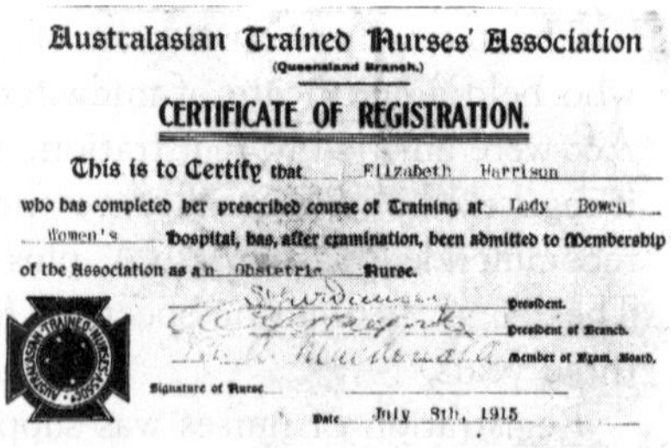

Australasian Trained Nurses' Association
(Queensland Branch.)

CERTIFICATE OF REGISTRATION.

This is to Certify that Elizabeth Harrison who has completed her prescribed course of Training at Lady Bowen Women's Hospital, has, after examination, been admitted to Membership of the Association as an Obstetric Nurse.

President.

President of Branch.

Member of Exam. Board.

Signature of Nurse

Date July 8th, 1915

ATNA, Queensland Branch, membership certificates of Mrs Elizabeth Harrison. The certificate of membership as a general nurse shows the signature of the long-serving Queensland Branch secretary, Miss Florence Chatfield. The other certificate contains a drawing of the ATNA badge, worn by nurses to signify their qualified status. (Courtesy of E. Jordan.)

registering uncertificated nurses who had worked as nurses in the three years before the introduction of the 1911 Act, in accordance with the concessional clause.[68] Employment of unregistered nurses was restricted in one way as registered nurses were given preference in employment for positions as qualified nurses in hospitals subject to the Hospitals Acts and in the asylum for the insane.[69] Thus the Act tied up hospital nursing in the hands of the registered but left private nursing open to all.

The monopoly on private nursing would come as the term 'registered nurse' gained greater currency in the community. The ATNA was concerned about non-nurses wearing nurses' uniforms as the practice had grown for shop assistants and unqualified workers in doctors' and dentists' rooms to wear uniforms and caps, creating the impression that a qualified nurse was in attendance.[70] An amendment to the Act in 1938 provided that no one should wear a nurse's cap unless she was a registered nurse, a provision which the ATNA had asked all state governments to enact.[71] The cap was that 'commonly worn by trained nurses consisting of a piece of white material so folded that when worn portion thereof hangs to or below the shoulder'.[72]

The involvement of the ATNA in the training of nurses did not cease with the establishment of the QNRB in 1912. It was involved in the operations of the board, influencing it to accept the standards of the association, and publicising the importance of the new registration provisions. The ATNA feared that if the regulations were not equal in standard to those already set by the organisation then Queensland State registered nurses would not be reciprocally recognised in the other states where the ATNA was the registering body. The council urged smaller

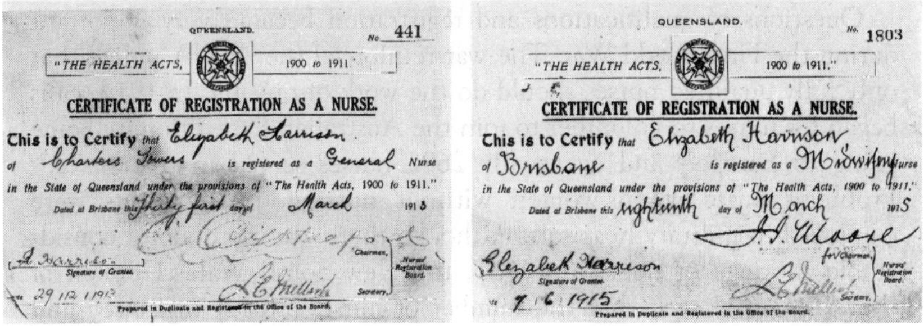
QUEENSLAND. No. 441

"THE HEALTH ACTS, 1900 to 1911."

CERTIFICATE OF REGISTRATION AS A NURSE.

This is to Certify that Elizabeth Harrison of Charters Towers is registered as a General Nurse in the State of Queensland under the provisions of "The Health Acts, 1900 to 1911."

Dated at Brisbane this thirty first day of March 1913

Chairman, Nurses' Registration Board.

E Harrison
Signature of Grantee.

29/12/1913

Secretary.

Prepared in Duplicate and Registered in the Office of the Board.

QUEENSLAND. No. 1803

"THE HEALTH ACTS, 1900 to 1911."

CERTIFICATE OF REGISTRATION AS A NURSE.

This is to Certify that Elizabeth Harrison of Brisbane is registered as a Midwifery Nurse in the State of Queensland under the provisions of "The Health Acts, 1900 to 1911."

Dated at Brisbane this eighteenth day of March 1915

Chairman, Nurses' Registration Board.

Elizabeth Harrison
Signature of Grantee.

7/6/1915

Secretary.

Prepared in Duplicate and Registered in the Office of the Board.

State registration certificates as a general and midwifery nurse of Mrs Elizabeth Harrison. (Courtesy of E.Jordan)

hospitals to retain the longer training period.[73] In December 1912 it sent a memo to hospitals pointing out that unless a nurse completed the full number of years of training she would not be recognised as a trained nurse by the ATNA or the RVTNA, which 'represent the Hall Mark of Nursing throughout Australia'. To avoid being penalised, a nurse was advised to complete the full period of training laid down in the ATNA regulations. The memo concluded that:

> the Council wishes to point out that the State Registration Board is simply a registering body; the names of the nurses are gazetted and each nurse receives a badge. The A.T.N.A. keeps up its connection and its direct interest in the nurses by means of the Journal, correspondence, social functions, etc., and strives in every way to further the interest of the individual nurse.[74]

Following this circular a number of hospitals throughout Queensland wrote to the ATNA expressing their continued allegiance to the association.[75] Despite State registration, hospitals continued to be registered with the ATNA as training schools, the majority of these having a training period of four or five years. The length of training of general and mental nurses was finally changed in 1916, incorporating the rules of the ATNA.[76]

A number of difficulties arose in connection with the supervision of training schools. Following a report that the five trainee nurses at the Alexandra Training School had not received any lectures during the previous two years, the council decided that in future training schools that did not comply with the ATNA rules would have their recognition withdrawn. In this case the matron was informed that all pupil nurses must attend the lectures in the prescribed schedule of study.[77]

Questions of qualifications and registration became very important during the First World War. The war reinforced the ATNA policy that only fully qualified nurses should do the work of nursing. In 1914, calls began for nurses to volunteer to join the Australian Expeditionary Force going to Europe[78] and eventually 2692 nurses served in the forces.[79] Problems arose when women without nursing qualifications were employed in military hospitals. Although there was 'no doubt a considerable shortage of nurses' in 1915, the New South Wales Council of the ATNA believed that the number of nurses already registered and those to be registered in the immediate future were sufficient to meet the needs of the military authorities. Shortages were more acute in civilian hospitals, particularly those in country areas, and in private work. The New South Wales Council did not want unregistered nurses employed in the services, or permanent registration granted to partially-trained women.

The most acceptable solution for the ATNA was the employment of the Voluntary Aid Detachments (VADs) as probationers and women orderlies. These detachments had received a certain amount of training in the duties they would be required to perform; were already organised and prepared to work hard; were offering their services merely for the special needs of wartime, and therefore would not be tempted after the war to presume on their experience in military hospitals to consider themselves trained nurses and thus act as a public danger.[80] Following conferences of the ATNA and BMA in New South Wales and Queensland, these views were submitted to the Director-General of the Medical Services of the Defence Department.[81]

Despite agreements to the contrary, however, the hospital ship *Kanowna* set sail with untrained probationers aboard.[82] An editorial in the *ANJ* responded that it was regrettable that the Defence Department 'should recently have departed from the attitude hitherto adopted and have roused the indignation of nurses, military and civil, all over Australia, by permitting a number of untrained girls to be taken on the Hospital Ship "Kanowna" '.[83]

The women were dressed in the uniform of staff nurses and received the same allowances as trained nurses. The ATNA protested strongly to the Director-General of Medical Services, but was told that the undertaking to send only trained nurses applied to transports, and not to hospital ships. The ATNA telegraphed an appeal for support to the Prime Minister and the Minister for Defence, interviewed federal parliamentarians in Sydney and Brisbane, and communicated with the RVTNA, which joined the ATNA in its protest. These measures had some effect when the Director-General of Medical Services gave an assurance that the incident of the *Kanowna* would not occur again.[84] The ATNA, for its part, hoped that the arrangement would not be repeated, and that it would 'be able to forget and even to forgive this little lapse of our Defence Department, and that Australia will never again see untrained girls masquerading in the garb of Army Nurses'.[85]

Seventeen years after the initial Act, the ATNA in Queensland gained the separate registration Act that it had originally desired. Once again the *Nurses and Masseurs Registration Act of 1928*, which introduced registration of child welfare nurses and masseurs (physiotherapists), was solely a government initiative, taking the ATNA by surprise when they learned from a newspaper report that the Bill was before Parliament.[86] A new seven-member board was constituted, including two qualified nurses or nominees of an association of nurses, one of whom was a current or former matron in a hospital training school.[87] The Act still retained a clause which allowed the minister to dispense with the need for certificates and examinations and register a person who had worked as a nurse or masseur for three years. A further amendment to the Act in 1933 provided for a board consisting of four members appointed by the Governor-in-Council as well as two nursing association representatives and one nominee of the masseurs' association. This change, which gave government nominees a more dominant position on the board, went 'virtually unnoticed' by the ATNA.[88]

Although the ATNA's policies had encompassed State registration of nurses, once this was enacted the Queensland Council 'made few demands on the government with respect to nurse training and registration over the ensuing forty years'.[89] The ATNA 'was satisfied to accept the status quo in matters of nurse training and registration' and until the 1960s 'did not utilize pressure group activities to any great extent'[90] to influence government policies. The ATNA in Queensland undoubtedly regarded itself as a professional association which represented the nursing profession and its prime concern in its first sixteen years was to have the trained nurse recognised as such and the training of a uniform and sufficiently high standard. It succeeded in this and State registration set the seal on its efforts.

Nursing's attempt to achieve professional status

The ATNA sought State registration of nurses not only for the protection of the public but also for the enhancement of nurses' status. Registration is bound up with the question of professionalisation which, in the case of nursing, is widely discussed in the sociological and nursing literature.[91] No generally accepted conclusion as to whether nursing is or is not a profession has come out of this debate.[92] A central question is not whether or not it is a profession, (for judging this is a debate which is frequently ahistorical[93] and sometimes clearly represents the vested interests of the established professions), but what role this goal and the striving for professional status has meant for nurses' image of themselves and the status of their occupation, and how this has affected the development of their occupation. Nursing organisations chose to pursue the goal of becoming a profession as a means of raising the status of their occupation and carving out specific occupational territory for trained nurses. Because professions did not engage in negotiations over pay and conditions with their employers or identify themselves with the activities of trade unions, nursing organisations carefully avoided such actions.

Inclusion in the elite group of professions can have very practical ramifications. The decision as to whether an occupation is a profession or not has been measured in industrial terms and nurses were hampered by the comparisons of trained nurses with tradespeople which were made by industrial tribunals. In 1958, the Federal Conciliation and Arbitration Commission decided that the classification of junior sister and male nurse were 'comparable in most respects with those covering tradesmen generally who had successfully served a period of apprenticeship [which] . . . was comprehensive and exacting'. The Commissioner concluded that 'the trained nurse—an employee of standing and exceptional talent in this industry—is equal in specialised status to the painter, the carpenter, and/or the mechanical fitter'.[94] This view persisted and in the early 1970s the Australian Public Service Board classified the nursing sister as a Tradesman (Second Class).[95] When the Industrial Relations Commission concluded that nursing was a profession in 1989, substantial pay increases were awarded on that basis.[96]

The origin of the categorisation of certain occupations as professions lies in the development and regulation of medicine and law in nineteenth century Britain. Standards were developed which regulated entry into the profession and limited competition from the formally untrained. These groups aspired to power and status and, once they had achieved this elevated position, they could define the characteristics of what was called a profession. The model of the professions which medicine and law exhibited was a very specific one, yet much of the literature has extrapolated from these groups to specific criteria which are perceived to apply universally to any group which wants to be called a profession. It is therefore hard for other groups to conform exactly to this mould and be labelled as professions. Much of the literature[97] starts

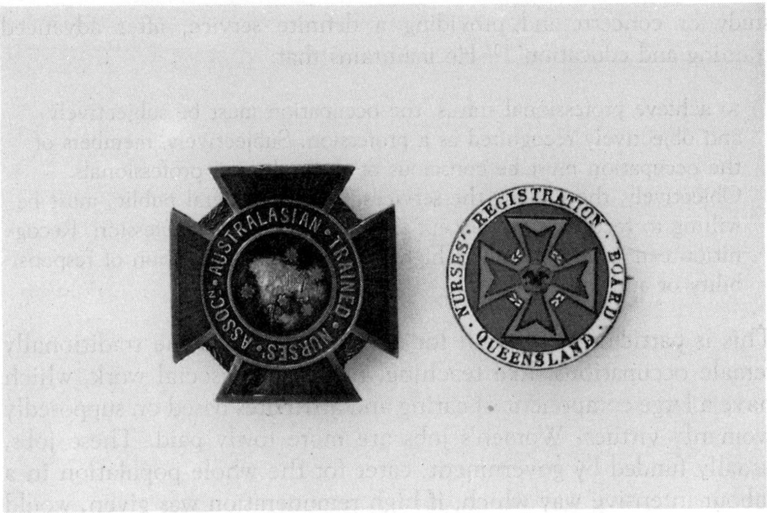

ATNA *badge and Nurses' Registration Board of Queensland badge which belonged to* Miss Eunice Paten, *first nurse president of the* ATNA *in Queensland. These badges were the hallmark of the trained nurse and proudly worn on nurses' uniforms.* (Courtesy of Queensland Nurses' Union.)

from the premise that certain occupations are professions (and therefore certain occupations are excluded) and delineates the characteristics of a profession by examining groups such as medicine and law which historically have achieved this status. Often the rhetoric of the professional groups themselves is used uncritically and the 'definitions of the content of these professional roles are based upon the official literature and ideology of the professions as developed by elites within those professional groups . . . the sociological perspective simply reflects the dominant view of the profession itself'.[98]

These 'attempts to treat the professions as unique are based on the assumption that there is some essential quality or qualities which mark off the professions from other occupations and provide a basis for a distinct body of theory and variant forms of analysis'.[99] The result has been many lists of 'traits' of what constitutes a profession.[100] For instance, although Millerson says that 'a mass of confusion stems from all analyses, which attempt to determine the occupational characteristics of a profession',[101] he defines a profession as 'a type of higher-grade, non-manual occupation, with both subjectively and objectively recognized occupational status, possessing a well-defined area of study or concern and providing a definite service, after advanced training and education'.[102] He maintains that:

> to achieve professional status, the occupation must be subjectively and objectively recognized as a profession. Subjectively, members of the occupation must be conscious of themselves as professionals. Objectively, those using the services, and the general public, must be willing to recognize and accept the occupation as a profession. Recognition can take the form of high remuneration, delegation of responsibility or authority.[103]

This is particularly difficult for nurses and indeed the traditionally female occupations, like teaching, nursing and social work, which have a large component of caring and attributes based on supposedly womanly virtues. Women's jobs are more lowly paid. These jobs, usually funded by government, cater for the whole population in a labour-intensive way which, if high remuneration was given, would disenfranchise a large proportion of the population from these services. At the time of the development of medicine and law as professions, paid employment was not accepted as a legitimate activity for middle and upper class women. They were not welcomed by the male practitioners and had to struggle to gain entry to university courses in medicine and law.

Women's occupations are in an impossible situation in relation to these definitions of professions. A woman's occupation in our society cannot meet these criteria, precisely because the characteristics of the jobs that have been open to and socially acceptable for women have not had the characteristics of exalted public status and high remuneration. The result of this historical development is that definitions of a profession are male-centred and professional status is therefore unattainable for female-dominated occupations like nursing.

Yet numerous writers have advanced lists of supposed criteria that nursing would need to meet to achieve professional status. For example, Katz suggests that nursing's 'corpus of knowledge . . . must be greatly refined and organized, with nurses themselves taking a leading part in this process' and 'nurses' caste-like status separation from physicians must give way to the colleagueship that now prevails among the various medical specialities'.[104] Twaddle and Hessler assert that 'it is not possible to say with confidence that nursing is a profession . . . Functional autonomy and societal prestige are not possessed by nursing to the extent necessary to propel nurses into professional status and roles equal to physicians and other similar health professions'.[105] Once again, these conditions mean that nursing cannot meet these criteria precisely because of the nature of nurses' work and its historical relationship to medicine. On the basis of these criteria, nursing is doomed to remain in a lesser position than medicine.

Nurses have been disadvantaged when trying to secure professional status by not being able to claim that they have their own body of knowledge, 'scientific knowledge', as against the experiential knowledge related to hygiene and caring. Nursing performed the caring role while medicine captured the province of curing the patient. As nursing developed in the nineteenth century the notion of care shifted from a definition of the nurse's role as an independent activity to one delimited by the doctors' orders.[106] Nurses' knowledge became limited to what was necessary to carry out the functions assigned by doctors. Colliere has commented that midwives were 'taught what doctors thought useful or necessary for the administration of cure and treatment which they prescribed but which they did not provide'.[107] General nurses were in this subservient position too. A high proportion of the lectures delivered to nurses in Australia prior to the development of nurse tutors in the 1930s were given by medical practitioners and they were often instrumental in the development of nurse training itself.[108]

In striving to achieve professional status medicine appropriated the notion of effectiveness, that is an ability to cure, and claimed that this was based on scientific principles.[109] In doing so it was able to gain 'the legitimacy of science itself'.[110] Nursing, by comparison, was not able to do this because its work was largely based on caring for the patient—frequent baths for fever patients for instance—a role which did not lead to dramatic recoveries but one which was critical for a return to good health in the days before much successful surgery or drugs. In nursing:

> everything dealing with care was never revealed as part of the work. It is just left to the nurse as a moral duty she had to perform. Notwithstanding that the content of care requires skill and competence to assess and evaluate patients' abilities, either to be compensated for or mobilized, and requires giving support to patients and their families, care itself was never taken into account as a specific activity.[111]

The idea of the central importance of this in the nurse's role is still evident. Katz writes that 'the nurse's nurturence . . . is probably the fundamental ingredient of traditional nursing, far more so than the harnessing of rational knowledge'.[112] This 'obligation to care has been at nursing's definitional core',[113] a notion which is illustrated by the number of histories of nursing that include the word 'care' in their title.[114]

Curing was rewarded with status and it was not chance that this was done by men and caring was done by women. The heritage of women performing the nursing role within their families plus the nature of the hospitals as charitable institutions resulted in 'no financial assessment of care value'.[115] The lack of value placed on caring, seen as a natural role for women and therefore for nurses, meant that no kudos in terms of status accrued from this. For 'nursing's transition to paid and trained labor did not change the assumption that the work was based on womanly duty requiring service to others and acquiescence to the authority of physicians'.[116] Nursing became increasingly dependent on medicine for its definition of itself. It was natural therefore that this position of professional subordination and subordination of women to men in society should be a major characteristic of the emerging nursing organisations where male medical practitioners played a prominent role.

In an attempt to deal with the problem that some groups aspire to professional status but cannot be judged to have achieved it on the standard criteria, a concept of professionalisation has been developed. It is seen as 'a process with an end-state towards which certain occupations are moving and others have arrived'.[117] This argument claims that:

> we must expect variation in the nature of professional practice, attitudes and organisation if only because not all those occupations scrutinised are equally professionalised. Certain occupations, such as social work, teaching and accountancy, are not highly advanced in the process of professionalisation, while others, such as law, medicine and architecture, are closer to the end-state of professionalism.[118]

Twaddle and Hessler, for instance, define nursing's 'struggle to attain functional autonomy and prestige on a level with physicians' as the process of professionalisation.[119]

Other writers developed a new category of 'semi-profession' into which teachers, librarians, social workers and nurses were put.[120] These are all areas of skilled employment in which women predominate. In the semi-professions practitioners are characterised as lacking autonomy, are more accountable for their performance, subject to numerous rules concerning their work and there is 'a great emphasis on hierarchical rank with duties differentiated by level'. Simpson and Simpson allege that these characteristics 'arise from the lesser knowledge and training of semi-professionals than of professionals'.[121] Thus the category of professional is generally reserved for men and women are once again placed in a lesser category, that of 'semi' or half the male rank. The other term which has gained wide usage is 'para-professional'. This term is currently used by the Australian Bureau of Statistics to include registered nurses while school teachers and 'health diagnosis and treatment practitioners' are placed in the professional category.[122]

One of the characteristics assigned to the professions is their humanitarian assistance to others. Yet the 'semi-professions' do this while at the same time receiving less income. This has led to some extraordinary conclusions: 'A fundamental orientation of semi-professionals is their desire to be helpful to others, to give humanitarian service. This must be distinguished sharply from the obligation to put the welfare of clients before personal gain which is regarded as a hallmark of the professions.'[123] Simpson and Simpson continue, saying that:

> the service orientation of semi-professionals . . . is an emotionally felt humanitarian urge to give of oneself, to relate in an intensely personal way to the recipient of the service. The act of service is its own reward, an expressive act, and it establishes a diffuse particularistic tie . . . Professional activity is sometimes expressive, but the rewards are derived more from the exercise of skills than from the response of the client.[124]

But as Melosh comments,

> commitment to service does not define which occupations become professions; instead a claim to altruism serves to legitimate professional prerogatives after the fact. Professionals are no more or less disinterested than any other workers, but because they claim power in such areas of intense cultural concern as sickness and health, they must justify their control and reassure their anxious clientele by seeming altruistic.[125]

The role of caring for others and giving of oneself to this end has been seen as natural for women and unusual for men. Because of this difference 'men in an aspiring profession had to declare their special commitment to service, reflecting the larger assumption that paid work is instrumental and self-serving in nature'. But when women perform these roles it is seen as an innate characteristic and not worthy of special recognition. Thus women have 'to escape the diffuse notion of womanly service' in order to achieve professional status.[126]

Turner has criticised the 'trait' approach to the definition of a profession on the grounds that it ignores 'the role of power and the privilege enjoyed by professional bodies which enable them to manipulate and control their clients and markets. The profession . . .

is an occupation which by licence has a monopolistic privilege over its particular practices'. Professionalisation should be regarded as 'a strategy of occupational control' between experts, patrons and clients.[127] This process of social closure will depend on university education as the basis for credentialism and require State backing. Turner concludes that 'the maintenance of this privilege requires the continuing exercise of dominance over allied and competing occupations', a process especially evident in health service occupations in relation to the medical profession.[128]

This control by the medical profession creates a significant obstacle to nursing's ability to define its own role. Melosh comments that:

> clearly, nurses never gained the large measure of control over their work that defines a profession. The relationship between doctors and nurses in itself poses an intractable obstacle to nursing's professionalization. If professions maintain their authority through controlling the division of labor related to their work . . . then doctors' own professionalization organizes and requires nurses' subordination.

In fact, 'doctors have consistently maintained and exercised the prerogative to define the scope of their own practice, and in so doing, they have claimed the right to set the limits of nurses' work'.[129]

Prior to the Second World War, health professionals in Australia achieved the legitimation of registration only with the consent of the medical profession.[130] Nursing gained registration with the assistance of the medical profession precisely because it did not offer any challenges to medicine. As Dr Sinclair Gillies, councillor of the ATNA New South Wales, said in 1913, 'after all, nursing is controlled by the medical profession'.[131] In contrast to midwifery, nursing had in no way offended doctors or usurped any of their work and did not compete with them for occupational territory. Nursing remained firmly in a position of subordination, and thereby gained medicine's strong support and assistance on the path to recognition. Forms of domination of the medical profession over other groups 'follow from the fact that medical dominance is typically exercised by physicians playing an important part in the official registration boards of such occupations. Registration Acts specify the professional competence of such groups within a narrow occupational territory, while also confirming the control of the medical profession over such terrain'.[132] The medical profession was represented on nurses' and dentists' registration boards in Queensland 'in a desire to have a controlling interest in allied professions as well as in its own'.[133]

The question of becoming a profession has been discussed widely by nurses. No other group seems to have been so concerned with gaining this status, while at every turn it appears to have been denied them.[134] The belief in professional status 'is a successful ideology and as such has entered the political vocabulary of a wide range of occupational groups who compete for status and income'.[135] This debate has to some degree influenced the actions of nursing organisations in their attempts to standardise practice and gain State registration. Nurses have strived to grasp the holy grail of professional status. But it has been difficult for them to achieve this because nurses are women, their work was seen as being based on womanly attributes and as a group they lacked power in society, especially when compared to the position held by medical practitioners.

If one consequence of a raised status is higher remuneration, as it is in medicine and law, then because large numbers of nurses are needed for today's health-care system and their employer is usually the State, there are additional forces militating against the achievement of professional status. State registration standardised and regulated nursing and acted as a barrier to the formally untrained. If registration was sought by the ATNA as a way of gaining professional status akin to that of doctors then nurses were to be disappointed. Yet again the forces which shaped nursing as a women's occupation have resulted in nursing only rarely being accorded the accolade of 'profession'.

CHAPTER 5

The working conditions of hospital nurses in the 1920s

'Except for the reduction of . . . hours of work . . . and increase of salaries, the nurse will gain nothing.'[1]

By 1920 the regulation of nurse training had been achieved. However, in contrast to many other workers whose wages and conditions were set by an award of the Industrial Court, the wages and conditions of hospital nurses remained unregulated, varying greatly from one institution to another. In 1920 Queensland became the first state where nurses gained award conditions. Moves to achieve this were not instigated by the ATNA but were initiated by another nursing association with industrial goals, the QNA.

Throughout the 1920s, the ATNA continued to avoid industrial activity, adhering to the view that nurses were unique and unusual workers not in need of the same conditions as other employees. This is very clearly shown in its desire for nurses to work longer hours than other workers. However, by 1925 the activities of the QNA together with changes to industrial legislation forced the ATNA to come to terms with the need for regulated working conditions for hospital nurses. Thus it became involved in the industrial arena, however reluctantly, as a trade union.

The wages and working conditions of hospital nurses in Queensland in 1920

The majority of Queensland hospitals in 1920 were overwhelmingly small and decentralised, making the co-ordination of uniform working conditions difficult. As well as their long and often irregular working hours, nurses were on call whenever needed because they lived at their place of work. No extra payment was received for night shifts, public holidays or, in most cases, overtime; all being regarded as a normal feature of a nurse's duty and not to be rewarded as exceptional. Apart from those few instances where a married couple formed the staff of a small country hospital, the nurses were, invariably, female and unmarried. Activity outside the hospital could only be a secondary and minor factor in their lives and the ideal of devotion to the service of humanity without huge reward was reflected in the salaries they were paid. Hence nurses' working lives set them apart, both physically and philosophically, from other workers.

In 1921 the Queensland Government conducted a survey of nurses' wages and working conditions in the 99 government-subsidised hospitals.[2] This provides a unique insight into the lives of the nurses, especially those in small country hospitals whose voices are rarely heard. The survey was undertaken as a direct result of the claim for an industrial award for nurses filed with the Industrial Court by the newly-formed QNA. The government obtained information about the number of nurses employed by each hospital, their salaries and working conditions and, if the hospital was a training school, details about the working conditions of trainees and their training.

Many of the conditions under which the nurses worked can be explained by the size of the hospitals they staffed. Almost one-third (25 out of 86) had an average daily number of patients of five or less. More than two-thirds (69 per cent) of the hospitals in Queensland cared for less than 20 patients each day. Only six hospitals averaged more than 100 patients a day, the largest being the Brisbane General with a daily average of 340 patients.[3] The government subsidised hospitals employed 869 nurses, with the Brisbane General Hospital employing the largest number of 127 nurses. Only eleven hospitals employed more than 20 nurses, with the average for the other 76 hospitals being five nurses. Seven hospitals employed one nurse only.

Although State registration of trained nurses had existed for eight years, not all nurses were formally trained and qualified. A few of the hospitals stated that their nurses had not undergone formal training or were not eligible for registration or membership of the ATNA, but no specific information was sought about this and no accurate figures of untrained nurses can be given. At Herberton Hospital none of the three nurses was trained, and Surat, Texas and Laidley all employed a number of untrained nurses.

Nurses in small country hospitals frequently worked unregulated hours whenever they were needed, as fluctuating patient demand produced very uneven work loads. In one-third of the hospitals (24 out of

71) nurses worked no regular hours. All these hospitals employed only one, two or three nurses. Adavale District Hospital (one nurse) replied: 'No regular hours: frequently no patients in the Hospital: extra assistance nursing engaged when required[.] Wardsman assists the Matron to watch patients, requiring constant attention'. Isisford District Hospital, with two nurses, reported 'we have no "hard and fast" working hours: sometimes we have eight or nine patients and at other times one or perhaps even none. Taking on average I do not think our nurses would average eight hours work each day'.[4]

In the 47 hospitals with more than two nurses which specified the hours worked, hours varied from 45 to 78 a week. The average working hours were 63 $^{1}/_{2}$ a week. At four institutions the nurses worked for 50 hours or less, with nurses at the Cairns and Torres Straits hospitals working a 48-hour week. At Cloncurry the staff nurses worked 45 hours per week (ten hours per day and two and a half days off) while the trainees worked 57 hours per week. At the Brisbane General and Children's Hospitals, nurses worked 56 hours per week. At the other end of the scale, nurses in five hospitals worked 78-hour weeks, usually made up of twelve hours per day with half a day off each week, often with one extra whole day off each month or every three weeks. These long hours, worked in shifts of ten to twelve hours, or hours that were regulated only by the demands of the employing hospital and patient intake, came at a time when most workers with an industrial award in Queensland worked a 48-hour week.

The length of the nurses' working week was not the only factor which set them apart from other workers. All nurses were boarded at their hospitals and led a cloistered life reminiscent of the religious and military origins of their profession. Annual leave varied from one to six weeks, with the majority of hospitals (46 out of 74) granting four weeks. A further fifteen gave their nurses two or three weeks leave, although six of these granted their matron four weeks. Thargomindah, Boulia and Adavale Hospitals had never had a nurse stay as long as a year so they had not been forced to consider annual leave, a comment which probably reflected the isolation of these hospitals, the harsh working conditions and the difficulty of obtaining staff. Annual leave was not always regarded as obligatory: Goondiwindi Border Hospital granted their nurses two weeks leave 'as an act of grace'. Sick leave was often similarly regarded but two-thirds of the hospitals (41 out of 66) readily granted paid sick leave. The amount of leave given varied greatly, with Atherton, Ipswich and Brisbane Children's giving four weeks sick leave each year compared with Townsville's two weeks. At seven hospitals paid sick leave was decided on the merits of the case, usually on the recommendation of the matron or medical officer, and in some hospitals the time had to be made up at a later date by the nurse. Several provided free treatment at the hospital.

By 1920, employees in most occupations received paid overtime but this was unheard of for the majority of nurses. In many cases, with the long and often irregular hours, there would not have been much time left in which to work any extra hours. For most hospitals overtime for nurses was an unthinkable concept and over three-quarters of the hospitals (56 out of 72) gave no extra payment for overtime. In other cases, informal recompense was given if excessive hours were worked, with eleven hospitals making some arrangement for the nurses to be compensated in some way for all or part of the overtime, usually with time off in lieu. As would be expected for nurses, no extra payment for work on Sundays or public holidays was given in all the 72 hospitals which answered this question. The survey revealed that nurses were expected to be shiftworkers, available on every day of the year, and not subject to any extra payment for duty at night, on Sundays or public holidays.

There was great disparity in the wages nurses received throughout Queensland. The salary of staff nurses, for example, varied from 52 pounds to 130 pounds.[5] All nurses lived at their hospital and all (except two who received board only) received board and lodging from their employer.[6] The hospitals argued that the value of this board and lodging was taken into consideration when wages were being determined as nurses were saved considerable expense by the provision of a roof over their heads and daily meals. Thus the provision of board and lodging kept nurses' wages lower than comparable workers. Even accepting that the provision of board and lodging reduced the weekly expenses of nurses to some degree, salaries, hours and lack of overtime payment meant that nurses' working conditions compared unfavourably with other areas of female employment. By 1920 other hospital staff were working a 48-hour week for wages determined by the Queensland Industrial Court.[7]

Nursing trainees formed the major part of the nursing workforce in hospitals and also worked long hours for low wages. Four hundred and thirty-two trainees were employed by 48 hospitals (excluding the Brisbane General Hospital) forming 68 per cent of the nursing staff. Training lasted from three to five years, giving the employer an extensive period of cheap labour. Many put in a full day's work and attended lectures in their own time, with fifteen out of 33 training hospitals giving lectures outside working hours. Of the remainder, half included the trainees' lectures in their hours on duty while half gave lectures at set times when both those on duty and those off duty were expected to attend. Salaries varied greatly, from 15 pounds for first year trainees at the Brisbane Children's Hospital to 82 pounds for a fourth year trainee at Winton Hospital. Generally, the more remote and outlying hospitals paid higher wages but in some hospitals the payment amounted to little more than pocket money.

The picture of the life of a trainee nurse that emerges from these statistics is one of long hours, little money and a demand for total dedication and obedience. At the Brisbane Children's Hospital the proportion of trainees to nurses was 65 to thirteen. The life of these 65 trainees was controlled by the demands of the hospital. They worked more than 70 hours a week, receiving about a penny an hour in payment. There was no extra payment for any overtime worked or for work on Sundays and public holidays. Out of their low pay, nurses had to provide their own uniforms, though the hospital eventually decided to refund 7 pounds 10 shillings for uniforms after a nurse had worked for one year. Trainees boarded at the hospital and their personal life and leisure time away from the hospital was limited. They attended lectures after duty hours 'as a rule'. They had three weeks annual leave, with an extra day off at Christmas, Easter and Exhibition (Royal National Association Show) time and for each month on night duty or duty in the infectious wards. One month's sick leave on full pay was allowed and free 'medical attendance and maintenance . . . Nurses who are unable to go to relatives for a change are allowed to go to the Sandgate Sanitorium (free) until fit to resume duty'.[8]

It was against the backdrop of these conditions that a new nursing organisation was formed in Queensland which viewed the regulation of nurses' conditions in a similar way to those of other white-collar workers.

The attitude of the ATNA to an industrial role

It was not until 1920 that the pay of nurses other than private practitioners came under scrutiny by the ATNA. A special general meeting of approximately 60 members endorsed a recommended set of salaries:

1. That £150 be fixed as the minimum salary for the Matron of any Hospital and that the minimum be increased to £200 for Hospitals with a daily average of 40 occupied beds.
2. That a Matron should receive at least 25% more than a subordinate domestic.

3. That the minimum salary for a Sister be fixed at £100 with increments of £10 per annum to £130.
4. That the minimum salary for a Staff Nurse be fixed at £80 with increments of £10 per annum to £100.
5. That one certificated nurse be employed to every five trainees in Hospitals with a daily average of less than 40 beds.
6. That Matrons, Sisters and Nurses be provided with board, residence and uniforms in Training Schools.[9]

Copies of these salaries were sent to public and private hospitals and the press, and the Queensland Branch of the BMA was asked for their 'sympathetic co-operation'.[10] However, as the council realised, these recommendations were not legally enforceable.[11] Atherton Hospital replied that when a demand was made by the matron and trained nurse for such increases the application would be given due consideration. The Mother's Hospital in Toowoomba stated that the new salary scales would apply from the ensuing year[12] and the Blackall Hospital said that it almost complied with the recommended salaries already.

Ironically, the secretaries of the Cairns and Walsh District hospitals suggested that the ATNA should apply for an award in the usual way.[13] However, the Queensland Council of the ATNA did not regard itself as a trade union or want to be associated with trade unions or the Trades and Labour Council. The council did not see a need to legally regulate and enforce minimum standards for the working conditions of nurses, even though this had been suggested by several employing hospitals. To gain an award setting a legal minimum for wages and conditions meant first registering as a trade union under the *Industrial Arbitration Act*, a move the ATNA steadfastly resisted.

Despite the ATNA's reticence, Queensland nurses, through the action of the QNA, gained the first specific award for nurses in Australia. This meant that the wages and working conditions of most hospital nurses in the state were legally regulated. Although many of these conditions were more onerous than those of other workers, most nurses' conditions were greatly improved. The ATNA's subsequent involvement in industrial issues was a direct result of the activities of the QNA, which was registered as a trade union with the Industrial Court in Queensland in February 1921. This impelled the ATNA to take action as it did not want to share any power with the newly-formed QNA and viewed it as a rival rather than as an ally in looking after the interests of nurses.

The registration of the ATNA would not have occurred without this stimulus, for in January 1921 the ATNA Council was still telling hospitals that the salaries set out by the association were only recommendations. No moves to have a ruling by the Industrial Court were contemplated.[14] A letter was tabled at the ATNA Council meeting stating that the QNA had been formed and was applying for registration in the Industrial Court.[15] In July the council decided to prepare a draft constitution and rules for registration as a trade union.[16] The Queensland Branch of the ATNA was registered on 8 November 1921 as an industrial union[17] able to cover registered nurses.[18] Thus in its application for registration the ATNA did not cover all categories in the award. This coverage was not changed until 1971, when the categories of nursing aid, trainee nursing aid, student nurse and assistant-in-nursing were added.[19]

Formation of QNA

The QNA was formed in 1920 by a small group of nurses and emerged as an organisation whose prime concern was the regulation of the wages and working conditions of nurses.[20] Its establishment was evidence that the ATNA did not fulfil the needs of nurses in Queensland as it had not considered the regulation of conditions.

Not much is known about the origins of the QNA, however towards the end of his life Mr Ken Laidlaw, QNA secretary from 1921, discussed the establishment of the association with Miss Bartz Schultz, an executive member of the ATNA. Already active in other white-collar unions, he was visiting friends whose daughters were nurses at the Children's Hospital in Brisbane. They complained about the working conditions and asked if he could do anything about it and a meeting was held at the Children's Hospital where Laidlaw, presumably drawing on his experience in forming a union for bank officers, explained that they could form a trade union. Signatures from nurses who wanted to form a union were requested, and dozens signed. The result was the formation of the QNA.[21]

Whereas the ATNA was run by senior doctors and matrons, the president and secretaries of the QNA were not nurses and held executive positions in other white-collar unions. Mr Vivian Partridge, inaugural QNA secretary, was secretary of the Public Service Association in Queensland until 1920 and secretary of the United Bank Officers Association from its inception in 1919 until August 1921. He saw the formation of a union and the regulation of working conditions through an award as the solution to the low pay of bank officers and their first award in 1920 increased salaries considerably. He played a large part in the preparation of this claim and brought this experience to his work with the nurses.[22]

His successor as QNA secretary was Mr Ken Laidlaw, who held this position from June 1922 until the demise of the association in the late 1930s. He had been instrumental in the founding of the United Bank Officers Association in 1919, president from its inception to 1921 and full-time secretary from then until his retirement in 1960. Through his work with the banking union Laidlaw gained a reputation as an industrial advocate and this, plus his industrial experience, meant his services were sought by other white-collar unions. He was secretary of five other unions at various times throughout the 1920s and 1930s, including the Commercial Travellers' Union, the Insurance Staffs Federation and the Municipal Officers' Association.[23] His success in bringing workers such as bank employees into unions related in part to his remaining outside political unionism and having no involvement with Trades Hall:

> He had no ideological commitment; he was not driven on by any sense of belonging to a broad trade union movement and he had no thought of backing his negotiation with strikes or industrial action. He was . . . a professional industrial advocate. Unionism, for him, was a means of providing increased pay and improved, regulated working conditions for his union members.[24]

Laidlaw's perspective on working conditions and his experience of comparing bank officers' salaries with those of other workers such as clerks gave the QNA a different outlook from the ATNA, which 'was reluctant to be drawn into the sordid business of wages, hours and a union for nurses'.[25]

Although its primary concern was industrial issues, the QNA did not identify with unions of unskilled or semi-skilled workers or those with trade qualifications and did not consider itself part of the wider trade union movement. Yet its concern with wages and working conditions was radical in comparison with the ATNA's steadfast avoidance of this area. The QNA aimed—

> (a) To protect the interests and rights of its members generally or in particular;
> (b) To discuss matters affecting the welfare of its members, and take such action as may be deemed necessary on their behalf;
> (c) To act jointly with any kindred Association on any matter affecting common interests;
> (d) To promote or assist in social gatherings.[26]

The association emphasised that action would be taken on behalf of members. It aimed to 'protect' their interests and rights whereas the ATNA chose to 'promote' the interests of trained nurses. Membership of the QNA was open to all nurses in Queensland for a fee of five shillings. The management was by a council of annually elected delegates with an executive elected by the council.[27]

The new association, under the name Australian Nurses' Federation,[28] initially applied for federal registration as a trade union with the Queensland Industrial Arbitration Court on 22 December 1920.[29] Information about the original application is scarce but in 1949 Mrs Mary Harper, secretary of the ATNA in Queensland, interviewed Miss Axelson, a member of the original council of the Australian Nurses' Federation and reported that as Miss Axelson 'remembers it, a group of these people were formed in 1921 to endeavour to better the nursing conditions. They had appealed to the A.T.N.A., but at that time the A.T.N.A. was unable to help them, so this separate group was formed and apparently registered themselves under the name of the Australian Nurses Federation'.[30]

In 1924 Mr Ken Laidlaw, then secretary of the QNA, replied to the Industrial Registrar that he could 'find no records dealing with the matter of the Australian Nurses' Federation. There has also been no correspondence returns received from the other States by this Association'.[31] Clearly the question of obtaining a federal award was not pursued by the QNA, which applied for State registration and a state award, a path that gave nurses an award without the potential legal wrangles over whether nurses could be covered by the Commonwealth *Conciliation and Arbitration Act.*

The QNA was registered on 3 February 1921 as a union covering nurses, except those employed in mental hospitals. When the QNA applied for registration it had a membership of 23 plus the president, John H.C. Sleeman and secretary, Vivian Partridge, who were not nurses.[32] By the time the list of members was filed with the court a year later, the association had grown to 221 nurses, most of whom worked in Brisbane.[33]

Miss E.M. Barron, who was joint honorary secretary of the ATNA from 1922 to 1933, joined the QNA on 24 March 1921. Miss Christense Sorensen, Matron of Rosemount Repatriation Hospital in Brisbane in 1921, subsequently Matron of the Brisbane Children's Hospital and Matron of the Brisbane General Hospital from 1928 to 1951, joined on 5 February 1921. Both women were active members of the ATNA so there was some overlap in membership between the QNA and ATNA.[34] Some QNA members were also members of the Queensland Professional Officers' Association (QPOA), with 20 trained nurses at five Brisbane hospitals belonging to the QPOA, in March 1922.[35]

The formation of a second nurses' association in the 1920s was not unique to Queensland as the Trained Nurses' Guild was formed in Victoria in 1921 with similar aims to the QNA. Once again there was an overlap in membership with the more conservative RVTNA which was not interested in pursuing better conditions through industrial activity.[36]

The QNA was only active until the mid-1920s when it disappeared as a force in nursing. In 1933 Laidlaw advised the Industrial Registrar that 'owing to the apathy of the members of this Association' no subscriptions were paid or meetings held in 1931. He added that 'I am endeavouring to work up further interest, but am not very hopeful of the result'.[37] Membership for the year ending 31 December 1932 totalled 30.[38] A year later there were 83 members in Brisbane hospitals, all except the president having joined in 1933.[39] By 1936 Laidlaw advised the Industrial Registrar that he had been unable to get a quorum to hold a meeting for twelve months, and no membership subscriptions had been paid. He added that 'although I cannot raise any interest in the Association, quite a number of nurses apply to me from time to time to have complaints under the Award rectified'.[40] This was the case for the next few years until the QNA quietly ceased to exist. Its registration was cancelled by the Industrial Court on 8 April 1940.[41]

The lack of documentation about the QNA means that little more can be learnt about its aims and activities but, given the executive personnel involved, it seems to have operated in a way similar to other white-collar unions at this time. The QPOA, for instance, which was formed in 1912, had both professional and industrial aims, and negotiated for better pay and conditions from its inception. Loath to engage in political or strike activity, it maintained a 'moderate industrial stance'.[42] The QNA adopted a similar position, while concentrating on industrial issues, apparently content to let the ATNA handle professional issues.

In Flanders' terms, the QNA had 'movement', that is a community of purpose, but it failed to develop an on-going organisation to sustain its efforts. The difficulty this union faced was how to evolve from a loose group and 'one way, usually the most important, was to secure recognition from employers so as to build enduring relations with them in the form of collective bargaining'.[43] But the ATNA had forged a more significant relationship with employers and handled training and professional issues. On gaining registration, many nurses joined their professional association, the ATNA, receiving its journal and, on occasions, participating in its activities.

Despite its short life, the QNA exerted a great influence on nurses' working conditions, giving Queensland the first industrial award for nurses, as nurses in Western Australia received their first award in 1935, New South Wales in 1936 and a Nurses' Wages Board was set up in Victoria in 1938.[44] Without the activity of the QNA it is highly unlikely that hospital nurses would have gained an award in the 1920s. Although the ATNA saw the QNA as a threat, many nurses clearly disagreed as they joined both associations. General pressure within the community for better conditions and inactivity on the part of the ATNA to deal effectively with this issue made room for another nurses' association.

With the formation of the QNA there were two courses of action open to the ATNA. It could co-exist with the new organisation and continue to handle educational and professional issues, while the QNA dealt with industrial issues, or it could insist that there should be only one organisation that looked after nurses. The course of co-existence would have placed nurses in a position similar to other professionals in government employment who belonged to their respective professional organisation as well as the QPOA, which negotiated awards and looked after other industrial concerns. The QPOA achieved its first award in 1918 and was represented in court by its full-time general secretary, Mr Henry Bond,[45] who assisted the ATNA with administrative duties.

The other alternative was to have only one organisation which represented both professional and industrial concerns, as the Queensland Teachers' Union (QTU) did for teachers. The ATNA chose the latter approach. It designated itself as the only organisation for nurses and saw the QNA as its rival. Indeed the honorary secretary, Miss Chatfield, characterised the QNA as 'our enemies'.[46] When its 'rival' gained registration as a trade union the ATNA felt forced to do likewise and thus entered the industrial arena.

QNA claim

The QNA claim, lodged on 8 February 1921, emphasised that nurses should have similar working conditions to other employees. The claim detailed salaries, allowances, hours, overtime payments and leave;[47] all conditions that existed in most awards. The most controversial point in it was a 48-hour week worked in eight-hour shifts. This was not radical when compared to existing awards but was revolutionary in the eyes of the ATNA and most hospitals, which strongly opposed the claim.

Dr McLean, speaking on behalf of the ATNA, maintained that if the QNA claim were adopted many difficulties would ensue. These included interference with the efficient training of nurses as a result of less time on duty. Private hospitals would either have to close or charge increased fees, he maintained, and this would force many to go to already overcrowded public hospitals which would have to provide increased nurse accommodation and their expenses would be increased by at least 25 per cent. Dr McLean concluded that 'with all this expense not one patient would receive any benefit'.[48] McLean played a dual role, answering the Queensland Government's queries from his influential position as Medical Superintendent of the Brisbane Hospital, the largest hospital in the state, at the same time as he was president of the ATNA.[49] This made him the most influential person speaking for the hospitals as employers and for the employees through their largest organisation. This was a remarkable situation, unthinkable for industrial unions, but commonplace for the ATNA where most of the executive were medical practitioners and nurses employed in management positions.

The ATNA emphasised the unique nature of the work of a nurse, especially her overriding dedication to the patient. Although the ATNA felt that 'the conditions of service require improvement in many hospitals',[50] it spoke disparagingly about the QNA claim saying it was 'based largely on other awards'. McLean emphasised that:

> the work of a nurse, whether she is in training or at a hospital, or in private work, is to attend the sick and ailing and the work is, more or less, of an emergency nature and goes on night and day. In the interest of the patient it is impossible particularly in midwifery, and any casualty work, to absolutely fix her hours.[51]

The special nature of a nurse's work was emphasised in an editorial in the *MJA*: 'nurses, like doctors, have obligations to the public which are paramount. The possession of special knowledge and skill in nursing and in medicine has a national significance and consequently the members of these two professions are not free agents to conduct their business to their own advantage in the manner best suited to themselves, but have to recognize a certain degree of servitude.' The *MJA* did allow however, that:

> it is one of the functions of the nurses' societies to take steps to prevent the management of hospitals from sweating . . . the young women undergoing training or the trained nurses employed for their

> skilled services. But this limitation of healthy work should not be driven too far . . . The probationer or trainee must also work hard and unselfishly if she is to develope [sic] into a highly trained and useful nurse.

It declared that 'a few trainees and dissatisfied nurses have taken the absurd and wholly unprofessional step of securing registration as a trades union. This misguided body of foolish virgins has sought a nurses' award'.[52] The allusion to 'foolish virgins' in the Gospel according to St Matthew (chapter 25) would have been recognised widely. These improvident maidens forgot to provide oil for their lamps, surely a reference to the image of Florence Nightingale, and, in the allegory, are denied entry to heaven.

The QNA claim sent ripples through the conservative hospital world. It led to the formation of a Country Hospitals' Association by the Roma, Tambo, Mitchell, Cunnamulla and Surat hospitals in western Queensland, established because the 'arbitration proceedings and trend of events make it necessary that Country Hospitals should combine, otherwise they are likely to be severely penalised since their special circumstances are little understood in the larger centres'.[53]

The employers who opposed the claim argued that hospitals were not run for profit and could not be compared with ordinary businesses as their work was the care of the sick. Dr E. Humphrey, who ran a private hospital in Townsville, maintained that:

> the only way to be certain of a regular day off and half holiday is for the court to grant an injunction restraining patients from passing water, or their bowels acting, especially if they have diarrhoea from noon on Saturday to eight on Monday morning. Also that no woman shall be confined during that time, and certainly not after sunset or before sunrise so that the nurse attending at nights shall be sure of rest. This should also apply on Saturdays and holidays.[54]

The Stanthorpe Hospital expressed the feelings of many of the hospital committees: 'It is impossible to conduct the hospital with stereotyped hours and allowing the sick to care for themselves on Sundays and holidays, whereas other walks in life can and are regulated to so work their respective businesses and the cost invariably passed on, one is a business the other more or less charity'.[55] The Gladstone Hospital committee felt that 'a public hospital, which is supported purely by voluntary donations etc and has no fixed income, cannot be considered an industry in any way, and so long as living wages are paid should not be forced into the market to raise funds possibly by questionable means'.[56] Some employers believed that nurses already enjoyed good working conditions. Dr Humphrey reported that the nurses he employed were 'quite happy and contented and don't wish to be interfered with in any way'.[57]

One of the most contentious points of the QNA claim was the hours of work. The claim requested conditions similar to other workers with a 48-hour week inclusive of 45 minute meal breaks and arranged in eight-hour shifts. Nurses were to be given one and a half days off each week. In the 1921 government survey, three-quarters of the hospitals (47 out of 63) felt that this would be 'impracticable', 'impossible', or 'not workable in their hospitals', and a number stated that they would be forced to close the hospital because they could not afford the extra expense of the additional nursing staff required. The small hospitals, those with less than two nurses, often expressed the view that working hours were impossible to regulate in a small hospital because of the unpredictability and irregularity of their patient loads.[58] Many committees replied that they would find it extremely difficult, if not impossible, to carry on if the hours of the QNA claim were enforced because of the extra nurses required. The Gladstone Hospital Committee stated this general view:

> There is no comparison . . . between the working of an ordinary business and an institution such as an hospital, for in the former case an employer can reasonably adjust and provide for the carrying out of his prospective business throughout the year, whereas with the latter the amount of sickness or accidents likely to occur cannot be estimated with certainty; at one period of the year the hospital may be full and at another period empty, and the committee of such an institution through their medical officers and matron should be allowed some discretion as to the working hours of their staff.[59]

Some hospitals objected to the arrangement of eight-hour shifts and the Hughenden District Hospital replied typically that:

> it will be quite hopeless to endeavour to work such institutions on a system of 8 hour shifts unless a surplus (and in our opinion unnecessary) staff equal to about 30% of the normal staff be employed . . . the heavy part of the work in the wards falls between 7 a.m. and 1 p.m. and during this period most of the Staff are required to be on duty. After say 1 p.m. the pressure is relaxed and fewer nurses at a time are necessary; and the adoption of a system of 8 hour shifts would mean that it would be impossible to so regulate the duties to ensure that each nurse would be reasonably fully employed throughout her shift.[60]

Nine hospitals favoured eight-hour shifts but felt that they would not be able to introduce them. Once again the reason was the cost. A few hospitals had tried the system of eight-hour shifts but had found it unworkable and only five hospitals thought these shifts were feasible.

The award did not cover members of religious orders but appeals to exempt hospitals run by some religious bodies, including the Mater Misericordiae Public Hospital in Brisbane, were not successful. Justice McCawley remarked:

> I am unable to see sufficient grounds upon which I should exempt such hospitals without exempting public hospitals generally. It was pointed out to me that the public hospital mentioned is in financial difficulties, and also that the nurses employed requested exemption. These circumstances are worthy of consideration; but the first of them, unfortunately, is of general application to all public hospitals, and it has weighed with me in fixing the Award and the date from which it is to apply, while the second is one to which the Court seldom gives effect, unless it is satisfied that the employees are better treated than they would be under an Award.[61]

The financial state of hospitals was a paramount consideration, not only for McCawley but also for the ATNA. This is clearly seen in the date of application of the award. The QNA asked that the award should operate from 1 January 1921 while the ATNA wanted the award to come into force three months after it was gazetted, making a difference of nine months.

Dr McLean believed that even though many sectors of the workforce had a 48-hour week, the situation within a hospital was such that this could not be granted to nurses:

> What strikes one most about this claim is the fact that in an already overcrowded hospital, with deficient equipment . . . there is not an increase of one bed or any accommodation for the sick poor.
>
> In fact, with all this increased expenditure, the unfortunate patient does not gain anything but probably loses with the frequent changes and loss of continuity of work.
>
> Except for the reduction of work from fifty-six to forty-eight hours of work per week and increase of salaries, the nurse will gain nothing and, I am sure, that under the conditions laid down in the claim that the trainee will not secure the experience and knowledge of the work, which, hitherto, has equipped her as an efficient and capable nurse.[62]

Thus the president of the ATNA opposed the reduction in hours. As medical superintendent of the Brisbane Hospital, McLean was primarily concerned with increased hospital costs. The Brisbane Hospital estimated that the QNA claim would cost 15 649 pounds extra for one year, including back pay and additions to the nurses' accommodation 'which must run up to many thousands of pounds'.[63] Similar sums of money were quoted for other large hospitals throughout Queensland, as well as a delay of up to two years to have the additional buildings completed. The smaller hospitals, though requiring less money, asserted that it would be extremely difficult to find the funds and some feared that they would be forced to close.[64]

1921 nurses' award

The first nurses' award came into operation on 1 July 1921. The conditions of the award differed from the proposals of both the QNA and the ATNA but were much closer to the more conservative views of the latter. In his judgment, Justice T.W. McCawley, president of the Arbitration Court, concluded that 'some of the provisions of this Award will be disappointing to the nurses, but it must be borne in mind that the Award is the first of its kind in the State, and to most hospitals will be a heavy burden, while upon most nurses it will confer considerable benefit'.[65] The poor working conditions of many nurses prior to the award are emphasised by the fact that most nurses would receive 'considerable' improvements.

The award applied to trainees, assistants in nursing, staff nurses, sisters and matrons working in hospitals, excluding mental hospitals, which had a daily average of six or more occupied beds. There were many nurses who did not receive any benefit from the new award. In Queensland, 34 per cent of public hospitals (31 out of 91) averaged less than six patients daily, and the 54 nurses they employed (5.3 per cent of hospital nurses) were not covered by the award.[66] Yet these were the nurses who were most likely to work long and unregulated hours and neither the ATNA nor the QNA had suggested that nurses in small hospitals should remain outside the award. Although the reasons for exempting these small hospitals were not stated in McCawley's decision, it is likely that cost was a major factor.

The award included assistants in nursing whose role was 'assisting in nursing duties in a hospital not registered as a training school'.[67] The inclusion of this category acknowledged the existence of untrained

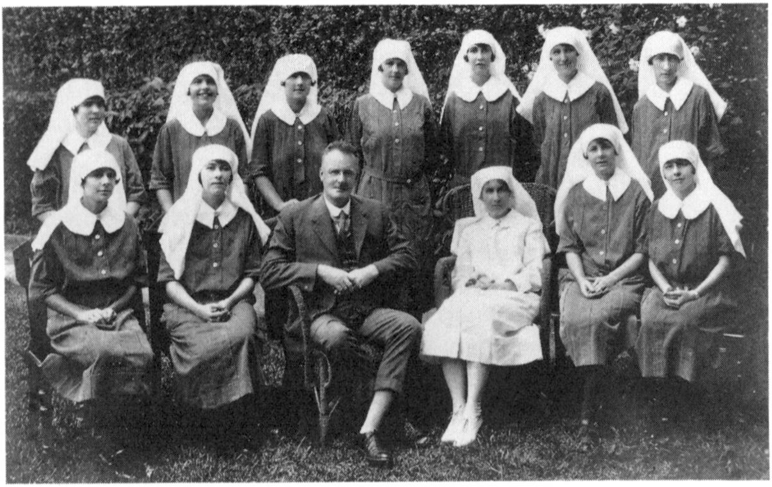

Staff nurses, Matron Effie Bourne (Matron from 1914 to 1928) and Dr John Barr McLean, Medical Superintendent of the Brisbane Hospital, photographed in 1928. Matron Bourne was an ATNA councillor from 1915 to 1916 and 1918 to 1933. (Collection: Royal Brisbane Hospital Graduate Nurses' Archive and John Oxley Library, Brisbane.)

nursing staff in hospitals, so although trained nursing had been recognised by state registration, hospital demands created a new category of hospital worker who was, in fact, an untrained nurse, working under the direction of a trained nurse. The first variation of the nurses' award, gazetted on 8 June 1922, extended the coverage of the award to all registered nurses in all hospitals but those on the lowest rungs of the nursing hierarchy, the assistants in nursing, were still not covered if they worked in small hospitals.[68]

Two categories of registered nurses, staff nurses and sisters, were included in the award. Staff nurses were defined as 'all registered nurses below the matron' in hospitals with less than 25 average occupied beds. In contrast, a sister had 'special responsibility connected with wards, special departments, and the training of nurses'.[69] Only 24 out of 91 hospitals had a daily average of 25 beds or more[70] which meant that in 74 per cent of hospitals a nurse could never be classified as sister and receive the higher wages. This gave them a short career path in small hospitals and a maximum salary as staff nurses of 110 pounds per annum.

The salaries awarded to nurses reflected the position of women's salaries generally in the labour market, although their long hours and other conditions set them apart from other workers. Women were not perceived as breadwinners, with paid work existing only until marriage. This view was reflected in the wage fixing principles: 'In the case of men, their occupation was their life's vocation; in the case of women, their occupation (beyond the domestic sphere) was, in most cases, transitory. It was the uncertainty of a woman's vocation that formed its chief difficulty.'[71]

By 1921, the system of unequal pay for female workers was firmly entrenched in the federal and state wage fixing tribunals. The 1907 Harvester decision by Justice Higgins in the Federal Court had determined the minimum wage for a man on the basis of 'the normal needs of the average employee, regarded as a human being living in a civilized community'.[72] With the acceptance of the 'needs' principle based on a man's position in society it followed that, as women were supported by men, they did not need the same amount of money. Men were seen as the rightful wage earners in society and 'fortunately for society', Higgins believed, 'the greater number of breadwinners still are men. The women are not all dragged from the homes to work while the men loaf at home'.[73]

While women in a few jobs where they were 'fairly in competition' with men were awarded equal pay in order to 'secure men in their employment',[74] work which was overwhelmingly performed by women received a much lower rate of pay. In 1919 Higgins set the female basic wage at approximately 54 per cent of the male basic wage after trying to ascertain 'what is the sum per week necessary to satisfy the normal needs of an average female employee, who has to support herself from her own exertions; and on the basis of the reasonably necessary requirements of a woman living in a civilized community'.[75] The *1916 Industrial Arbitration Act* in Queensland enshrined the principles of the Harvester judgment in law. While an adult male had to receive a wage sufficient to support a family of five, women only needed to support themselves.[76] Like other women workers, nurses were not regarded as needing a wage which would be sufficient to support a family. The Stanthorpe Hospital Committee upheld this view, stating that:

> ninety-nine per cent of the Nurses and Matrons have nobody but themselves to maintain and provide for either in life or after death . . . their respective salaries are their property free of all responsibility as to household expenses, sickness expense, insurance against sickness and accident . . . their whole earnings which are quite up to the average of the earnings of other walks of life already, go to them for their sole personal use in 99 per cent of cases.[77]

The Queensland Act also endorsed the principle of equal pay when competition from women's cheaper labour might mean that men would lose their jobs. Section 8 provided that 'the same wage shall be paid to persons of either sex performing the same work or producing the same return of profit to their employer'.[78] The standard which women workers had to meet was work as it was performed by men. Any differences would mean that the job a woman did was not the same and therefore was unworthy of equal pay, even if the work done by women could have been judged to be more valuable.[79] Yet because of the extreme degree of segregation of the labour market by gender, few women did exactly the same work as men. Power's study of census data from 1911 to 1971 shows that, throughout this period, the majority of women worked in occupations where at least half the workers were women, while most men worked in occupations that employed very few women.[80] It was never necessary to consider if the work of female general nurses was in competition with or more valuable than male general nurses, as the latter did not exist.

Until the latter half of the 1960s most workers' wages were a composite of the basic wage plus margins for skill or other particular characteristics of the work. This extra payment was given when the job demanded training, as in the case of a skilled tradesperson; or if the worker had to have exceptional physical strength, such as a stoker; or if the worker had responsibility for human life, such as winding engine drivers who raised or lowered human beings in mine shafts.[81] Many female wage rates were determined without the same arguments as to skill and responsibility which characterised male workers. Responsibility for human life was never considered a factor in evaluating nurses' wages. Despite the fact that a nurse's training could have been equated with those of other professions or trades, and other features of her work such as responsibility for human life differentiated her from an unskilled worker, this skill and responsibility was not used in arguing rates of pay for nurses in the first award in Queensland.

The rates of pay set by the court were close to the proposals of the ATNA and the wages that the hospitals were prepared to pay. In fact, McCawley stated in his judgment that 'the salaries awarded do not differ greatly from those which the parties were willing to pay'. Salaries ranged from 36 pounds a year for a first year trainee to 160 pounds for a sister with four years experience and up to 370 pounds for a matron of a hospital with more than 300 beds.[82] These rates were generally at least 10 per cent higher, and in the case of trainees 30 per cent higher, in the award than in the rates proposed by the ATNA. However the

ATNA proposed wage rates for most matrons that were higher than both the QNA claim and the award.[83]

The salaries awarded to hospital nurses were below those of other comparable groups of workers. If the value of their board and lodging was added to the value of their wages, as employers argued, their wages approached those of other female employees. The lowest paid workers in the hospital were the first and second year nurse trainees and the first year assistant in nursing. The salary of the third year nurse trainee and the assistant in nursing with two years experience equalled that of the pantrymaid, housemaid, waitress and general servant in the hospital. The ATNA likened the trainee nurse to an apprentice and industrial courts accepted this classification.

The low educational entry standard was an additional point in favour of not raising the salaries of nurses. The hospital committees of Hughenden, Cloncurry, Richmond and Winton expounded this view:

> It is true that the trainee nurses are required to work longer hours than the female public service clerk, but against this may be set the fact that the clerk is required to pass a competitive and somewhat exacting examination, namely the University Junior whereas the educational standard of the average trainee nurse is much lower.[84]

Nursing trainees were poorly remunerated when compared to women less than 21 years old in other female occupations and McCawley noted in his judgment that 'there are some trainees whose parents can afford to supplement their earnings, but I am satisfied that this does not apply in the case of the majority, nor is it a circumstance which I can consider in framing an Award'.[85]

The training of midwifery nurses was viewed differently and salaries in the award did not apply to trainees in midwifery. Despite the fact that the *1900 Factories and Shops Act* prohibited the payment of a premium to an employer,[86] midwifery trainees at the Lady Musgrave Hospital in Maryborough and the Mothers' Hospital in Toowoomba made such a payment (15 pounds at Toowoomba). Although the payment of a premium to an employer was uncommon by the 1920s[87] and the QNA asked that all premiums in hospitals be abolished, this was not included in the award. At the midwifery training hospitals at Maryborough, Rockhampton and Toowoomba in 1920 the course was of twelve months duration and no salary was paid to the trainees. At the Rockhampton Women's Hospital there was only the matron, one staff nurse and eight trainees, providing a considerable saving on wages to the employer.[88] This meant that only those women who had some other source of income could train as midwifery nurses in these hospitals, and they provided the cheapest of labour—free. However conditions remained unaltered as McCawley decided that 'qualified midwifery nurses are insufficient in number, and, after a short period of training, trainees . . . are eligible for certificates which enable them to practise as fully qualified midwifery nurses'.[89]

In most cases it is difficult to envisage any adequate supervision of trainees, many of whom must have had substantial responsibilities placed on them. Indeed, in the smaller country hospitals with one matron and one trainee or up to six trainees with one nurse and the matron, there must have been many times when no qualified nurse was on duty. Although the ATNA had shown great concern for the standards of training it had not addressed this issue in relation to accredited training hospitals. There were no regulations from the Nurses' Registration Board on the ratio of trainees to trained staff, and nurses never came under the jurisdiction of apprenticeship boards. In the ratio present in the hospitals, the emphasis was on the labour provided by trainees, and not on the transmission of knowledge and skills to new members of the occupation. McCawley himself was concerned about midwifery trainees at the Lady Bowen Hospital as 'the proportion of staff nurses to trainees seems extraordinarily small, and is a matter which may require consideration under some subsequent Award'.[90] Yet the award standard of eight trainees to one trained nurse (as requested by the ATNA, compared to the QNA claim of five trainees to one registered nurse) fell far short of the general regulations for apprentices of one trainee to three qualified workers.[91]

Trained nurses earned more than female unskilled workers but less than other female skilled workers. The wages of qualified nurses were low compared to other adult female skilled workers including teachers, clerks and public servants. A female clerk took home as much pay as a matron of a hospital of up to 35 average occupied beds (*see* Table 5.1).

Female salaries within the hospital were significantly lower than those for male employees, even when the value of board and lodging is deducted from the male rate of pay.[92] The lower paid nurses and female hospital staff received less than the normal percentage of at least 50 per cent of the male rate for the same or comparable work, even when the value of board and lodging is considered. It was only at the level of matron that a nurse achieved the actual salary of a dresser or head laundryman.

Under the 1921 award, nurses worked longer hours than most other employees. The ATNA had opposed the QNA's claim[93] of a 48-hour week with eight-hour shifts, arguing that continuous shifts were unworkable because of the emergency nature of the work and the impossibility

Table 5.1 Salaries of nurses and other workers, 1921

Occupation	Female salaries (pounds per annum)	Male salaries (pounds per annum)
Nurses		
Nurse trainee	36–75*	—
Assistant in nursing	46–85*	—
Staff nurse	110*	—
Sister	120–160*	—
Matron**	160–370*	—
Other hospital workers		
Pantrymaid, waitress, housemaid	65	—
Laundress	78	—
Head laundress	91	—
Laundryman	—	221
Head laundryman	—	227/10/–
Junior wardsman	—	78–182
Wardsman, theatre & mortuary	—	221
Attendant, dresser	—	—
Porter, yardman & general hand	—	221
Female cook	117	—
Shop assistants		
18 to 21 years	65–83/4/–	92/6/– to 137/16/–
over 21 years	93/12/– to 176	143–247
Clerks		
18 to 21 years	76/14/– to 170/6/–	115/14/– to 240/10/–
over 23 years	189/16/–	260
Qld Public Service clerk & typist, up to 5 1/2 years service	87–157	90–190
Qld Public Service clerk, after 5 1/2 years service	172–232	210–275
Qld Public Service typist, after 5 1/2 years service	172–192	—
Teachers		
up to 4th class	60–108	72–120
Teacher, class III	135–255 (195 at age 21)	155–285 (225 at age 21)

* Annual salaries include the payment of board and lodging.

** Matrons' salaries were determined by the size of the hospital, measured in terms of the average daily occupied bed number. Matrons of hospitals with less than 11 average daily occupied beds earned 160 pounds; 11 to 35 beds, 170 to 200 pounds (annual increments of ten pounds); 36 to 150 beds, 200 to 230 pounds; 151 to 200 beds, 230 to 270 pounds; 201 to 300 beds, 270 to 320 pounds; over 300 beds, 320 to 370 pounds.

Source QGG, vol. CXV, no. 164, 23 Sep. 1920; vol. CXVI, no. 104, 23 Mar. 1921; no. 159, 13 Apr. 1921; no. 187, 21 Apr. 1921; no. 290, 23 Jun. 1921.

of fixing definite hours for the matron. The ATNA recommended a 56-hour week, exclusive of meals, with one and a half days off each week. The award provided for 112 hours a fortnight, inclusive of meal times, close to the ATNA's proposal and giving the employer the greatest amount of flexibility in arranging hours. In hospitals with a daily average of not less than 25 beds, nurses were to have one and a half days off, the latter commencing not later than 2 pm. Smaller hospitals were to comply with this if possible, but if this could not be arranged, three whole days off per fortnight were to be allowed. Only 26 per cent of hospitals in the state had more than 25 occupied beds, so the clause relating to time off each week was not mandatory in the majority of hospitals.[94] As well as this, the clause did not apply to matrons.

By 1921 it was usual for workers under an award to have a standard working week of 48 hours, with some employees working 44 hours.[95] Hospital workers other than nurses enjoyed a 48-hour week with one day off in every seven. The hours of nurses exceeded those prescribed by the Queensland *Industrial Arbitration Act of 1916* which stipulated a maximum of 48 hours a week except where the court certified that 'for reasons of paramount public interest such greater number of hours should be worked in the calling'.[96] The court agreed with the prevailing view of the ATNA and the employers that the care of the sick involved work that was different from most other industries. Justice McCawley decided that the public interest required a longer working week and concluded that:

> it cannot be doubted that the sick, especially the sick poor, would be very greatly inconvenienced if the Court were now, on the first occasion when the hospital conditions are subjected to an Award, to require all hospitals to establish a forty-eight hour week. Indeed, it would be impracticable to establish a forty-eight hour week at present, as the requisite number of nurses is not available, nor could the requisite accommodation be provided. However, I think that a reduction to 112 hours per fortnight, inclusive of meal hours, is reasonable and practicable.[97]

Many clauses in the initial nurses' award differed from other awards. For instance, nurses who worked in country areas did not receive a district allowance under the award, even though this was a common feature in other awards. Although requested by the QNA,[98] the ATNA opposed the payment of these allowances.[99] The award specified the rate of time-and-a-half for all overtime,[100] despite the fact that the *Industrial Arbitration Act* stated that overtime was to be paid at not less than double time in jobs which required shiftwork.[101] In lieu of time-and-a-half or double time for work done on statutory public holidays (as provided in the Act), nurses were granted four weeks annual leave.[102] The QNA had proposed that nurses should have one month's annual recreation leave as well as the higher rates for public holidays. The ATNA had wanted three weeks annual leave and commented that the QNA claim would mean that 'the nurse would have 12–13 weeks (if Sundays are included) plus sick leave and weekly day and a half'. The award granted four weeks annual leave in lieu of payment for statutory holidays.

The result of these provisions was that nurses worked longer hours than the majority of other workers and the four weeks annual leave that they received replaced twelve gazetted public holidays or additional payment for working on these days. However, one provision that was more beneficial than that in most awards was sick leave. One can speculate that this amount of leave was needed when the chances of infection and the longer hours of the nurse are considered. Paid sick leave for a period not exceeding three weeks was provided for nurses in their award with nursing treatment supplied by the hospital for any illness contracted in the course of a nurse's duty.[103]

Adequate accommodation for nurses was an on-going problem. Nurses invariably lived at the hospital. An *ANJ* editorial protested that 'perhaps the idea of the nurse being a ministering angel has so imbued those in authority that the provision of suitable sleeping accommodation for her has been lost sight of'. The journal felt that the solution to this problem was for ATNA members to 'work together and unite in all matters affecting the welfare of nurses as a whole' so that 'their influence must be felt and the desired good attained'.[104] But the clause dealing with accommodation followed the ATNA recommendation that nurses should have separate rooms or cubicles rather than the QNA claim of separate rooms.

In general, the award included most of the clauses requested by the QNA but the level of salaries and working conditions within these clauses was closely related to the counter claim of the ATNA. If the ATNA itself had instigated the award it is likely that nurses would have received even less salary than the amounts they actually obtained because the court awarded higher amounts than the ATNA had proposed.[105]

Unlike the QNA, the views of the ATNA were almost identical with those of the hospitals. The question of the financial difficulties of hospitals and the needs of the patients were always the prime consid-

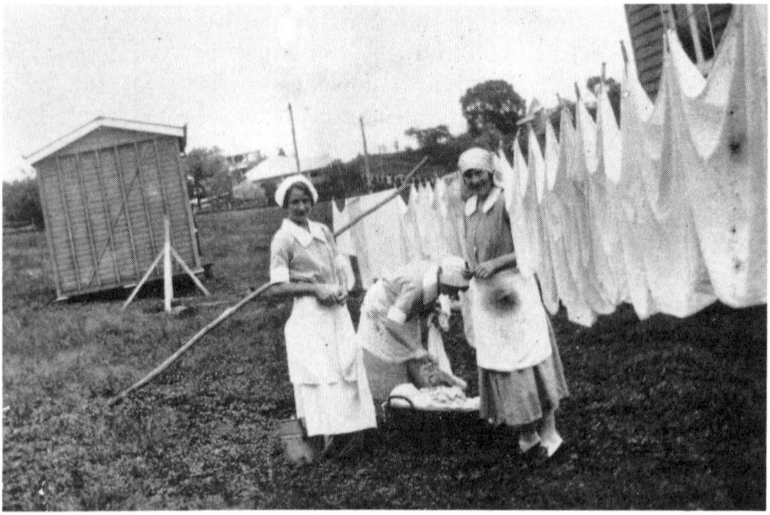

Nurses' work usually involved many domestic duties, especially in country hospitals. Here nursing staff are hanging out the washing at Boonah Hospital, west of Brisbane, about 1920s. (Collection: John Oxley Library, Brisbane.)

eration and created a set of conditions with which a nurses' award should comply, something that did not occur for other groups of workers. The ATNA and the employers argued that nurses should be paid what the hospitals could afford, and although other hospital staff had an award similar to most workers, nurses came into a separate category. The ideal of service to humanity was central to this argument, and payment and conditions similar to other workers contradictory to this notion. Their feelings of satisfaction in the service of the sick were often seen as sufficient reward for their devotion to duty. Indeed, their conditions reflected:

> the convenient social virtue [which] is widely important for inducing people to perform unpleasant services . . . [It has] helped obtain the charitable and compassionate services of nurses, custodial personnel, and other hospital staff . . . the resulting merit in the eyes of the community served as a partial substitute for compensation. (Such merit was never deemed a wholly satisfactory substitute for remuneration in the case of physicians.) But the ultimate success of the convenient social virtue has been in converting women to menial personal service.[106]

Nurses themselves helped perpetuate the uniqueness of nursing with its strong emphasis on devotion to duty above all else. For instance, the nurses at the Mater Misericordiae Public Hospital requested exemption from the award when the hospital experienced financial difficulties.[107] Yet this award, which came into operation on 1 July 1921, provided Queensland hospital nurses with their first set of uniform working conditions. The change it brought was recognised by Justice McCawley: 'Upon most nurses it will confer considerable benefit.'[108]

Reduction in working hours, 1925

During the 1920s there were two variations of the nurses' award, once again initiated by the QNA. Minor changes were made in 1922 and a significant reduction in working hours achieved in 1925, bringing nurses almost into line with other workers. Once again the ATNA objected to the major changes, particularly the reduction in hours to 88 a fortnight, on the grounds that nurses were not like other workers, hospitals could not be run like other businesses and the training and work of a nurse required dedication but not high monetary reward. It was supported in its argument by the major hospitals.

In its application to vary the award in 1922 the QNA reiterated its claim for a 48-hour working week. Despite the fact that if this claim was granted it would merely bring nurses into line with other workers, the ATNA still regarded it as radical and the potential cause of great financial distress to hospitals. It did not want to alter the clause from its existing 112 hours a fortnight. Hospitals reiterated their arguments of the previous year, saying the shorter hours were 'unworkable and impracticable'. The major argument against reduced hours was once again the cost of extra accommodation at the hospitals. While three hospitals already had a 48-hour week, the Children's Hospital Committee stated that they would be compelled to consider reducing the number of patients, as they did not have the means to increase the staff.[109] In the face of this opposition and the views of the ATNA, the 112-hour fortnight was retained in the award.

In the years between 1921 and 1925 there were several changes to the clauses covering hours of work in the Queensland *Industrial Arbitration Act*, culminating in the 1925 amendment which reduced the working week from 48 to an obligatory 44 hours.[110] A general meeting of QNA members in 1925 resolved to submit a claim to the Industrial Court with the sole request of a 44-hour week, a claim which was supported by the QPOA.[111] The ATNA, in an answer submitted by the President Dr A. M. Marks, and the respondent hospitals made claims that asked for the longest hours legally possible and gave the hospital the greatest flexibility in setting shifts with hours calculated per fortnight.

Various hospitals had been circularised to obtain the views of the nurses and these were 'practically unanimous in favour of no alteration in the present hours being made, in view of the detrimental effect it would have on their training and on the patients owing to the continuous change of nurses required'. Therefore the council had decided to oppose the QNA claim.[112]

The arguments against the QNA claim had not changed since they were first voiced in 1921. The Brisbane Hospitals Board alleged that:

> it is not good for patients to have the continuity of attention and supervision broken as must happen with shorter hours. The efficient training of nurses will not only be reflected in the treatment of the sick in the Public Hospitals, but will be reflected in the treatment of the sick when the nurse leaves the Hospital to embark upon the practice of her profession.[113]

Another memorandum expressed this point of view more strongly saying that 'the constant changing which must ensue with shorter shifts will be detrimental to the patients' welfare, which should be the first consideration in a hospital'.[114]

Without the specific Act of Parliament the ATNA and the employers would undoubtedly have opposed the QNA claim more vigorously. The court had no option but to reduce the hours, but followed the wishes of the majority of respondents in its decision. The change in the nurses' award, effective from 7 July 1925, varied the hours from 112 per fortnight to 88 per fortnight, exclusive of meal times.[115] Once again this arrangement provided the greatest flexibility to the hospitals in their organisation of the nursing workforce while complying with the *Industrial Arbitration Act*.

The Queensland Branch of the ATNA 'approached the area of legal determination of wages and conditions with extreme reluctance. This area of the association's activities was forced on it by circumstances beyond its control and was regarded as not as important as the professional activities of the ATNA'.[116] Trembath and Hellier have criticised this conclusion, claiming that I have assumed that 'the only possible model of industrial activity for nurses' organisations . . . [is] the trade union. They concluded that because 'nurses chose to remain outside the arbitration system, it has been argued that nurses' associations did not pursue any economic activities'.[117] For hospital nurses in Australia however, this was the only way that they could be guaranteed certain conditions because, as the 1921 survey of nurses' working conditions in Queensland showed, vastly different conditions applied. Recommendations to hospitals carried no legal weight and it was up to the hospital, already working on a tight budget, to implement better conditions. In fact, as Trembath and Hellier conclude, 'dislike of being classed with factory workers took the form of opposition to the growth within nursing of what can be called "the trade union spirit"'.[118] This was obviously the case with the ATNA Council in Queensland, yet by 1920 this did not reflect the views of all nurses, otherwise the QNA would not have gained support. Trembath and Hellier add that 'nurses rejected any industrial activity which resembled that undertaken by trade unions. This is not to say that nurses spurned all forms of industrial activity or completely shied away from discussion of their material interests'.[119] There is no evidence that nurses did engage in industrial activity prior to 1920, even though private nurses discussed their income and working conditions. The ATNA certainly rejected all forms of industrial activity although groups of members did on occasion force the council to discuss their material interests.

Distinction must be carefully made between the ATNA Council and nurses generally, although it is difficult to ascertain the views of the latter group. The only action taken by the ATNA Council on industrial issues was to make recommendations to employers which had no force in law. Trembath and Hellier have concluded that, because the working conditions of private nurses were discussed and those of hospital nurses were not, 'the location of a nurse's work determined whether her conditions were suitable subjects for investigation by the R.V.T.N.A'.[120] Why, when both groups underwent the same training and socialisation, should the location of the nurse be the determining factor? Trained nurses in private practice were a more numerous group than trained nurses employed by hospitals. Private nurses successfully pressured the council to consider their plight for, not living in at a hospital, their wages had to meet their living needs. The size of the group may have been important in determining the amount of activity and debate of issues. Trained nurses in hospitals held supervisory and management positions and were a major part of the socialising process for newer nurses. Most hospital nursing was performed by trainees, who could not even belong to the ATNA and, effectively in the position of apprentice, were beholden to their employer for their future livelihood. Legal determination of working conditions was the only way most of these nurses could achieve better working conditions, yet the ATNA never actively pursued this.

Trembath and Hellier appear to place too much faith in alternative methods of improving wages and conditions for it is clear from the variations shown in the 1921 survey that the ATNA's recommendations of fees, salaries and conditions were not universally complied with by employers.

With the impetus of nurses who had formed the QNA, the ATNA Council felt compelled to challenge this new organisation's existence. The ATNA had been forced by the activities of the QNA to enter and remain in the industrial arena. In order to further the interests of nurses, as the association perceived them, it became a party to the nurses' award in 1922 but remained a steadfast opponent of most changes in working conditions.

Many of the changes in nurses' working conditions at this time were remarkable, and in the space of less than five years some nurses' working hours were reduced from over 140 hours per fortnight to 88 hours. Standardised and regulated conditions were available to most hospital nurses with the introduction of the first award in 1921. The 'dedicated, capable angels of mercy'[121] had, unwittingly for the most part, entered the world of trade unions.

CHAPTER 6

The working conditions of hospital nurses in the 1930s

'. . . the pendulum has now swung too far in the opposite direction, and present working hours are too short.'[1]

In the 1920s, hospital nurses in Queensland achieved award wages and greatly improved working conditions. Hours were reduced to 88 a fortnight, a change that occurred because the Industrial Arbitration Act had specified a maximum of 44 hours a week. This had left the court, the ATNA and the employing hospitals with little room for movement and had forced them to comply, bringing some of the working conditions for nurses into line with those of other workers. But the progress that had been made with increased wages and reduced hours of work was halted in the 1930s. With the severe economic Depression bringing high levels of unemployment throughout Australia, most workers received a cut in wages, some worked longer hours and others faced reduced working weeks.

During the early 1930s many unions encountered problems including a drop in membership and funds. However Queensland's level of unemployment was significantly lower than that in other states with approximately 30 per cent of the state's workforce unemployed in 1931[2] and the state maintained a higher level of real income per person.[3] In 1932 18.8 per cent of trade unionists in Queensland were unemployed, compared with a national average of 29 per cent.[4]

Assessment on the overall impact of the Depression on trade unions varies. Costar has concluded that it is surprising 'how little the depression altered the essential fabric of the Australian and Queensland trade union movements'.[5] The effect on most unions in the short-term was dramatic, with a rapid decline in membership and a low level of industrial action, but 'there is little evidence of . . . longterm structural change within the union movement'.[6] On the other hand, Louis comments that 'unions found awards difficult to enforce even among unionists, and virtually impossible in the case of non-unionists'. In Victoria there was 'a serious deterioration of union organisation and effectiveness. Although the different unions experienced varying degrees of decline, over all they suffered greatly'.[7] The impact on individual unions varied, depending on the economic circumstances of the industries concerned, but public employment was only slightly affected. Members of the QTU suffered a wage cut but their employment as state public servants meant that, with the exception of married women, they could not be easily retrenched. The QTU suffered only a small decline of four per cent in membership between 1927 and 1932. The State Services Union, covering state public servants in the clerical ranks, experienced a slight increase of four per cent in membership. However other unions' membership declined by more than 30 per cent during this period.[8]

Women who remained in work were relatively unaffected by the Depression for, 'while there was female unemployment in the areas of domestic service, teaching, and nursing, for many women these jobs provided relatively stable employment'.[9] Maintaining a job as a nurse meant receiving accommodation and food and an income which provided the necessities of life. 'We were so thankful to have a job' was the sentiment shared by trainees at Wollongong Hospital.[10] Another nurse recalled that 'training as a nurse during the depression years had its compensations as I had a job and the hospital was my home for four years'.[11] With the unavailability of many areas of employment for women during the early 1930s, training and work as a nurse had an added significance in providing on-going employment for many single women.

During the Depression years community attitudes towards women working outside the home were generally negative:

> working women were blamed for male unemployment and, if married, often faced open hostility . . . It seemed obvious to the unthinking that the low wages paid to women made them attractive employees in order to cut costs. It was not considered obvious that these low wages made it almost impossible for women to be self-reliant . . . Man was the provider, woman the helpmate and homemaker, only working temporarily between school and marriage.[12]

For this reason, and because women comprised the less organised sector of the workforce, they were 'the obvious scapegoats'.[13] In Queensland, trade unions campaigned against married women working and asked the Labor Government to legislate against this, an issue the government refused.[14]

Views that women were taking men's jobs did not apply to nursing. Those trained nurses who remained working in their profession were seen as performing a unique function in society, one which was not carried out by men. Women's incomes were low, but hospital nurses did not face the additional problem of keeping a roof over their heads. With members working in an essential service, many in government employment, the ATNA did not suffer the large loss of membership characteristic of unions in manufacturing and building nor did it suffer any 'serious deterioration of union organisation and effectiveness'.[15] Like the QTU and the State Services Union the drastic problems of mass unemployment did not affect it. Members in hospitals received a cut in wages and a lengthening of hours, while private practitioners faced some decline in their income if clients could not pay for their services. The ATNA reported no extraordinary problems with the enforcement of their award or a drop in membership or funds and the Depression did not have a significant impact on the internal politics and machinery of the ATNA.

Forced into the industrial arena in the early 1920s by its 'rival' organisation, economic Depression gave the ATNA an opportunity to reiterate its largely non-industrial stance and embrace lower wages and longer hours of work. But the Depression destroyed the QNA, and its demise allowed the ATNA to revert to its original anti-union stance and lack of involvement in industrial activities. Once again there was little pressure for the council to take notice of the industrial concerns of ordinary nurses. The ATNA Council welcomed the extension of working hours for hospital nurses in 1930 because it had not wanted them to be so short in the first place.

In the climate of the early 1930s financial considerations were paramount and hospital boards and committees were advised by the state government that they had to exercise the strictest economy. Hospitals were asked to cut their estimated expenditure to the bone and only provide for essential requirements. The government reduced their maintenance expenditure grant by five per cent and deleted all items of estimated extraordinary expenditure. The rate of endowment to hospitals was reduced from four shillings to three shillings in the pound and grants were reduced from the Golden Casket, a lottery conducted by the Queensland Government. Hospital boards were informed that it was absolutely essential to balance their budgets for the financial year. The government:

> realised that the Hospital Boards and Committees will have a very difficult problem in balancing their budgets, especially as during periods of financial depression more people are compelled to avail themselves of the services of the public hospital, and the number of patients unable to pay for their treatment increases.[16]

The boards wanted some assistance in doing this and pressed for changes in working conditions.[17]

Most Australian workers received wage cuts during the Depression. All workers under federal awards suffered a reduction of 10 per cent from 1 February 1931,[18] and this, combined with a reduction in the cost of living, meant that the federal male basic wage declined from 4 pounds 15 shillings in 1929 to 3 pounds 7 shillings in 1933.[19] The basic wage in Queensland was reduced from 4 pounds 5 shillings per week to 3 pounds 17 shillings, with a further reduction to 3 pounds 14 shillings in May 1931.[20] State public servants, including teachers, were removed from the coverage of the Industrial Court in 1930 and suffered a cut in wages ranging from 10 to 15 per cent, according to their classification, and a further 5 per cent reduction in July 1931. Hours were increased to 48 a week, some allowances reduced, other conditions downgraded and retrenchments occurred in some departments.[21] Teachers' salaries were first reduced by 6 per cent in August 1930 and between 1929 and 1932 their income was reduced by 21 per cent to 26 per cent, compared with an 18 eighteen per cent fall in prices and rents. Married female teachers who were not sole breadwinners were automatically retrenched.[22]

In 1930 nurses also had their wages lowered. On 5 September Mr Henry Bolton, Manager of the Brisbane and South Coast Hospitals Board, applied to the Industrial Court for a reduction in nurses' wages for hospitals under the board's jurisdiction. Neither the ATNA nor the QNA approved of this claim as it did not cover all Queensland hospitals, and it was considered that there should only be one award for all hospitals.[23] On 2 October Bolton put a second claim on behalf of all hospitals which requested a reduction in annual salaries ranging from 5 pounds for most trainees, assistants in nursing, staff nurses and matrons of small hospitals, to 20 pounds for matrons of the largest hospitals.[24] The percentage reduction in wages would have ranged from 3.1 per cent for some matrons to 16.7 per cent for first year trainees. The government argued that trainees would still be well rewarded, and emphasised that their status was similar to apprentices. Once again this comparison was important in keeping wages low: 'The trainees are practically apprentices, and if the Claim is granted their emoluments will be 95 pounds to 135 pounds with uniform in addition—a rate much in excess of that usually paid to apprentices.'[25]

Misses Paten, Dunne, Chatfield and Bourne comprised the ATNA sub-committee which drafted a reply to the government's claim.[26] They represented hospital management as Miss Chatfield was Superintendent of the Diamantina Hospital and Miss Bourne had been General Matron of the hospitals administered by the Brisbane and South Coast Board until 1928. The ATNA objected to any reduction in salaries, as nurses had received no wage increases since the 1922 award had come into operation.[27] Yet Dr Marks, who represented the ATNA in the court, said that 'we object to the reduction on principle more than anything else. We recognise salaries will have to come down and if so we are agreeable'.[28]

The QNA, represented by its honorary secretary Mr Ken Laidlaw, objected to the reduction in salary for trainees who would suffer the highest percentage cuts if the claim were granted. This was different from other occupations 'where the higher paid officials are reduced the greatest'.[29] The QNA wanted the reduction for trainees to average 5 per cent, the same as senior nurses would suffer. The court granted a reduction in salaries. In the case of trained staff the reduction was the same as the government had requested, but the salaries of trainees were reduced by only 3 pounds a year, a 4 to 8.3 per cent reduction.[30] The wage cuts of less than 10 per cent were lower than those of many other groups of workers, particularly those under federal awards, but this was offset by a low initial wage rate.

In July 1930 there was a reduction in the basic wage in Queensland but the court refused to alter the rates of pay of nurses because the basic wage component of their salary had not been increased in 1925. No application had been made for an increase in nurses' salaries and their rates of pay had remained the same until the reduction in wages in November 1930.[31] But nurses' rates of pay were reduced in accordance with the state basic wage decision of 21 May 1931, with a reduction of one pound per annum on all wage rates.[32] This meant a further 2.9 per cent reduction for first year trainees and a reduction of 0.3 per cent for the highest paid matron. Thus the overall reductions in salary were less for nurses than for many other workers, because of the low wage which they earned at the beginning of the Depression, one which had not been adjusted by the basic wage increase in the mid-1920s.

The main feature of the government claim to change the nurses' award in 1930 was an extension of working hours from 88 to 96 a fortnight.[33] Bray and Rimmer have concluded that 'unions had offered a spirited defence of the award standards built up in the 1920s, but lost',[34] but the ATNA welcomed the diminution of award conditions by the extension of working hours. The application for the longer hours was possible because a new *Industrial Conciliation and Arbitration Act* had been introduced in December 1929. With the election of a Country Progressive National Party in May 1929, moves were made to give the state's workers less favourable conditions than they had received during Labor's time in office. The new Act excluded many rural workers and many in domestic service from award coverage, including 'an employee engaged in domestic duties in any hospital whose daily average of occupied beds does not exceed nine'. The court had jurisdiction to fix the maximum weekly hours to be worked but all reference to what these should be (44 per week in the previous Act) was removed. In arranging the spread of weekly hours and overtime the Industrial Court was now bound to take into consideration 'any circumstances which make it essential or desirable for the efficient carrying-on of an industry'. In addition, the court had to consider the probable economic effect of its basic wage and hours decisions.[35]

The changes to the Act together with the economic Depression provided hospital management and the ATNA with an opportunity to extend the hours of nurses. Employers, the union and nurses themselves were in favour of longer working hours and there was widespread opinion that shortening the working hours to 44 each week had been a detrimental move, with harmful consequences for both patients and nurses. These views were expressed by a 1930 Royal Commission on Public Hospitals in Queensland which inquired into certain matters relating to public hospitals, and included an investigation of nurse training. The commission asked 'whether under present conditions the facilities for the training of nurses in public hospitals are satisfactory'[36] and placed advertisements and notices in hospitals inviting nurses to give evidence. The commissioners concluded that 'the evidence submitted tends to show that the limitation of duty to 44 hours per week is detrimental to the training of nurses, and is not in the interests of the patients'.[37]

Miss Florence Chatfield, joint secretary of the ATNA from 1922 to 1933, gave evidence to the commission in her capacity as Superintendent of the Diamantina Hospital in Brisbane. Her opinions were crucial, for the commissioners 'were much impressed by the evidence of Miss Florence Chatfield . . . whose general experience on this subject is unsurpassed, and whose evidence is substantially supported by all the evidence submitted, with one or two minor exceptions'. Miss Chatfield expressed the view that as nursing was a 24-hour a day task it had been the experience of all hospital administrators that the 44-hour week

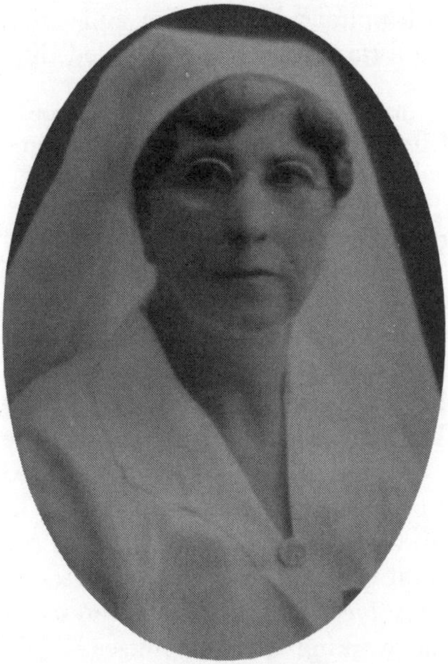

Miss Florence Chatfield was active in the ATNA from 1904 until 1945, holding positions as councillor, secretary from 1912 to 1935 and vice-president from 1937 to 1943. She was appointed Patroness of the association in 1945. Matron of the Diamantina Hospital in Brisbane, her views that hospital nurses should work longer hours were seriously considered by the Royal Commission on Public Hospitals in 1930 and nurses' hours were increased. (Courtesy of Royal Brisbane Hospital Graduate Nurses' Archive.)

'inevitably' involved numerous broken periods of duty. She felt that the frequent staff changes did not allow a nurse to become familiar with her duties 'and thus the suffering of the patients, both mental and physical, is increased'. She considered that the shorter hours were detrimental:

> From the point of view of the patients, many of whom, owing to prolonged illness, are in an exhausted condition, the frequent changing of nurses necessitated by the 44 hour week is definitely a nervous strain. Further, it is only by regular repetition of a duty or treatment that both patient and nurse can learn how the necessary work can be accomplished with a minimum of pain, discomfort, or fatigue to the former. In the case of the sick and suffering that is, I consider, a matter of great importance.

In Chatfield's view, the hours were 'equally harmful' for the nurse:

> The lack of continuity in her work not only prevents her obtaining the necessary knowledge of the technique of her duties . . . but prevents her acquiring the keen interest in her work which is so essential if the best ideals of the nursing profession are to be reached and maintained. This lack of interest, which I am not alone in observing, is not the fault of the nurse as much as of the conditions under which she labours.

From Chatfield's dual position as hospital administrator and union official, though speaking from the former role, she concluded that:

> while realising very fully that, for many years, the working hours of nurses were unduly long, I am definitely of the opinion that the pendulum has now swung too far in the opposite direction, and present working hours are too short for both the efficient training of the nurse and the welfare of the patient.[38]

Miss Chatfield was not troubled by a conflict of views or interests between her work and her union activities and the ATNA did not object to the proposed extension of hours. Dr Marks, representing the ATNA, pointed out that the association had objected to the shorter hours in the first place.[39] In the face of this testimony the report of the Royal Commission on Public Hospitals recommended that the hours of nurses should be altered to 96 per fortnight. In doing this they were running with a forceful tide of opinion in the industry and profession. The federal conference of nursing associations held in March 1930 had resolved that, in the interests of nurses and patients, the minimum working hours of nurses should be 96 per fortnight.[40]

In accepting a lengthening of hours, however, the views of the ATNA were different from the opinion of the majority of trade unions:

> To organised labour, casting around for explanations of the unprecedented high levels of unemployment, it seemed that . . . the factor aggravating the current economic catastrophe was the displacement of labour by machinery . . . Hence the work available must be spread amongst as many employees as possible by a drastic reduction in hours.[41]

In 1930 the Australian Council of Trade Unions (ACTU) 'Key Industry Conference' called for the introduction of a 40-hour week and 'from this date on all sections of the industrial labour movement campaigned for work spreading through a shorter working week'.[42] The ATNA had never regarded itself as a trade union or part of the union movement, and its views on hours of work contrasted starkly with those of the ACTU.

In their approach to the regulation of the hours a nurse worked, the ATNA emphasised service through dedication and self-sacrifice. In 1925 the *ANJ* reprinted an article from the English *Nursing Mirror*, entitled 'A Question of Ethics'. It spoke about the spirit of voluntary service in nursing which 'not only meant the giving of time, energy and work without just adequate payment in return: it embraces a spiritual element, permeating all these, but infinitely above them'. The article warned that:

> it must be remembered, however, there is always a lurking danger lest, while insisting on just rights for the worker, the work itself should suffer. It is true that the payment of an adequate salary need not necessarily destroy the spirit of voluntary service, but it is possible it may help it do so unless the nursing instincts and ideals held by the worker are very fine.[43]

Perhaps the spirit of dedication could be retained, even in the face of receipt of an adequate salary, if longer hours were worked.

During the 1920s and 1930s writers to the *ANJ* expressed similar views, linking these to the difficulty in financing hospital services. These correspondents were firmly opposed to involvement in trade union activities. A matron of a small private hospital wrote that 'nursing has always been a noble profession; it seems a shame to see it brought to the level of an ordinary trades union. I feel sure that if the nurses as a body were consulted it would be found that most of them would deplore it'. She commented particularly on hours: 'It is just . . . impossible to bring nurses under award hours . . . We are not dealing with so much merchandise, but human life, and any true nurse does not mind what energy she puts forth in this cause'.[44] Another writer commented that 'nurses pride themselves on belonging to an honourable profession and refuse to join a union which workers in other spheres have done in self defence. Hospital authorities realize the sacrifice made by the nurses, but are faced with the difficulty of finance when seeking a remedy'.[45]

These views were the same as those put by employers in the case for a variation of the nurses' award in October 1930. Mr R.S. Mackay, speaking for the Brisbane and South Coast Hospitals Board, said that the lower hours were not in the best interests of either patients or nurses. This view was reiterated by many others including Miss Chatfield, Miss Sorensen, the board's General Matron, and Miss Bourne, her predecessor, all of whom were prominent ATNA councillors. It was the central argument presented in the case for lengthening working hours. Mackay submitted that it had not been possible to arrange a suitable timetable in the board's hospitals since the 44-hour week had come into force, so the trained nursing staff had worked four hours overtime each week. In a comparison with five hospitals in other states, only Sydney Hospital trained nurses worked less than 96 hours a fortnight. The majority worked from 96 to 102 hours per fortnight, with

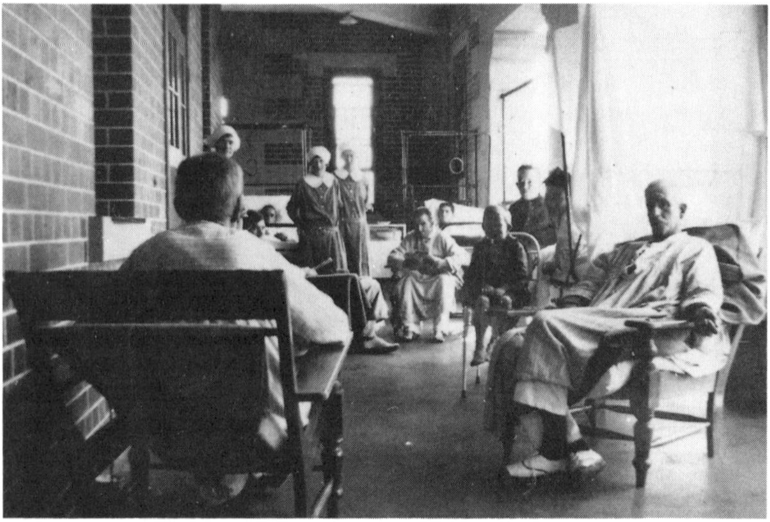

Student nurses and patients on a verandah adjacent to a male ward at Brisbane Hospital in the 1930s.
(Collection: Royal Brisbane Hospital Graduate Nurses' Archive and John Oxley Library, Brisbane.)

Adelaide Hospital nurses working 111 hours and Sydney Hospital trainees working 114 hours each fortnight.

In his arguments, Mackay differentiated the work of nurses from that of other employees. He felt that hospital nurses had distinct advantages in their work. They lived close to their work, spent no time in travelling, ate meals already prepared and did no household duties outside working hours.[46] The unique qualities of a nurse's work—dedication, dealing with human suffering, the cloistered, live-in nature of the work, the in-hospital training system—all served the argument well for the extension of hours.

The only voice raised against the extension of hours was that of Ken Laidlaw, speaking on behalf of a small and inactive QNA. He objected to the lengthening of nurses' hours, 'owing to the strenuous nature of their duties'. He stressed that 44 hours was long enough to work each week:

> At the present time their duties are such that they have on occasions to work through their meal hours without meals, and that is a great strain on the system. They are on their feet the whole of the

time, and in outside callings the female employees are allowed rest times, but nurses in hospitals are not allowed rest periods.[47]

The views of the ATNA however, were the most important influence on the court, which noted that the ATNA, with a membership of 1454, supported the extension of hours. In contrast the QNA had only 85 members, although Laidlaw claimed to have enrolled 150 new members.[48] The Industrial Court ordered that the hours should be 96 per fortnight. The shorter hours had been granted 'when conditions were more favourable', the judges maintained, but the changed economic climate and new Act necessitated alterations to the award: 'We, of course, are bound by the Industrial Conciliation and Arbitration Act to have regard to the economic effect of an Award on the particular industry and on the community'.[49] In addition to these points, the longer hours worked in other states and the question of adequate training of nurses were cited in the decision as reasons for lengthening nurses' hours.

A lowering of standards was proposed in other award clauses, representing a significant loss of conditions for nurses. Annual leave was reduced from four to three weeks and sick leave was reduced by one week. The ATNA agreed to the change in sick leave, while the QNA opposed all reduction of conditions.[50] The new award, with longer hours, less leave and lower salaries, took effect on 1 November 1930.[51]

Questions of equal pay, addressed by the QTU, did not touch the ATNA. Muriel Heagney, advocate for the New South Wales Council of Action for Equal Pay, emphasised that equal pay was a possibility and 'because jobs were sex-typed, women would not lose their jobs'.[52] But general nursing was an exclusively female occupation and the ATNA once again stood apart from movements like this. In reality, they would have had little hope of achieving higher wages this way as the QTU were unsuccessful in their attempts to gain equal pay in 1934 and 1936.[53]

Lone voices of protest were rare, although 'Disgusted' wrote to the *Daily Mail* complaining about the small amount of food at meals: 'Our meagre salaries reduced, hours lengthened and holidays reduced and our morning tea cut out, we had to grin and bear it on the pretext of essential economies, but is it necessary to starve us out of our positions?'[54] One traditional working practice was eroded at the Brisbane General Hospital when, from 1 October 1930, the morning and afternoon tea periods were cut out. The nurses' main objection was that these were occasions when they could enjoy a few minutes rest off their feet: 'Now, it is work from starting time to ceasing time, and it is hard going all the time . . . Whilst we realise that the present time is time for economy we feel that the economy should not be thrown upon such people as the nurses, who are so practically inadequately paid for their work'.[55] Nurses were told to sign off at four o'clock 'but they do not stop work until four thirty or five. We have had the inspector down several times to try to stop this'.[56]

The ATNA thought that nurses should have a quarter of an hour off for morning and afternoon tea[57] and the QNA felt that this should be incorporated into the award as many privileges were being taken away from nurses and this might also disappear. The time should not be taken out of the weekly hours.[58] Mackay said he had no objection to a morning and afternoon rest as nurses received it already but the time taken was added to their hours.[59] But Judge Webb, President of the Court, said it was beyond his province to order morning and afternoon teas. It was not one of his functions 'otherwise the Watersideworkers may want me to award them whisky'. It came under the heading of refreshments and this was for the hospital boards to decide.[60]

At a time when most unions faced the threat of a falling level of working conditions and felt powerless to maintain existing standards, the ATNA barely tried to stem the tide of changing conditions. They were willing to accept most aspects of the claim put forward on behalf of the hospital boards. They accepted that financial stringencies were necessary on the part of hospitals and that changes in nurses' wages and working conditions could reduce hospital expenditure.

A number of councillors were in positions of authority in public hospitals while others ran private hospitals and, as the views of Florence Chatfield show, they were readily able to see the government's and employer's point of view. In many cases in fact they would have helped to shape this view. In contrast the QNA often compared the working conditions of nurses with other female employees, and was not as apt to regard nurses as a unique group of wage earners. But the QNA was not a large organisation and the views of the ATNA were much more influential in determining award conditions. The ATNA continued to make industrial decisions concerning nurses, thus reinforcing its role as their industrial representative. When the Country Women's Association asked for an exemption from award conditions for their employees, including nurses, the ATNA objected.[61] When Mt Isa Mines Limited applied for a consolidated award which would include nurses, the ATNA expressed the view that 'there should be one Award to cover all hospitals in Queensland governed by such Award, as the conditions of all hospitals should be uniform'.[62]

1937 award variation

It was not until 1937 that the ATNA actually initiated changes in the nursing award when they made a claim for the restoration of the wages lost during the Depression. By this time other workers were gaining wage increases. Salaries had been increased in the Basic Wage Case of 22 March 1937[63] and the ATNA asked that rates be returned to those awarded in 1922, which was little more than trainees already received following the 1937 basic wage adjustment.[64] Although the wage increases asked for by the ATNA were not great, the court awarded no increase beyond the basic wage adjustment.

Once again employers objected on the grounds that nurses' conditions were more than adequate. Mr Charles Chuter, representing the Brisbane and South Coast Hospitals Board and the Public Service Commissioner, also opposed the increase in salaries stating that the present rates were 'ample and generous'.[65] His position was particularly influential as the *Hospitals Act of 1936* had given the state department authority over all expenditure in public hospitals, placed the administration of hospitals with the state public service and firmly consolidated the public hospital system under state control.[66] The state government, through direct control or regulation, was the largest employer of hospital nurses.

Miss M. Dowling, representing the Private Hospitals' Association and the North Queensland Employers' Association, felt that 'the girls are adequately paid now. We cannot find any other case where they are trained and are kept from the moment they begin work and where uniform and laundry allowances are paid'. These organisations wanted the ATNA to agree to a three-month probationary period for trainees at a nominal wage of ten shillings per week as, in their opinion, the new nurse was of practically no use and was a great anxiety to those training her.[67] Dr Quinn, ATNA advocate, countered by pointing out the longer working hours of the trainee nurse and the lack of ordinary public holidays. Living-in was not only a benefit for the nurse, he argued, it was in the hospital's interest as they preferred that nurses live on hospital premises.[68]

One major feature of the 1937 award variation was the retention of the 96-hour fortnight. The ATNA did not ask for any change and were happy to retain the longer hours. The Private Hospitals' Association had brought a case before the court on 21 June 1933 protesting against a reversion to 44 hours a week for nurses and domestics and the ATNA had decided that the hours should not be shortened.[69] In a decision which clearly shows the disparate ways in which the work of a nurse

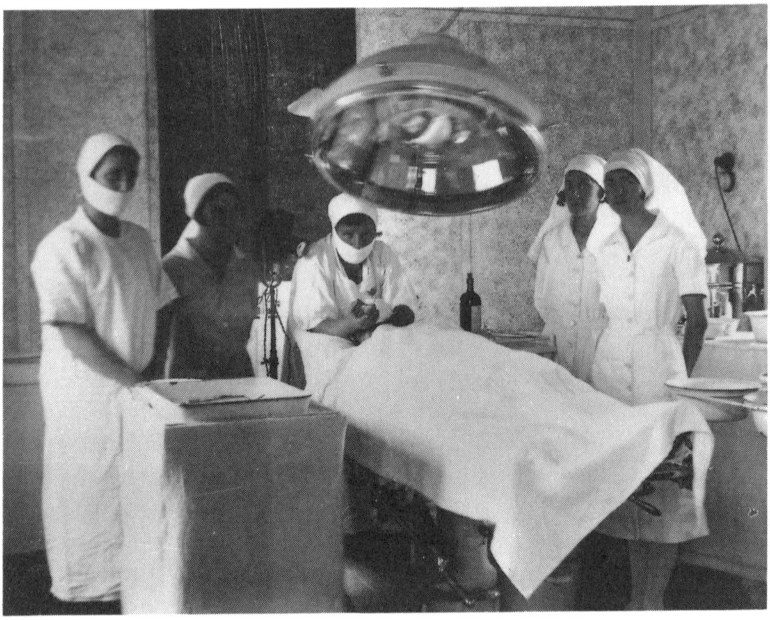

Nurses working in the operating theatre at Rixon's Hospital in Kingaroy, north-west of Brisbane, in 1933. (Collection: John Oxley Library, Brisbane.)

and other hospital staff, who were also predominantly female, were viewed, the court decided that the hours of hospital nurses should remain at 48 per week, while, at the same time, it reduced the hours of hospital domestic staff to 44 per week.[70]

Although the weekly hours were not reduced, at the request of the ATNA the court restored the four weeks annual leave of the 1922 award.[71] Dr Quinn stated that four weeks were necessary for nurses to recuperate. With no public holidays a nurse had no long weekends and 'therefore needs a very much longer spell when she does get her annual holiday and on the grounds of health we feel that four weeks is the minimum that is desirable'. Dr Quinn agreed that there was a difficulty concerning training but it would be better to extend the training period than to wreck their health. The employers opposed this on the grounds of the added expense for hospitals and the detrimental effect of shortening the training period.[72]

The 1937 award variation was not a radical departure from previous awards. It was the first time the ATNA had lodged a claim for a variation, but the claim was very conservative. It asked for a restoration of pre-Depression wages but not pre-Depression working hours, and for a few other minor improvements. These were often justified in terms of a nurse's health, rather than argued on the grounds of equity with other workers. The decision of the court was even more conservative than the ATNA's claim, often picking a middle ground between the ATNA and the respondent hospitals. Nevertheless, the ATNA regarded the award as 'very satisfactory' as they felt all the major points they had requested had been granted.[73]

The economic Depression, which was the overriding feature of the 1930s, had little impact on the operations of the ATNA. Their members did not suffer drastically in terms of unemployment and many enjoyed the security of government employment in a much needed service industry. The ATNA continued to reject the idea of trade unionism, and proudly regarded itself as a professional organisation only. With the decline in membership and activities of the QNA and its eventual demise, the conservative views of the ATNA were pre-eminent and unchallenged. The ATNA welcomed the lower standard of working conditions that the Depression brought. They particularly embraced the longer working hours and did not seek to have these changed to pre-Depression conditions in their 1937 claim for variation of the award. The longer hours fitted well with the ATNA's view of nursing as a unique job, and hence it believed that it was quite acceptable for nurses to have conditions that were very different from other workers, even other hospital staff. The longer hours were seen as necessary both for the benefit of nurses, giving them continuity of practice and better training, and for the benefit of patients, who would not have so many changes of staff. It served well the ethic of dedication without high remuneration. These views corroborated those of the employers, both government and private, for whom the dedication ethic meant a cheaper means of staffing hospitals. Given that the ATNA Executive and Council still predominantly comprised the elite within the nursing and medical professions in Brisbane, this unanimity of views was not surprising. The overlap in personnel, and therefore in ideas, policies and allegiances, remained.

CHAPTER 7

The work of private nurses

' . . . leave it to them to take the initiative.'[1]

Private nurses made up the bulk of the trained nursing workforce until the 1930s[2] and most nurses spent at least part of their career nursing in private homes. When training began in hospitals only a very few of the graduating nurses remained at the hospital and most undertook work as private practitioners. As hospitalisation became a safer option than it had been in the previous century a wider section of the community, even the wealthy, were nursed in hospital. Moves such as the *1925 Maternity Act* in Queensland, which provided free pre- and post-natal clinics run by the state as well as maternity hospitalisation,[3] encouraged this trend. Hospitals were staffed by a few trained nurses and a large number of trainees as well as untrained assistants in nursing. Greater status was accorded trained nurses working in hospitals and private work was 'seen even within nursing as often no more than domestic service or a mother's work, [and] bestowed little status'.[4] As hospital-based care grew in the early 1900s and became an acceptable alternative to care in the home, the status of private nursing declined even further.

The attitude of the ATNA Council to the working conditions of this group of nurses was similar to the position it adopted in relation to hospital nurses. Once again it was caught up in the ethos of self-sacrifice which had been translated into the idea of long hours of work without high remuneration. The ATNA in Queensland considered these industrial issues only when it was forced to do so, either by outside circumstances, like the formation of a 'rival' nurses' organisation in the 1920s, or when there was substantial pressure for change exerted on the council from within the association. This occurred only in the case of private nurses and in order to achieve the changes that they wanted, these nurses had to struggle for a long time and overcome obstacles purposely put in their way by the ATNA Council. Nursing organisations did not often acknowledge the fact that the overwhelming majority of nurses needed to earn a satisfactory living. The case of the private nurses and their desire to increase their fees is a prime example of the extreme reluctance that the Queensland Council showed in dealing with questions which directly affected their members' livelihoods.

Private nursing was exhausting work and in America shifts of twelve to 24 hours were the norm until the 1920s, which meant that the nurse would be working from 84 to 168 hours a week.[5] Similar conditions were experienced in Australia and discussed in letters to the nurses' journals. In a lecture about private nursing given in 1903 Sister Lena advised nurses, especially younger nurses who were leaving hospitals and entering private nursing and were 'not seasoned to long irregular hours', to 'consider yourselves as to rest and food. You will find that people are apt to think that as it is only for a few weeks, any makeshift will do; they forget that a nurse's whole year is comprised of a few weeks here and there'. Sleeping arrangements could be a problem and she advised nurses on night duty to make sure they had a room where they could sleep undisturbed for six hours. If a nurse had to sleep in the patient's room, she should have 'a comfortable bed or wire stretcher to sleep on, instead of putting up with a sofa or that worse abomination a box couch'. She added that:

> I know it is the boast of many nurses that they can sleep anywhere and anyhow, and watch for countless hours at a stretch. I have done it myself, but I know now how unwise it was, and though you may go on for three or four years under these circumstances, in time you will find yourself breaking down, and I assure you that a nervous breakdown in a nurse is a very serious thing.[6]

She felt that ten months nursing a year was the maximum that a private nurse could do if she wanted to keep nursing for 15 or 20 years. However, Reverby reports that it was frequently assumed that a nurse would only last ten years in private duty before her inevitable collapse.[7] The work was so tiring that Sister Lena recommended that after several years of private nursing, a nurse should work on the staff of a good private hospital as the 'regular routine is a great relief to mind and nerves'.[8]

The work of the private nurse had its good and bad points. It gave her autonomy and she worked with little supervision. As one nurse put it, she was acting on her 'own responsibility, no doctor to be had at a moment's notice if anything serious goes wrong. No ward sister to be applied to, no fellow nurse to help lift or move the patient, nor to keep one company during the long nights'.[9] She was not subject to the rigid hierarchy and discipline of the hospital but she was locked into the relationships of personal service, for 'to keep herself at work, the freelancer had to satisfy doctors and patients according to standards that might be remote from her training school's definition of good nursing'.[10]

A doctor had enormous power over a nurse's career, and could recommend her for cases or have her informally barred from work in a community. Nurses 'were still supposed to be submissive to higher authority and morally committed to their work. In private duty, a nurse was working for a *doctor's* patients'.[11] Yet because she was hired by the patients she also had to meet their standards. Personal characteristics and social demeanour were often critical with private employers who set exacting social standards. Others tried to treat the nurse as a domestic servant, wanting her to do the cooking, laundry, cleaning and child-minding. This even resulted in a plea by nurses in Queensland in 1922 that those who had general plus obstetric training should not be expected to do domestic work.[12] The nurse was not usually from the same class as her frequently upper class employer and was often resented by domestic servants for her intrusion into the household.[13] Often segregated from others in the patient's home, she frequently ate her meals in her own room. She was advised to 'adopt a conciliatory tone as much as possible', so that the family could see that she was a help to them.[14]

Private work could be a very isolating experience, with long and irregular hours disrupting social life and contact with friends. Living at the home of the patient gave her little 'normal' life and even between cases the nurse had to be ready to take the next case to secure her livelihood. An American nursing leader in 1926 characterised private work:

> Its irregularity breaks down her health, its seclusion tends to narrow her interests . . . she is unethical if, after ten years of hard work, she charges any more than does the newest graduate in the field. Yet she must be all things to all people, she must remain human though she cannot live like most humans.[15]

Free from the hierarchical supervision of hospital nursing and in a position to give total bedside care, the result could be a low income, constant tiredness, fear of a poor old age and a lack of recognition by the public and doctors that she was doing highly skilled work.

Private nurses found it very difficult to participate in the activities of nursing organisations because of their long and unpredictable hours and their isolation from each other in individual workplaces. In the first years of their existence the nursing organisations in Australia recommended the fee that nurses should charge. Mrs Amy Mercer Smith who ran Walmer, a Nurses' Home at New Farm, Brisbane, where private nurses lived between cases, submitted a scale of fees that she wanted adopted by the nurses who stayed at Walmer.[16] This was the first Nurses' Home registered with the Queensland ATNA and all its members were therefore ATNA members. The council decided that the matrons of the two Registered Nurses' Homes should submit a scale of fees for ATNA approval[17] and this was accepted by the 1905 annual general meeting.

The recommended fee for ordinary, influenza and midwifery cases was two guineas a week and three guineas for other cases, including infectious cases.[18] However, letters to the journal *Una* show that nurses frequently charged a lower fee if patients could not afford to pay. One nurse observed that every nurse would have reduced her fee at some time.[19] Another nurse described her most recent case of nursing a patient with an infectious disease, where because the parents were 'in narrow circumstances', she could not charge the three guineas a week for the three and a half weeks she nursed him. This case required constant day and night nursing:

> the only sleep I got was between 8 p.m. and 12 midnight, frequently then disturbed. On more than one occasion during those three and a half weeks I worked 36 hours without any sleep. My patient required the most unremitting attention, and, as the only person able to share the nursing was his mother, who had besides to do all the house work, you well understand that in this instance self-sacrifice was inevitable.[20]

She accepted a fee of two guineas a week for two and a half weeks and worked for one week without payment. Another nurse detailed a case where the people could not afford the usual fees:

> so I reduced mine, for they have had two years of constant sickness through consumption in the family. After six weeks, though they were anxious to keep me, they said they could not afford it, so I reduced my fees again. The doctor was anxious for me to stay if I could, for he said I had been a help and a comfort. I certainly have helped the overworked mother and daughters to make the home more comfortable for the young sons who are trying to fill a dying father's place on the farm, and I am sure, in the long run, a nurse never loses by being sympathetic and womanly.[21]

There were also cases of nurses not being paid by their former patients. By 1920 a number of these cases had reached the ATNA and some were put into the hands of the association's solicitors. In one case a nurse, whose solicitors had advised her to sue her employer for fees not paid, asked for assistance from the council. The council gave 10 pounds to assist in her legal action.[22]

It is difficult to ascertain the overall earnings of nurses in private duty as their income depended on how frequently they obtained work and whether they collected the full fee. A nurse working ten months of the year and collecting a weekly fee of two guineas would earn 92 pounds. This was twice the average annual earnings women in manufacturing in Australia gained in 1912, although women in Queensland averaged only 41 pounds.[23]

Nursing was seasonal work and evidence from America shows that nurses took on other work between cases or returned to their families if they could.[24] In America the Burgess Report documented the harsh working conditions and economic marginality of these nurses in the 1920s. They worked longer hours than other nurses, lost more time in fatigue and illness and had a lower income than hospital or public-health nurses. Out of this income they also had more expenses because they had to maintain a home to live in between cases, and had transportation and telephone costs. Many private nurses 'lived uncomfortably close to the margin of economic security'. Yet 'compared to the labor force as a whole, private-duty nurses still commanded a respectable income'. As single wage earners they may have occupied 'a relatively privileged position'.[25] Private nurses in Queensland were in a similar position.

Private nurses had little representation on the executive or council of the ATNA in Queensland but lobbied the organisation for better earnings. It was this agitation that forced the council to consider the question of nurses' earnings, but prolonged efforts were needed before the council would accept that the majority of members wanted changes. Nurses' rationale when asking for fee increases was almost always linked to their own welfare, and only rarely did any nurse justify her income by comparison with that of other workers.

By 1911 there was dissatisfaction with the recommended fees and some private nurses raised the issue with the ATNA and RVTNA. In New South Wales, ten nurses called a special general meeting of the ATNA to discuss the hours worked by private nurses and the possibility of overtime payment. They wanted nurses on night duty to have nine hours out of the sick room during the day for sleep and fresh air. If the nurse took both day and night duty she should have four hours away from the sick room during the 24 hours, in addition to what rest she could secure in the night. If these conditions were infringed, one shilling an hour overtime should be charged in addition to the usual fees.[26] Unfortunately, none of the letter's signatories attended the special meeting held in June 1911. This meeting voted against the proposals, expressing the view that it was impossible to lay down any hard and fast rules about the hours a private duty nurse could work. One of the councillors, Dr Blackburn, said that 'his experience had been that Nurses were generally more anxious about the welfare of the patient than about their hours off, and this was the true spirit of nursing'.[27] Another councillor, Miss Gould, felt that nurses 'always had the Doctor to appeal to, and he could generally insist on proper rest for the Nurse'.[28] The ideal nurse was once again seen as a woman who would sacrifice herself for her patients and therefore could not work specified hours like other workers.

Although the meeting was unanimously against the idea of fixed hours and any overtime payment, the hard life of many private nurses was discussed. Nurse Davies admitted that 'her work gave her great pleasure, but she had often been forty-eight hours at a stretch on duty, and had once had as little as nine hours sleep in a week'.[29] Miss Gould said that she 'had seen Nurses leave Hospital at the end of their training looking fresh and well, and after a year of private nursing they were wrecks'. She felt that 'private Nurses deserved much sympathy', but the solution to their problems was not payment for overtime.[30]

Over the next few years the plight of the private nurse and her income was debated in the *ANJ* and *Una*. The prime theme, the need to save enough money for retirement, was expressed by 'Sympathiser' when she said 'Private Nurses—or, indeed, most nurses—never are able to earn enough to put away sufficient for the old age that will come in time or the ill health that may meet one half-way there'.[31] One article expressed the view that it was impossible for a nurse to have small pleasures and leisure as well as provide for her old age, pay into a Nurses' Home, take a yearly holiday, keep her uniform immaculate and sometimes help support her family, out of 2 pounds 2 shillings a week.[32] 'Puck' agreed: 'It is plainly the duty of every nurse to put by as much money as she can in her young days; and, here, in Australia, it is only on "three guinea" cases she can afford to bank money without having to stint herself of every pleasure and comfort in doing so.' It was absurd, the writer maintained, to say that the Australian community could not pay more than 2 pounds 2 shillings per week for a trained nurse: 'Will the public ever come to her assistance and offer her fair thing for fair thing? I am afraid she will have to help herself—turn some of that strength with which she so capably helps others towards her own interest.'[33]

It was readily admitted in an *ANJ* editorial that 100 pounds a year was the extent of a private nurse's income, 'an income, in inverse proportion to the hours worked, and the skill required in her calling, and an income less than that paid to the cook of a third-class hotel or a girl on the telephone exchange'.[34] Comparisons with the earnings of other workers were made, but the element of sacrifice in nurses' work was emphasised. The *ANJ* reiterated this point saying that nurses whose—

> lives are devoted to the care of the sick have for many generations given so much time and intellect to the assistance of the sick poor without reward, that patients have come to look on nursing as something to be had for nothing, or very little. Consequently nurses' work is never estimated at its value.[35]

The overwhelming majority of correspondents wanted to increase the fee to three guineas.[36] Arguments in favour of this centred on comparisons with other wage earners, with nurses inevitably receiving lower pay for longer hours and more responsibility. One correspondent felt that the current conditions amounted to 'white slavery'.[37] Nurses had charged the same fees since the 1890s and one non-nurse forcefully said that if the public could afford 2 guineas 27 years previously, they were better able to afford 4 guineas in 1913.[38] 'Nurse' wrote to *Una* that:

> prosperity, that magic word, is written all over Australia at the present time; the splendid seasons enjoyed of late years have directly or indirectly resulted in wealth to both town and country dwellers. Almost every industry has benefited. Improvements have taken place, and in the condition of all workers, skilled or otherwise . . .
>
> We nurses are workers; skilled workers, with long hours and unhealthy surroundings. We do not derive anything from this tide of prosperity now rolling through Australia from end to end; it does not roll our way, though it is calling to strangers across the sea from other lands to share in it. Why should there not be a change with us as with other workers? Our work is more arduous, more self-sacrifice is exacted from nurses than any other body of women on earth, or men either.[39]

There were a few letters which did not favour an increase, one writer saying that 'nursing is not supposed to be a money-making profession. As long as a woman is imbued with the true nursing instinct, i.e., to go about doing good, and following in the footsteps of the late Florence Nightingale, her fees should not be the object of her visit.'[40] The editor of *Una* replied: 'Hearken unto good counsel'.[41]

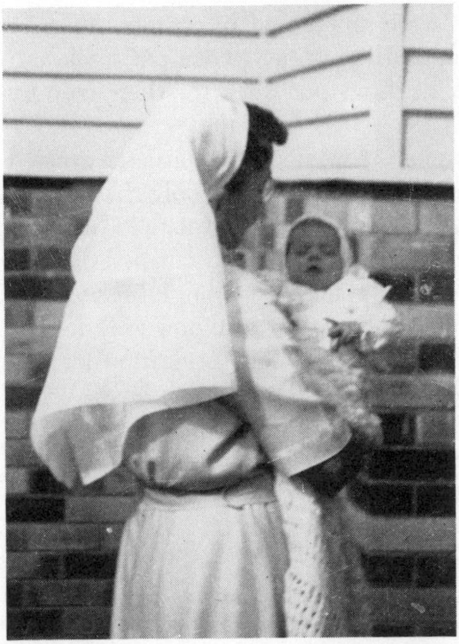

Sister Moores looking after a baby in a Brisbane home in 1951. The baby was born in hospital but because of the mother's illness, Sister Moores was employed to work for the family for two weeks. Photographs of private nurses at work are rare and are usually only found when they were nursing infants. (Collection of author.)

Occasionally a correspondent to the *ANJ* suggested specific action to ease the nurses' plight. Waitresses earned as much or more than nurses, said 'Oberon', 'because the Waitresses' Union fights on their account for all it can get'.[42] Another correspondent suggested working through the ATNA for better wages: 'Use the Association (or Union) to get the best conditions in Hospital, Public and Private, for both trainees and trained. The better these conditions are the better will be those in private nursing.'[43]

While this debate was raging in the pages of the journals, steps were being taken to increase the fees. In 1912 a resolution came from the RVTNA stating that the ATNA and its branches should consider the advisability of increasing the fees of private nurses. The Queensland Council resolved that:

> in view of the fact that many nurses have to provide for old age out of their earnings and that their employers are frequently wealthy; and of the greatly increased cost of living and of wages and salaries in general, the fees of private nurses might be raised without injustice or detriment to the public and with a further advantage to the nurses and that this rise should be on the basis of a sliding scale allowing for a smaller fee for long cases or when two nurses are employed or other special circumstances.[44]

But minimal increases only were made, with obstetric nurses allowed to charge 2 pounds 12 shillings and 6 pence per week and all nurses allowed to charge 5 shillings per week for their laundry allowance.[45]

In New South Wales, a referendum of members held in 1912 decided that the fees should not be raised in that state, and only the laundry allowance increased to 5 shillings a week.[46] However, the following year a special general meeting of the New South Wales Association decided to raise the fees of private nurses to 3 pounds 3 shillings. Miss Gould, in seconding the resolution, said 'no tradesman would now work for the same wage he worked for years ago'.[47] The major justification for this was not a comparison with other workers however, but worry about being destitute in old age.[48] The only point of objection was a fear that the increased fee would mean that people would employ partially qualified women. This was of particular concern to the vice-president, Dr Dansey, who believed that it would be best if all members of the association could vote on the question of increased fees.[49] An editorial in the *ANJ* also felt that it was 'injudicious' for nurses to raise their fees without taking a referendum.[50] Meanwhile, the RVTNA also ran a ballot which resulted in a small increase in fees.[51]

Dr McLean, president of the Queensland Branch, who did not favour an increase in fees, supported the idea of a referendum: 'Country members have very little opportunity in taking part in discussing the affairs of the Association, and it is a constant complaint that the Metropolitan members do not consider the country members'.[52] These views about the involvement of all ATNA members in their association were very unusual and only happened over an issue that was initiated by ordinary members.

At a special general meeting in Brisbane on 18 December 1913 the majority of speakers strongly favoured the increase in fees, especially since the higher fee was charged, by this time, in New South Wales, Western Australia and New Zealand. Those against it objected on the grounds that a large number of patients would not be able to pay the new fees. The meeting resolved to conduct a referendum of all members about a possible increase in fees to 3 pounds 3 shillings a week.[53] Of those who voted, 83 per cent (296) were in favour of raising the fees of private nurses.[54] The new scale, operative from 1 April 1914, set a recommended fee of 3 pounds 3 shillings a week, one pound one shilling for 24 hours work and 10 shillings and 6 pence for twelve hours, with a 5 shilling laundry allowance in infectious cases. A nurse was to have eight hours rest and at least two hours daily for exercise when the patient could be conveniently left. The fees were the recommended maximum amount that members should charge and the council specifically stated that nurses could reduce their fees when desirable.[55]

The example of the private nurses' fee increases shows that the Queensland Council of the ATNA had to be forced into taking any action related to nurses' incomes, for the ATNA believed 'the pursuit of economic goals to be incompatible with their principles of disinterested service to the sick'.[56] But it is clear from letters to the nursing journals and the result of ballots and votes at meetings that not all nurses felt this way. Those who remained in nursing were unmarried and their work usually provided the sole source of income for their lifetime. They did not fit the stereotype of women working only until marriage brought financial support from a husband; a view of women's position which justified wages that were approximately half those of men.

Most trained nurses worked as private practitioners at some time in their career and their own testimony shows that their long, unregulated hours and isolation from other nurses were great problems. Many private nurses were concerned with their earnings and conditions, even if they only took action when they felt that conditions were so bad that it resulted in ill health and led to a precarious financial position in their old age. Despite the isolation and the difficulty of participating in the association's affairs because of their working schedules, it was the strength of opinion from these nurses that led the ATNA to discuss the question of fees, the first time it had seriously considered the wages and working conditions of nurses.

Private nurses' fees, 1920–1945

In the period between the wars the process of setting private nurses' fees mirrored the pre-World War I pattern. When changes occurred it was because the council had been driven by the overwhelming tide of membership opinion. Once again, the question of fee increases was raised by private nurses themselves and was dealt with very slowly and with extreme reluctance by the council. Initially a request for discussion of an increase in fees was made by members in 1921, but in a long drawn-out process, including two ballots of members, the recommended fee was not raised until 1929. It took eight years to achieve this but, two years later, in the midst of the Depression of the 1930s, members voted to reduce their fees to the 1921 level. Discussion of raising fees began again in 1939 but was interrupted by the outbreak of war. The higher fee was charged briefly from 1929 to 1931 and its restoration was delayed by the Second World War.

In January 1921, fourteen members asked the council to call a special meeting to discuss the question of raising their fees from 3 guineas to 4 guineas a week.[57] The council decided not to call the meeting because private nurses' fees had been included in the QNA claim to the Industrial Court.[58] The ATNA opposed the claim to include private nurses' fees in the first nurses' award and the court agreed that their fees should not be regulated by an award.[59]

The following year proposals were put forward at a council meeting to include private nurses in the industrial claim which the ATNA itself was preparing.[60] At a meeting in January 1922 approximately 33 private nurses listened to the claim prepared for discussion by Mr H. Bond, the ATNA's paid secretary, and councillor Miss E. Barron. The major point of the claim was that the fee of 4 guineas a week should be paid for infectious cases only, with all other cases collecting the existing fee of 3 guineas. Contrary to this proposal, the meeting resolved, by a narrow vote, to increase the fees for all cases to 4 guineas.[61] The private nurses had called for higher wages than those proposed by the officials and succeeded in having them accepted by the meeting of private nurses.

In the face of these initiatives by members, the ATNA Council countered with deliberate procrastination. A further meeting of private nurses was held on 7 February and defeated a motion that all members of the ATNA be allowed to vote on the fee rise. The draft claim was again discussed and several objections were expressed at raising the fees from 3 guineas to 4 guineas. On a show of hands 'a large number' favoured the old rates and 'a large number' wanted the proposed new rates. Finally the meeting decided to ask the opinion of private nurses through the *ANJ*.[62] Further delays occurred as the Sydney office did not approve the insertion of a ballot paper in the journal so an advertisement which included a ballot paper was prepared for the April issue.[63] But the council was not content with this action and again considered the draft claim. This time it adopted a course of action with which it felt very comfortable and consulted the most influential members of the private nursing area, the two matrons of the Nurses' Homes. The council decided, contrary to the wishes of the meeting of private nurses, that if the two matrons agreed with the original claim prepared by Bond and Barron, it would be filed with the Industrial Court.[64] Thus the opinions of these two influential women could outweigh the views of numerous members.

The ATNA filed a claim with the court but it did not contain the recommended schedule of fees of previous meetings. Although no result of the nurses' ballot is in the journal or minutes, the higher fee of 4 guineas a week was requested for infectious and mental cases only, with

3 guineas for general and obstetric cases.[65] It had taken from January 1921 till October 1922 to finalise the scale of fees for nurses and then the fee for general and obstetric cases had not been increased. But the Industrial Court judge, T.W. McCawley, refused to include private nurses in an industrial award because it would mean an intrusion of the court's regulations into private homes and domestic arrangements. Domestic servants were explicitly excluded from the Industrial Arbitration Act, and—

> though nurses would not be engaged in domestic service within the popularly accepted meaning of that term, there is no doubt that the nurse's duties necessarily involve some work of a domestic nature. That work, it was contended, is of minor importance. The main duties are of a professional nature, in the performance of which, according to the evidence of Dr. Marks, the nurse exercises professional skill, acts under the directions of the doctor and not of the patient and is responsible to the doctor. But the fact that the employer has not complete control over the nurse weighs against subjecting the employer to an Award.[66]

Work in private practice was the crux of the issue. McCawley argued that there was no place in Australia where wages and conditions for work in private homes were governed by an award of an industrial tribunal. The employer was an individual patient and not a business. As well as this, no prospective employers were represented at the court hearing to give their views and the employers' circumstances varied so greatly 'that no universal rule could be laid down which would not entail hardship in some cases'. Legal concerns over representation of potential employers and the perceived similarity of nursing with domestic work coincided and the outcome was no legal regulation of private nurses' earnings. McCawley made the additional point that trained nurses were 'apparently well organised' and their charges were already regulated by a general understanding amongst themselves. In addition, he reminded the ATNA that they had opposed the inclusion of private nurses in the QNA claim the previous year.[67] All the agitation by private nurse members had achieved very little. The Industrial Court declined to enter into the debate and the council was not eager to increase the recommended fees for most cases. It was to be eight and a half years before changes were made to all fees.

In 1928, a member again raised the issue of revising the fees, this time because other states had higher rates.[68] The council investigated and found that the prevailing rate in other states was 4 guineas.

However this evidence was not sufficient for the council to take action and once again it decided to refer the matter to the matrons of the Nurses' Homes, requesting them to form a committee to advise the council on the matter.[69] The matrons did not want to take any active part in it, so the council decided that 'as the question of increased fees is one which concerns the nurses engaged in private work, it was thought advisable to leave it to them to take the initiative'.[70] The council thus forgot about the issue.

Several months later, the matron of the Brisbane Private Nurses' Home forwarded an appeal signed by twelve ATNA members requesting an increase in the fees to 4 guineas. The council replied that such a matter had to be decided by members of the branch, so a special general meeting was organised for January 1929 to discuss it.[71] Thirty-two members attended and a majority voted for a fee increase. But this was still not sufficient evidence of a desire among private nurses for the council to move in this direction. Members at the meeting were asked to ascertain from friends in southern states the effect of the higher fee and the council decided it was necessary to take a ballot of all members.[72] The result was a vote of 470 in favour of raising the fees and 57 against.[73] The new recommended scale of fees with the rate of 4 guineas per week, finally came into force on 12 July 1929, almost a decade after the first moves had been taken by ATNA members.

By the 1930s, the community was using hospital services more frequently and this, combined with the economic Depression, reduced the clientele of the private nurse. The decline in the diseases that private practitioners had nursed in the home, such as typhoid, influenza, diphtheria and pneumonia, also contributed to the lack of work available and with the advent of the Second World War, private work came to be seen as nursing's backwater.[74] The Depression led to a review of fees as private nurses were more affected by the economic downturn than other nurses. Fewer people in the community could afford the nurse's fee and in Western Australia, for instance, 'the doctor's surgeries were empty and pharmacists were forced to close, while the out-patient clinics and dispensaries of the public hospitals were full to overflowing as more and more people qualified for the means test'.[75] Also at this time the birthrate was falling,[76] further decreasing demand for private nurses.

In 1931 a group of obstetric nurses appealed to the ATNA Council in Queensland regarding the advisability of reducing fees. Unlike earlier requests from nurses to increase fees, the council responded swiftly and called a general meeting to debate the issue.[77] Opinion at the meeting was divided on whether fees should be reduced but 'the fact that the supply exceeds the demand' was one reason in favour of changes. The fee charged by obstetric nurses for a confinement and visits for the following ten days was reduced from four guineas to 4 pounds, the amount of the Baby Bonus. Once again, it was decided to hold a referendum.[78] The majority of nurses favoured the lower fees[79] so the ATNA Council acted swiftly to reduce them. The feelings of ordinary nurses can be construed from the referendum result, with the economic necessity of the Depression forcing them to reduce fees in order to retain a livelihood.

The working conditions and payment of private nurses were not discussed again by the council until 1937 when one of the councillors suggested that private nurses on a long case have one day off a month and one week's leave when a case lasted more than a year.[80] The matter was referred to the matrons of the Nurses' Homes for their comment and the proposal for time off was added to the scale of fees.[81] A few months later, this was amended to one day off a month or payment in lieu on a long chronic case.[82] Thus in 1939, the basic fee charged by private nurses was the same as it had been in 1914.

Private nurses suffered problems during the Second World War, including shortages of women for this work. Hospitalisation was becoming more common and free treatment in public hospitals was introduced in 1944.[83] The ATNA Council's attitude to this section of its membership mirrored its attitudes to the problems of hospital nurses during the war. It did not wish to see any increase in fees or be concerned with these issues, and the war provided the perfect excuse for delaying the issue. In February 1939, the question of increasing fees for private nurses was discussed at a council meeting but the reaction was typical, and the issue was put off for several months until the annual meeting.[84] Like the salaries of hospital nurses, the council resolved that 'the time is inopportune' to look at fee increases.[85]

The method of increasing fees for private nurses which had existed before the war, continued. Requests for increases invariably came from the nurses themselves. In 1942 members of the Alstonville Nurses' Club requested that the council consider increasing the fees from 3 guineas to 4 guineas per week. The nurses informed the council that the 3 guinea fee existed only in Queensland, as other states had increased their rates.[86] The nurses argued for the rise on the basis of the higher cost of living after the Depression, and that other workers had received basic wage increases since that time.

However, letters were received from fourteen members who were opposed to the increase, compared with three letters in favour. Debate ensued and a special meeting of private nurses finally resolved by a vote of five to three that the fees be increased to 4 guineas.[87] This did not, of course, mean that the recommended fees would rise. A report of the meeting was given to the council[88] and it was decided to discuss the matter at the annual general meeting. Members attached to registered Nurses' Homes were contacted giving them the opportunity to appoint a proxy to vote for them on the fees question if they were not able to attend the meeting.[89] This meeting, with about 50 members present, voted 'by a large majority' to increase the fees to 4 guineas a week.[90] But the saga was not yet over, as the Deputy Commissioner of Prices wrote to inform the ATNA that under the Prices Regulations the maximum charges for all services had been pegged to those which operated on 15 April 1942. To increase the fees, an application to the Deputy Prices Commissioner had to be made. This was done[91] and at the end of 1942 this approval was received.[92]

The case of the private nurses and their fee increases illustrates the power of the ideal of the self-sacrificing nurse and the reticence with which the ATNA Council considered ways of alleviating her poor working conditions. It also illustrates how the council viewed its role. It was clearly not interested in representing the views of groups of members if their ideas went counter to those of the majority of council, let alone actively seeking out the wishes of members. Queensland nurses gained fee increases later than nurses in southern states and even the argument that the higher fee was being charged south of the border did not induce the council to act quickly. The ATNA in Queensland did not initiate the debates about the earnings and conditions of private nurses, just as it did not do this in relation to hospital nurses. It was not particularly interested in industrial issues, and often used stalling tactics to delay discussion and resolution of the issue. When changes occurred it was because the council had been led by the overwhelming tide of membership opinion.

CHAPTER 8

Nursing conditions during World War II

'The remuneration now paid to qualified nurses is so inadequate that to secure their future they must leave the profession.'[1]

The 1939–1945 war posed a direct threat to Australia. The war in the Pacific reached Australian shores with the bombing of Darwin in February 1942 and the sinking of the hospital ship *Centaur* on 14 May 1943 when it was a mere 65 kilometres east of Brisbane. This caused the loss of 268 lives, including eleven of the twelve nurses on board.[2]

Nursing held an essential place during the Second World War. The demands of a nation at war and the needs of the civilian population, the changes in working conditions and the position of women in the workforce, had profound effects on the nursing labour force. The period was characterised by extreme shortages of nurses, caused by the demand from the military services for nurses to work overseas and the increased competition for jobs from other occupations and industries in Australia.

The attitudes and actions of the ATNA in Queensland must be seen against the backdrop of the demands on labour during this time and its extensive regulation, including the regulation of hospital and nursing services. Gradually, as the threat to Australia became greater and the requirements of the armed forces and war-supply industries increased, women's labour became indispensable. They entered industries in which they had not worked previously and took up jobs which had been unacceptable for women and were subject to extensive powers of direction. Wages for women working in wartime industries were increased and the consequent disparities between these new levels and those of women employed in traditional female jobs widened alarmingly. This in itself did not force a general reconsideration of women's wages. Only when sufficient numbers of women could not be found to do the traditional lowly-paid female jobs essential to the war effort, such as nursing or work in clothing factories, was the government forced to examine women's wage rates. Even then, nurses' wages were not increased in line with many other women's occupations.

Shortages in the number of nurses emerged and committees flourished, discussing ways to alleviate this problem. Inquiries revealed that the major obstacle to the recruitment and training of more nurses was their low pay and poor working conditions compared to other women workers. The remedy, agreed to by government committees, hospitals, and reluctantly the ATNA, was to increase nurses' wages and improve their working conditions. However, despite opinions that wages were insufficient, there was little real activity to remedy the situation during the war.

The effect of the Second World War on the activities of the Queensland Branch of the ATNA was more dramatic than that of the First World War. Being at war was an excuse for the council to continue its habit of attending to wage rises with extreme reluctance. The council ceased to be concerned about the wages and conditions of nurses and the president, Dr Alex Marks, stated that during the war the activities of the branch should be confined mainly to matters of national service which could be performed by nurses.[3] The council unanimously resolved in November 1940 that 'the present time is not opportune to approach the Industrial Arbitration Court for an amendment of the Nurses' Award'.[4] It replied to the Charleville Branch of the ALP, which complained that nurses were underpaid, that the matter would be considered 'when our national position is improved'.[5]

Finally, in 1943, when the shortage of nurses was extreme and the ATNA Council conceded the need to increase nurses' wages, these activities were justified solely in terms of their necessity to provide an effective nursing service capable of meeting the needs of a nation at war. In fact, hospital nurses had not received a wage increase, except for the cost of living increases on the basic wage component of their salary package, since their first award in 1921.

Wartime need for women workers

Labour force demands can be divided into three broad periods: from the outbreak of war in September 1939 until December 1941, labour force growth was largely met by the addition of the male unemployed; from 1942 until mid-1943, the threat to Australia demanded more defence personnel and munitions and war-related equipment and provisions; and from the latter half of 1943, the direct threat lessened and American troops were stationed in and near to Australia, making demands for food and provisions for these troops paramount.

These phases all made particular claims on female employment. In the first years of the war the employment of women in areas directly related to the war effort proceeded slowly. Up to the beginning of 1941 women constituted only a small part of the workforce which produced munitions and had seen service in the Army only as nurses.[6] In fact, the efforts of women to serve their country, through, for instance, the formation of military-like women's corps, embarrassed the Federal Government and the Labor Opposition, who were both afraid women would take men's jobs.[7] Work involving heavy machinery and factories (but not clothing) and work in the armed forces (apart from nursing) were seen as solely men's work.

With the entry of the Japanese into the war, the defence needs of Australia intensified and massive increases in the services, munitions and other war-related industries were needed. Tighter restrictions on employment and the movement of labour were instituted culminating in the establishment in January 1942 of a Manpower Directorate, responsible to the Minister for Labour and National Service, which had a mandate to organise 'the resources of manpower and woman-power in Australia'.[8] The regulations enacted in 1942 gave extensive powers to this Directorate which could allocate and direct labour to areas judged to be most in need. This came very close to total civilian conscription for industry of those regarded as available labour (married women with dependants, for instance, were excluded).[9]

The release of men to enter the fighting services was dependent on women entering the paid labour force. During 1942 the policy was to bring women into the services in non-combatant roles to replace men in many occupations, to remove obstacles to women's civilian employment and to induce women to seek employment.[10] A contemporary newsreel exhorted viewers by saying, 'if the cautious see major post-war problems growing out of the wholesale transfer of women to male jobs, there can be but one answer to them: war stands on no ceremony, and this war we must win—no matter how our social structure may suffer in its winning'.[11]

Some workplaces, including hospitals and health facilities, were designated as protected undertakings and the rights of employers and employees were severely circumscribed, including the right of the employee to leave the job and of the employer to dismiss a worker.[12] The engagement of labour was so severely circumscribed by the manpower regulations that Mr W. C. Wurth, Director-General of Manpower, commented that, 'by the end of August, 1942, practically all labour movements were subject to official sanction, as the flow of workers was canalised through the National Service Office organisation'.[13]

Regulations were strengthened in January 1943 when powers were given to the Director-General of Manpower to direct anyone to work for a specified employer or to perform specified work. Women were a major target of this order. Voluntary transfers were encouraged with a variety of jobs being offered to the individual. Directions were to be given if the person failed to avail herself of any of these, but not if hardship would occur. Civilian Registration Cards were examined for single women aged 18 to 45 and married women aged 18 to 35 without dependent children who were 'not gainfully-occupied'. Then single women aged 18 to 30 employed in the entertainment, sport and recreation, domestic and personal service areas and sales and commerce and finance areas were assessed.[14]

The Manpower Regulations temporarily challenged the beliefs about women and their place in society, a change which would have been unthinkable without the urgent necessity of the war and all its demands on labour. The convention that single women could remain at home and not be employed in outside work was challenged by regulations in the latter half of 1942. Single women under 45 years had to explain why they were 'not gainfully occupied'. Employment in the paid workforce was seen as acceptable, suitable and necessary for women without children to care for, even if they were married. It was even seen as acceptable that women with children could work outside the home, and many were encouraged to do so.

The nature of the work done outside the home changed for many women. Some went to the women's auxiliary forces and at the beginning of 1942 approximately 7000 women were engaged in the services, including the nursing services.[15] From 1942 some women worked in factories which had previously been barred to them or replaced men in some industries but many others worked in traditional women's jobs. Although women formed the essential component of the workforce that provided additional labour during the war, their work was largely menial and unskilled and few emerged with qualifications for skilled jobs.[16]

By 1943 the direct threat of an invasion of Australia had ceased and an offensive war was being fought in the Pacific. American forces in Australia and the Pacific needed supplies from Australia which produced food, clothing and other goods for these troops.[17] The demands on labour changed as a result of this. The most serious labour problem was in the rural industries, as many farm workers had been attracted to factory employment by the higher wages and better working conditions. The Women's Land Army was formed in July 1942 and its numbers rose to about 4000 in the 1943–1944 harvest season. In October 1943 releases from the Army and munitions and aircraft

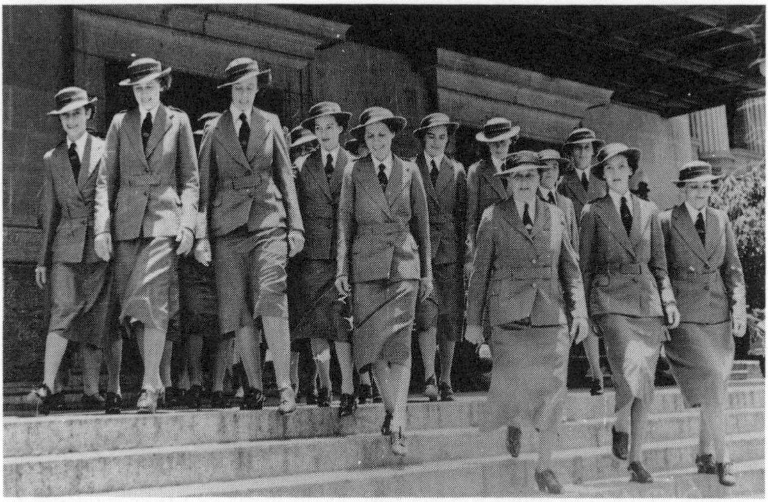

Queensland nurses attached to the Second AIF leave the Brisbane City Hall after attending a civic farewell on 17 January 1940. Miss Eunice Paten is third from the right in the front row. The following day the Courier-Mail *reported, under the headline 'Nurses May Use Lipstick, But No Nail Lacquer' that 'except that they are forbidden to use lacquer on their fingernails, 1940 Australian Army Nurses are under no restrictions in the use of cosmetics. When they were entertained by the Lord Mayor . . . yesterday at morning tea several admitted having used lipstick, but, like the touch of rouge, it was so discreetly and artistically applied that no objection could have been raised by the most fastidious'. Commenting that the seventeen nurses were an 'attractive group' the article quoted one nurse as saying: '"it's rather hard to get used to doing without a handbag . . . Where do we keep our powder-puffs? In our pockets," and she lightly tapped the buttoned hip-pocket.'* (Collection: John Oxley Library, Brisbane.)

factories were approved by the War Cabinet to meet the demands of rural industries, but these occurred very slowly.[18]

The number of women employed rose to 855 000 in 1944, compared with almost 644 000 in 1939. By 1944 women formed 25 per cent of the workforce, with almost one-third of all women aged fifteen to 65 in paid employment, 5 per cent more than 1939.[19] However, by 1944 labour shortages had limited the production of food, primary products, clothing and services such as transport. The health industry was severely affected and the Acting Commonwealth Statistician stated that 'hospital staffs were so short as to seriously embarrass provision of hospital services'.[20]

The government faced grave difficulties in increasing the numbers of women in the workforce. Direction was the final method used to move labour to the areas most in need of staff. Between August 1943 and July 1944, almost 10 000 direction orders were issued, 697 of these to women in Queensland. Direction meant accepting the job one was sent to or, if a satisfactory excuse was not forthcoming, being prosecuted for failing to turn up at the designated employer. The power of direction was not, in Wurth's opinion, used extensively, with approximately one per cent of those placed in employment for the eighteen months from January 1943 to July 1944 being directed.[21] Yet the efforts of the authorities in directing women to jobs gave diminishing returns. More success in gaining labour in essential areas was achieved through continuing efforts to improve labour productivity and conditions in factories.

Although Manpower Regulations required women who did not have the primary responsibility for the care of children or other relatives to work outside the home, even if they were married and keeping house, the dominant ideology and the belief that women's primary place was in the home did not change. On numerous occasions governments and trade unions stressed that, in peace time, society would return to the way it had been before the war. The reality for the last three years of the war however, was different. Lake has said that during the war Australian men faced the prospect of three invasions—the Japanese, the American and 'worse still, women's "invasion" of "men's jobs" '.[22] But it was an incursion that was successful for the duration of the crisis only, because it was authorised by men in positions of power. The 'women's "invasion" of "men's jobs" ' was propounded, sanctioned and encouraged by the government and officials who had to organise labour to meet the needs of the war. This was done only after all other available sources of surplus labour had been exhausted. Without the acceptance of those in power, this temporary invasion would not have occurred.

Most women still worked in traditional jobs and 'the structure and nature of the female workforce remained largely unaffected by the war and was made particularly inflexible by the effects of Manpower Regulations preventing women in traditional occupations from moving into higher-paid defence work'.[23] In fact, government policy 'rigidified both the gender division of labour and the occupational hierarchy of the female labour market'.[24] After the war, only small gains remained. By 1947 the percentage of women in the workforce had dropped to the pre-war level of 23 per cent.[25] The consolidation of many of the wartime changes such as the availability of work in a wide variety of jobs and industries took many decades. Although equal pay with men was gained in limited areas during the war, most women workers had to wait at least another 25 years to achieve this.

Women's wages during the war

The differences in rates of pay for women, from the low pre-war rates in traditionally female jobs and industries to the equal pay awarded in a few areas, created major problems in the distribution of female labour. There were enormous ramifications for the occupation of nursing, as low wages meant it was not a very attractive option for many women. Special regulations were enacted to set the wages and working conditions for women in newly created wartime jobs and in work which released men for the forces and in 1942 a Women's Employment Board (WEB) was established and continued until October 1944. Its guidelines provided that female wage rates were to be set at 60 to 100 per cent of the male rate for substantially similar work. By 1944 the board had made 288 decisions affecting the lives of between 70 and 80 000 women or about 9 per cent of the female workforce[26] and awarded a variety of rates of pay, but most frequently 90 per cent of the male rate.[27] Of course, the state and federal industrial tribunals continued to arbitrate on the wages and working conditions of other women including nurses using the traditional criteria which had kept women's wages at about 54 per cent of the male rate.

Wage rates clearly had an effect on the dispersal of female labour. A 1941 survey of 800 women commencing work in a munitions factory found that they were:

> obviously attracted by the higher wages offering in munitions work . . . When asked why they were taking up the work, some said that they wanted to do something to help the war effort: but, if questioned directly, the majority admitted that the relatively high wages had also affected their decision.[28]

Many could earn more than twice their previous wage in the munition factory. While the majority had been domestics and factory workers, 38 or nearly 5 per cent had been nurses.[29] WEB decisions increased the disparity in wage rates, giving rise to a great deal of discontent among women working outside war industries and those who had been employed in munitions work before the war. Women in the metal industry could earn up to 9 pounds a week with overtime while in food processing, with the same overtime, they could earn only 4 pounds a week.[30] Low wages and the disparity of wages in traditional female industries led to strikes of women workers, particularly among textile workers.[31] Women wanted jobs at the higher WEB rate. In 1942, Sydney County Council advertised twelve positions at rates ranging from 4 pounds 8 shillings and 7 pence to 6 pounds 7 shillings and 6 pence and received 2000 applications. But when Manpower authorities called up 2000 women for work in fruit canning factories, 1800 did not attend the interview. Some even came with borrowed babies to prove they were occupied.[32]

By 1943 women's wage rates were 'a mess'. It was possible that women in the one workplace could be doing similar kinds of work but be receiving three different rates of pay, for example 90 per cent, 75 per cent and 54 per cent of the male rate. There was 'a growing resentment that work which was as vital to the war effort as any other, such as clothing and textile manufacture, food processing and light metal work, was still low paid just because it was 'women's work'. The Arbitration Court in 1943 was forced to award wage increases of 75 per cent to women in the clothing and rubber industries in an effort to keep them at work.[33] This serious problem led to a re-examination of the position of women's wages. The Commonwealth Arbitration Court conducted a review of female wage rates and in May 1945 a majority of the judges concluded that the rates paid in the investigated industries were not unreasonably low. However, because women's work was vital to the war effort the Federal Government stepped in and disregarded the court's judgment in an effort to raise female workers' morale. In August 1945, the National Security Regulations provided that the remuneration of women in vital industries should not be less than 75 per cent of the corresponding male rate.[34]

Long working hours, few days off, suspension of annual holidays and an increased rate of industrial accidents characterised wartime work.[35] Conditions at work were 'often primitive' and a code of minimum conditions in factories was only mandatory in government establishments. In October 1942, weekly hours were limited to 56 for those aged eighteen and over and 48 hours for juniors.[36] The work many women did was so arduous that one factory worker complained that men in the armed forces were much better off.

The option of better working conditions was not used by governments. Rather the labour shortages and disinclination of women to work in some jobs was addressed by increasing the power of the government to direct women to take up these undesirable jobs. It was not contemplated that the dire labour shortages could be overcome by raising women's wages to attract them to jobs.[37] Despite the government's direction powers, women deserted low-paid jobs when they could to take up the 90 per cent war work. This was recognised by those in power, yet a solution to the labour shortages was never sought in the widespread use of higher rates of pay. Wurth stated that:

> obviously, women have been attracted into the higher wage occupations rather than into the low ones . . . Of course, other motives besides the opportunity for earning attractive wages have induced many women to offer themselves for employment, but the influence of higher wages was probably the most significant.[38]

This had disastrous consequences for the staffing of hospitals. Nursing suffered due to its low rates of pay and this was the cause of many problems encountered during the war. However, just as the raising of women's wages in other traditionally female occupations had been resisted as a means of solving the labour problem, this also happened in nursing. Powers of direction were used, often without the desired result.

Regulation of nursing

The regulation of health workers, obviously essential in the event of war, commenced early and continued via various committees throughout the war. The Central Medical Co-ordination Committee (CMCC), which first met in July 1938, regulated labour to meet the medical needs of the armed forces and the civilian population. It was estimated that there were 13 000 trained nurses in Australia at this time.

In September 1939 the *National Security Act* required medical personnel, including trained nurses, to practise or place their services at the disposal of the Commonwealth.[39] In the early months of the war, nurse volunteers for the military far exceeded requirements, and by 1940 about 4000 applications had been received for overseas service. Recruits had to be registered trained nurses, preferably with several years experience and an additional nursing certificate, British subjects, single, widowed or divorced without dependants, medically fit and of good character. For overseas service, sisters and staff nurses had to be aged between 25 and 35 years, with matrons below the age of 40.[40]

Miss Eunice Paten, the first nurse to become President of the ATNA in Queensland, was called up as Principal Matron of Northern Command, and held this position until she retired in February 1941. She was a veteran of the First World War and had been appointed Principal Matron 1 Military District in July 1923, accepting this part-time appointment while engaged in civilian nursing. Rates of pay for members of the AANS ranged from 19 shillings 6 pence per day with 3 shillings per day deferred pay for the Matron-in-Chief, to 8 shillings 6 pence per day with 2 shillings deferred pay for staff nurses. The public reacted to this with 'immediate newspaper criticism' of these salaries and uniform grants.[41] There was also discontent over pay among female members of the Australian Army Medical Corps, including pharmacists, physiotherapists and dietitians, who did not receive male rates of pay.[42]

The first members of the Australian Army Nursing Service (AANS) embarked for the Middle East on 9 January 1940. Nurses served in many locations overseas, including the United Kingdom, Greece, South-East Asia and New Guinea. AANS nurses serving in Australia worked in base, general, camp and women's hospitals, at casualty clearing stations, convalescent depots, internment camps, on ambulance trains and in medical research and training. In locations such as the Northern Territory and Torres Strait they provided a civilian hospital service. From 1939 to 1947, 3477 nurses served in the AANS, including 552 from Queensland. Deaths due to enemy action totalled 53. The Air Force and Navy developed their own nursing services with 616 nurses in the Air Force in December 1945 and up to 60 nurses serving in the Navy during the war.[43]

These nurses were Australia's collective heroines. *The Australian Women's Weekly* lauded them with headlines like, 'In tropical heat and hardships they cheerily help heal the battle-worn', 'A.I.F. [Australian Imperial Forces] Nurses Inspired Besieged Singapore: Rescue squad found night sister calmly dusting bombed hospital' and 'Nightingales of the 9th Division'.[44] In 1944, under the headline 'Devoted nursing saves thousands of lives: Lady with the lamp', the *Weekly* published a large photograph of a nurse on duty with her kerosene lamp in 'an Army hospital under canvas'. The caption read: 'Inheriting the great tradition of the original lady with the lamp, members of the Australian Army Nursing Service and the Australian Army Medical Women's Service have given devoted care to the sick and wounded of the A.I.F. in this war.'[45] Such images of Florence Nightingale were frequently invoked. One poem, by Private X, was dedicated to nurses overseas:

> The modern Nightingale
> Is every whit as frail
> As the Lady with the Lamp of long ago;
> But of such metal she is made
> To walk with fear—unafraid,
> And the soldiers call their blitz-worn Angel, 'Flo!'

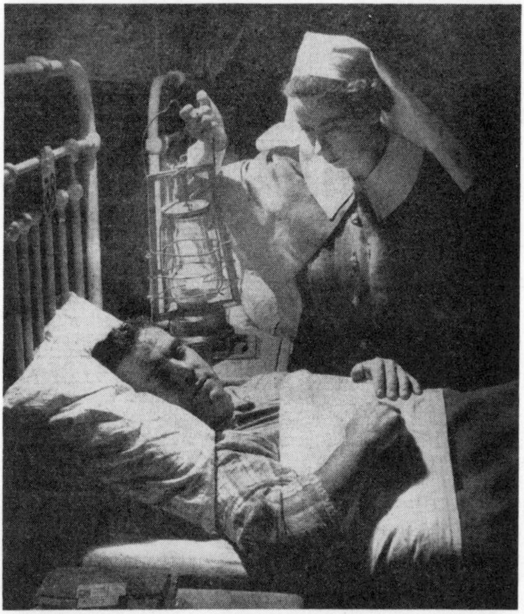

Military nurses were frequently portrayed as heroes and images which conjured up the work of Florence Nightingale a century earlier were used. This photograph in The Australian Women's Weekly *of 10 June 1944 was captioned 'Lady with the Lamp'. 'This picture', the article began, 'is symbolic of the devoted care of sick and wounded men of the A.I.F . . . These courageous women face danger and hardship cheerfully, doing monotonous routine work and knowing that on them depend thousands of precious lives'.* (Courtesy of Australian Consolidated Press.)

She makes sunshine out of rain,
Can camouflage your pain
With a smile framed in a halo stiff with starch . . .

It ended with the stanza:

Now wherever I may go
I am certain that my Flo
Will watch over me and guard me with her Lamp;
And if God takes my advice,
In a soldier's Paradise,
He will give to Flo the freedom of HIS Camp.[46]

In Australia, shortages of nurses, especially in the areas of midwifery and child welfare, were experienced as early as 1940. Some hospitals experiencing difficulties requested that double and triple certificated nurses be retained for civilian work and not be permitted to join the services,[47] however no action was taken to enforce this. In September 1941, a conference was held to discuss the position of nursing in Victoria which Sir Alan Newton, deputy chairman of the CMCC, hoped would give an indication of the state of nursing elsewhere. Documents were tabled from hospitals which detailed 'acute' shortages. The Country Hospitals Association represented seven hospitals which continued functioning only 'by the overworking of the Hospitals' permanent staff. In some instances, nurses, after having worked twelve hours a day have to attend urgent operations at night'. Sr M. Aloysius, Mother Superior of the Mercy Hospital, East Melbourne, said the maternity section was 'well-nigh unmanageable'. She added that 'for the past six months, the cause of suffering humanity and intense demand on hospital beds have urged us to cope with the situation and this has been accomplished by working our permanent staff twelve hours daily without the usual day off'. The Secretary of the Community Hospitals Association wrote that 'constant overwork at high tension is not likely to endure, and we feel ere long, the nurses who are bearing "the heat and burden of the Day" will succumb to their labour'.

The conference chairman concluded that 'a shortage of nurses did exist'. The single most important reason for this was felt to be the poor pay and conditions of nurses which compared unfavourably with the service hospitals. Miss Jane Bell, president of the ANF, declared that she was 'constantly' hearing of nurses leaving to work in munitions and other occupations. Various suggestions were made including shortening the training period, improving working conditions and asking retired nurses to return to the profession. But the immediate remedy, the chairman felt, was that 'the hospitals concerned would have to revise the rates of pay for nurses'.[48]

Miss K. Caldwell, Principal Matron, Northern Command, and an ATNA Councillor in Queensland, attended the Melbourne conference[49] and reported to the ATNA in this state. Council agreed that there was a shortage of nurses in Queensland and 'that the civilian hospitals should consider the question of increasing the pay and improving the conditions of nursing staffs'.[50] Yet the annual meeting the previous year had agreed that the ATNA would not make any attempt to do this.[51] Although better pay and conditions were seen as a major way to alleviate the shortage of nurses, the council felt in no way involved in this process and did not make any suggestions about how to bring about these changes, except to say that hospitals should consider this. To increase nurses' wages would mean that hospitals paid above award rates, an impossible practice in government employment.[52]

The CMCC decided on further investigations and in June 1942 resolved that a nursing sub-committee should be formed[53] and Miss Doris Bardsley, honorary secretary of the ATNA in Queensland, represented nurses in this state. No general picture of the position in

Queensland was reported to the meeting but the dire staff shortages in some country hospitals were recorded. Monto Hospital in western Queensland said their usual staff was a matron and four sisters, but they only had a matron and one sister. Cloncurry reported that they would lose three sisters soon and would be left with no qualified sister on the staff despite extensive advertising.[54] Once again this committee resolved that:

> a major cause of the shortage of nurses for civilian requirements is the inadequate salaries paid to nurses in public hospitals and other institutions requiring the services of nurses. Civilian nurses' pay compared unfavourably with that of nurses in the services and most unfavourably with the pay ruling for other occupations in which women were engaged.

One of the keys to change lay in increasing nurses' salaries. The sub-committee believed that 'representations for an increase in nurses pay could be made with more dignity by a body such as the Central Medical Co-ordination Committee and that that committee should be asked to take steps with a view to securing an increase in pay to nurses'.[55]

The Nurses' Sub-Committee report was considered by the CMCC at their meeting on 30 September 1942, which resolved that the control of nursing should be a Commonwealth responsibility directed by the CMCC and state MCCs. Nurses' salaries should be fixed by government regulations.[56] The ANF, the national organisation of ATNA branches, supported the idea of Commonwealth control, telling the Prime Minister that it was:

> much concerned regarding the need during the present national crisis for co-ordination of nursing services throughout the Commonwealth to avoid overlapping and waste of effort whilst providing fully for the needs of the civilian population should an emergency arise, and also to deal with the present shortage of nurses which is becoming very acute.

The ANF agreed that this control should be exercised by the Commonwealth through State Advisory Committees, the personnel of which would be nominated by the recognised nursing organisations in each state. These committees would have 'expert knowledge of matters concerned with hospitals and the nursing profession would be in a position to give sound advice and make informed decisions upon the very important matters brought before them'.[57]

Both the ATNA in Queensland and the ANF federally felt that they should be the sole representatives of civilian nurses.[58] Miss Bell strongly expressed the belief that nurses should be making the decisions about their profession:

> The nursing position appears to be becoming more and more chaotic in Australia, and the methods adopted to deal with this important National service do not appear to be the wisest or most helpful approach to the solution of the difficulties. That the responsibility of advising the Central Medical Co-ordination Committee, which presumably acts under the Commonwealth Government, as to the full control and powers over the entire nursing profession, numbering over 15,000 nurses, throughout the Commonwealth, has been vested in a nursing sub-committee, consisting of one person from each State, selected in a more or less arbitrary manner, one of whom is not even a nurse, has given rise to the greatest dissatisfaction here.
>
> Trained nurses, who have in their work to accept the gravest responsibilities in their share of the Nation's work, not only in peace, but in war, are shocked that they should be slighted and treated in this inconsiderate way and not allowed to know what is being done, or to express their views in matters vitally affecting them, as this is not in accordance with the principles of the freedoms and democracy this world-wide conflict is being waged to uphold.[59]

There was disagreement about the form that Commonwealth control of nursing should take. The upshot was that, at a meeting on 16 January 1943, the CMCC resolved that the legal and administrative control of nurses should pass to the Manpower Directorate.[60] An executive matron was appointed in each state to deal with administration matters concerning nurses and hospital personnel and nursing advisory committees were set up in each state. Miss Christense Sorensen, ATNA councillor and Matron of the Brisbane General Hospital, served as the representative of the nursing profession.[61]

From February 1943 the engagement and transfer of nurses and domestic staff were made by National Service Offices and all female nurses were required to register with the Manpower Directorate. In March 1943 there were 48 374 registrants, 8542 of them in Queensland. Of this group, 45 per cent were in nursing work and 4 per cent were employed in other jobs. The directorate took immediate administrative action to examine the cases of nurses who were not working as nurses and Wurth reported that this 'brought about an immediate improvement' in staffing hospitals. In March 1943 the shortage of trained nurses for hospitals was estimated at 1900, and this was reduced to 1100 by the end of June 1943.[62]

In addition, there were shortages of nurses and domestic staff in hospitals and institutions for the aged, and an acute shortage of nurses to work in private homes. Wurth saw enlistments in the nursing services as the major cause of the shortage, although 'many civilian nurses had been attracted to other occupations by higher wages and generally more attractive conditions in other employment'. Another problem was that 'the supply of trainees had also dwindled, many suitable girls having entered attractive employment before attaining the entrance age and being unwilling to enter the profession'. Further difficulties in gaining and keeping domestic staff were 'largely due to problems of differential wages, and generally the more favourable opportunities in industry for women' and 'this further aggravated the nursing problem, as nurses had to do domestic work'.[63]

On 3 June 1943, Wurth instructed his deputies that sufficient opportunity had been given for nurses and domestics to come forward voluntarily and, 'after a well-publicised final appeal, steps should be taken to direct single women to hospital work'.[64] By August that year, however, there was still a serious shortage of nurses and domestics in some state hospitals and institutions. In some cases the staff shortage was so desperate that patients were being refused admission and denied urgently needed treatment.[65]

Lack of trainees was a continuing problem[66] because there were so many avenues of employment open to young women, for 'unless nursing as a war time job and a future career is very definitely brought to the notice of girls they will choose some other calling in life'. Therefore Wurth urged that 'full use should be made of active propaganda by means of press, radio and films'. He also suggested that preliminary training courses should be conducted, so that girls between the ages of sixteen and eighteen could be secured for the nursing profession, before they became engaged in other activities.[67]

Other measures were tried. Surveys of nurse registration forms showed that there were large numbers willing or able to do part-time duties but many matrons and hospital managements were reluctant to use part-time assistance. Wurth suggested steps should be taken to convince hospitals of the necessity of using such assistance.[68] Married nurses were called into service. Wurth wrote to his deputies that 'marriage should not in itself be sufficient to justify refusal on the part of nurses to engage in active nursing duties for the duration of the war'. Yet there were taboos about the employment of married women, as 'certain religious organisations have asked whether the Directorate, is "assisting to break up the home" '.[69] On marriage, nurses were released for the purpose of setting up a home, but if they entered paid employment they had to return to nursing. Married nurses not keeping house for their husbands were treated as single for the purposes of direction.[70]

There had been a limited amount of extra labour available to alleviate the dire shortage of nurses and the Powers of Direction were used to flush this out. By 1944 however, these labour reserves had been exhausted and the armed services were forced to release women for civilian hospital employment[71] as happened in other industries that were desperately short of labour. By June 1944 the shortage of trained nurses in civilian hospitals was assessed at 257, assistant nurses 509, and trainee nurses 521.[72] The problem of the shortage of nurses was compounded by a shortage of domestic staff in hospitals. The directorate found that satisfactorily staffing hospitals with nurses depended largely on a sufficient domestic staff and Wurth urged his deputies to try to supply hospitals with full-time and part-time domestics and hospital aids.[73] In order to conserve their scarce resources, trained nurses were not to perform domestic duties.[74] But all attempts by the Manpower Directorate, the State Advisory Committees and other organisations did not succeed in remedying the nurse shortage. An analysis of the staffing position of hospitals in June 1944 showed that 'little further reduction of shortages could be anticipated, as available supplies of civil workers had been fully exploited'.[75]

While it was obvious and freely admitted that the problems of staffing hospitals related to the unattractiveness of the employment, no steps were made to change this and thus encourage more women to work in hospitals or train as nurses. Instead, the remedy was authoritarian. Thus hospitals and institutions were gradually protected and instructions were given so that 'hospitals received priority of treatment in allocation of women suitable for domestic work'.[76] Frequently women had to be directed to work in hospitals, particularly mental hospitals. Many did not turn up for work and some were prosecuted. There was no concerted effort to raise the wages of nurses or domestic staff so that they competed more equitably with other areas of work open to women or to reduce the arduousness of the work.

In Queensland some hospitals were so short-staffed that nurses took strike action in an effort to improve their conditions. The picture of docile, compliant, obedient servants of the hospitals taking such drastic action is out of character with their tradition and training. At this time, it was acknowledged that higher levels of pay were enticing women into wartime jobs. In July 1944 Major General S.R. Burston, Director General of Medical Services, noted that:

> the pay of munition workers, clerks and stenographers, in fact almost any class of work open to women, is better than nursing and when the long period of training, the poor pay, compared to the high degree of professional responsibility a nurse must accept are taken into account, it is not surprising that the supply of trainees is not equal to the demand.[77]

Thus it was recognised at the highest levels that amongst all women workers, nurses were among the worst off in terms of their wages and conditions.

In January 1945 another committee was appointed by the Minister for Defence to enquire into the shortage of nurses to serve the civilian population. The committee's report was submitted on 4 June 1945, a month after Germany had surrendered in Europe but two months before the war in the Pacific ended. Again the thrust of the report was that the pay and conditions for nurses were totally inadequate. The committee emphasised that:

> all the evidence supports the view that there will not only be no improvement in the nursing situation in Australia, but that the present position will rapidly deteriorate unless all Governments are prepared immediately to improve vastly:
>
> 1. Rates of pay for all classes of nursing;
> 2. Conditions under which nurses live;
> 3. Nursing Education.

The evidence that the committee took from trainees and trained nurses was that salaries were 'hopelessly inadequate'. It believed that:

> the remuneration now paid to qualified nurses is so inadequate that to secure their future they must leave the profession. The Committee came across instances where prospective trainees went out to work in other occupations in an endeavour to secure sufficient money to enable them to enter the nursing profession, and in all the lower paid States the trainees frequently said that they could not live without parental assistance on the wages they received during their training period.

Some trainees were earning as little as 14 shillings per week, leaving 11 shillings after tax had been deducted. There were great discrepancies in the amounts deducted for living allowances and 'in view of the appalling staff accommodation seen in a number of hospitals it would appear that there is little justification for the amounts deducted'. The committee commented that 'under such circumstances, the causes of discontent are self-evident'. Thus young women whose parents did not have sufficient funds to keep them throughout their training were frequently unable to enter the profession. As there were more avenues of work open to women at much better rates of pay, many young women chose this over a life, at least in the short term, of poverty and restriction. The committee also commented on nurses' education, saying it was urgently in need of an overhaul. Because of the policy of using trainees as a form of cheap labour, too much of the nurse's time was taken up in domestic work. Once again, in the face of three years of nursing shortage, the low pay of nurses was identified as the major problem.

Looking to the future, the committee did not feel that there would necessarily be a sufficient number of nurses when the war ended,

> because during the war tens of thousands of young women have been living under better conditions . . . From the Committee's investigations nothing was heard to indicate that when the war ends any of these young women are likely to enter nursing. At the present rates of pay and conditions Service personnel are receiving, they regard a nursing career as economic retrogression.

The committee concluded that 'the shortage of nurses cannot be improved until the nursing profession is made worthwhile to the trainee and trained nurse, and until conditions become sufficiently attractive to hold suitable trainees, and likewise, to hold the nurse when she has qualified'.[78] Shortly after this report was released the war ended and all legislation that had been passed to cope with the wartime situation was gradually rescinded.

Yet the question of increasing nurses' salaries had been voiced two years earlier and no action had been taken on an Australia-wide basis. Several committees with senior personnel had deliberated for many years over the problems of staffing hospitals during the war. The solution was seen as better pay and conditions for nurses but recommendations which actually achieved this were not forthcoming.

What was so disconcerting about raising nurses' wages or giving them better working conditions? This was acknowledged as the cause of the shortages. Increased nurses' wages would have added considerably to the cost of running hospitals and this could have been a significant disincentive. Were the authorities afraid of equal pay with its implication of giving women an equal place in society or recognition that their labour was equal in worth to that of men? The composition of the various committees, with senior medical and nursing personnel, may have led to an acceptance of the place that nurses held within the hospital hierarchy. Better pay could have disturbed this relativity. The practical problems in implementing these changes were complex. Problems of state and federal regulation of pay and wartime wage regulations meant that a simple solution could not be found. Instead of enticement, force was used in an attempt to staff hospitals adequately. The methods of the Manpower Directorate which applied to other areas of employment were transposed to hospital employment.

Wages of nurses

The first meeting of the Central Nursing Sub-Committee in 1942 had identified the inadequacy of nurses' salaries as the reason for the shortage and decided that the sub-committee should attempt to secure an increase in pay for nurses. But there were difficulties in adjusting the rates of pay for, while the central sub-committee could make recommendations to the Minister, the Minister could give effect to them only by regulations under the *National Security Act*. This would have been relatively easy if the rates of pay for nurses had varied only slightly from state to state, but the difference in salaries was great, especially for trainees. Salaries for first year trainees, for instance, varied from 10 shillings 10 pence per week in Victoria to 17 shillings 10 pence per week in New South Wales. The Central Nursing Sub-Committee faced a dilemma. Unification of trained and trainee nurses' salaries at the highest level would involve extra expenditure of approximately 200 000 pounds to 250 000 pounds annually. A further difficulty was that there was no award in South Australia and Tasmania and, in default of a federal award, there would have to be an arbitrary fixation of salaries for those states. But how was this to be done?

One solution that the sub-committee contemplated was that the ATNA should apply for registration with the Federal Arbitration Court and obtain a federal award.[79] With the lack of government action in regard to salaries the extraordinary recommendation was made that the union gain a federal award. This suggestion shows a highly unusual view that the union should be the vehicle for remedying the situation when government regulation had been used in other instances. It indicates that the image of the ATNA was that of a professional organisation rather than a trade union, and probably the expectation that its claims would be moderate. The overlap between nurses in senior positions in military and civilian life, and positions of power in the ATNA, would also have helped sub-committee members feel comfortable with this idea.

The suggestion of a federal award also exhibits a complete lack of industrial knowledge on the part of those committee members, nurses and medical practitioners, who thought that this was the way to proceed. The ATNA in Queensland was a registered union of employees with the State Industrial Court and had carriage of the nursing award but the national federation, the ANF, was not registered with the Commonwealth Arbitration Court. The process of registration would be lengthy, taking a minimum of many months, if not years. More important, though, was the question of whether nursing was an 'industry'. Section 51 (xxxv) of the Constitution gives the Federal Government its major industrial relations powers and allows it to legislate for 'the prevention and settlement of industrial disputes which extend beyond the boundaries of any one state'. Until 1983, the High Court interpreted the meaning of 'industry' in a way which limited it to production and associated areas such as banking. Teachers and firefighters, for example, were not able to gain a federal award because they did not work in an 'industry', with the result that these groups were restricted to operating under state industrial legislation.[80] Any attempt to gain a federal award could have been challenged successfully in the High Court, a process which would have extended over several years, so it would not have brought immediate relief to the problem it sought to solve.

Moves for a federal award did not proceed but the ANF consulted branches about the possibility of registering as a federal union. The branches approved this at the end of 1942.[81] However, legal opinion provided to the ANF stated that it would be unable to obtain registration as its membership included employers. The suggested remedy was a separate organisation of employees only.[82] But the issue of federal registration was not pursued and lay in abeyance until the end of 1944. By this time the Queensland Branch thought the matter was urgent as 'other organisations such as Hospital Employees and Professional Officers Unions have come into operation and could be considered as rivals therefore making it necessary to strengthen the position of the A.N.F'.[83] By the end of the war however, federal registration, a necessary precursor to a federal award, had not been achieved. This goal had meant that other means of securing changes had not been pursued vigorously. Without government regulation to increase wages and with the impossibility of a federal award (which was achieved for nurses in public hospitals in Queensland in 1991)[84] the only means of increase was via a state award. The mirage of a federal award prevented any real solution being attempted.

Because of the difficulty in remedying the wide discrepancies in salaries, the problem of central regulation of salaries was set aside. The only alternative was for salary changes to occur on a state basis. Nurses' salaries in Queensland were relatively low in comparison with other states. First year trainees were paid 13 shillings 1 pence per week, with lower salaries being paid in Perth and Victoria. Matrons, staff nurses and sisters in Queensland earned less than their counterparts in other states.[85] From the time these recommendations were made in October 1942 until late 1943, there was no change in the nurses' award in Queensland, even though Miss Doris Bardsley was on the sub-committee which made these recommendations. A log of claims had been drawn up in 1940[86] but the claims did not reach the court.

The changing situation of nurses during the war was largely responsible for award changes in August 1943. The dire shortages prompted the ATNA to approach the court for an award variation. The ATNA representative, Mr Richardson, stated that over 800 trained nurses in Queensland had left the profession and sought employment in other more remunerative areas of commerce.[87] This argument was substantiated by most of the employer respondents. Reasonably attractive salaries needed to be offered to retain an adequate staff of nurses and induce new trainees to enter the profession. The Brisbane and South Coast Hospitals Board even proposed a scale of increased salaries.[88] The Industrial Court judges, T.A. Ferry and W.J. Riordan, pointed out that there had been no change in the salary scale of nurses, apart from basic wage fluctuations, since the first award in June 1921. The commissioners concluded that 'after consideration of the salaries prescribed for nurses in other states of the Commonwealth and the wages fixed by this Court for other callings in the State, we are of the opinion that . . . an all-round increase in salaries is called for'.[89] The court judged the position of nurses' wages to be anomalous, and therefore could order an increase while still adhering to the Commonwealth regulations which severely restricted wage increases.

These increases still left nurses financially behind other workers. A staff nurse earned 3 pounds a week after completing a four-year apprenticeship while a female shop assistant over the age of 23 earned 3 pounds 10 shillings. A female clerk of the same age earned 4 pounds 4 shillings and 6 pence per week. Both these workers had a 44-hour week, compared with the nurse who worked 96 hours per fortnight. Females over 21 doing any unskilled work earned 2 pounds 14 shillings and 6 pence for a 44-hour week compared with 1 pound 10 shillings plus board and lodging for an assistant in nursing in her first year. Assistant mistresses in non-government schools earned from 178 pounds 10 shillings to 407 pounds in their fourteenth year compared with a first year staff nurse who earned 156 pounds and the matron of a hospital of over 300 beds who earned 434 pounds 4 shillings for unlimited hours.[90] Women workers, of course, earned substantially less than men, and the variety of wage rates for women during the war resulted in women's wages averaging only 59.5 per cent of male wages in 1943.[91]

The new nurses' award in 1943 did, however, include a more careful delineation of the categories of nurses and the payment of special allowances. Reflecting the increasing specialisation of training within a hospital, the new categories of tutor sister and assistant tutor sister were introduced. A new payment of 2 shillings per week per certificate was made where a trained nurse was required to hold more than one certificate in connection with her duties. The rates of pay were further regulated by the inclusion of the clause that the total certified experience of a nurse had to be taken into consideration when deciding the rates to be paid on commencing a fresh engagement which meant a nurse would not lose pay if she changed employment. The award variations were also notable for their extension to cover nurses working outside the hospital environment. Rates of pay were prescribed for registered nurses and assistants in nursing working in industrial and munition establishments, creches and kindergartens, mothercraft hostels, day nurseries and doctors' rooms.[92]

On 2 November 1944 in a further award variation, the ATNA was granted a preference clause. There were no objections and it was granted by consent. The clause stated that:

> all employers subject to this award shall, in employing a registered nurse, give preference of employment to members of the Australasian Trained Nurses' Association (Queensland Branch), Union of Employees.
>
> No registered nurse shall continue or be continued in employment for more than one month after the coming into operation of this clause unless she has made application to join.[93]

This amendment further acknowledged the position of the ATNA as the organisation representing nurses. The ATNA accepted one of the benefits of being a trade union, receiving fees without having to personally sign up members, without seeing itself as a trade union and only reluctantly bargaining for better wages and conditions.

The 1943 variation of the award marked a turning point in ATNA activities during the war. The council could no longer afford to excuse its inactivity on the industrial front in terms of helping the war effort.

The poor conditions of nurses were acknowledged by virtually all parties and the ATNA had justified its case in terms of the war effort. The shortage of nurses, clearly apparent by mid-1943, could only be overcome by improving the conditions of nurses and making the profession more attractive to newcomers.

In failing to recognise the seriousness of the shortages, the unhappiness and disquiet felt by nurses and even the feelings of some hospital boards, the ATNA showed itself to be lagging behind the needs and demands of its members. Its major preoccupation, and the way in which the council saw the organisation's role, was as a professional association, without the additional role of protecting and enhancing the working conditions of nurses. Despite all the evidence to the contrary, the council could still say in 1945 that 'in Queensland it is considered that the salary paid to nurses is satisfactory'.[94]

Nursing situation in Queensland

The shortage of nurses during the war forced the ATNA Council in Queensland to rethink some of its conservative views concerning wage increases. Before the war there were no problems attracting women into the nursing profession,[95] but by 1940 the annual report noted that 'the war has accentuated the shortage of trained nurses in Queensland, and country hospitals, in particular, are being affected'.[96] Dr R.G. Quinn, ATNA president, felt that 'the conditions for nurses in these places should be made as attractive as possible, instead of which some [hospital] Committees were inclined to endeavour to even evade the provisions of the Nurses' Award'.[97]

By 1942, when government committees were busy enquiring into the nursing shortage, several country hospitals wrote to the ATNA outlining their difficulties in gaining staff. In emergencies the matron of Quilpie Hospital had called on the assistance of married nurses living in the district.[98] The matron of Kennedy Hospital, Bowen, asked whether trainees could be retained on the staff after their marriage, to which the council replied that it was a domestic matter to be decided by a hospital's management committee, but added that the Brisbane and South Coast Hospitals Board did not permit this.[99]

Nurses at the Brisbane General Hospital reported working long hours during the war. One nurse said that 'ward conditions of 1938–42 era xtra [*sic*] busy—always on early off late—many hours o'time—(o'time not mentioned that I know of)'. Another nurse who trained during the war recalled the overtime worked at the Children's Hospital:

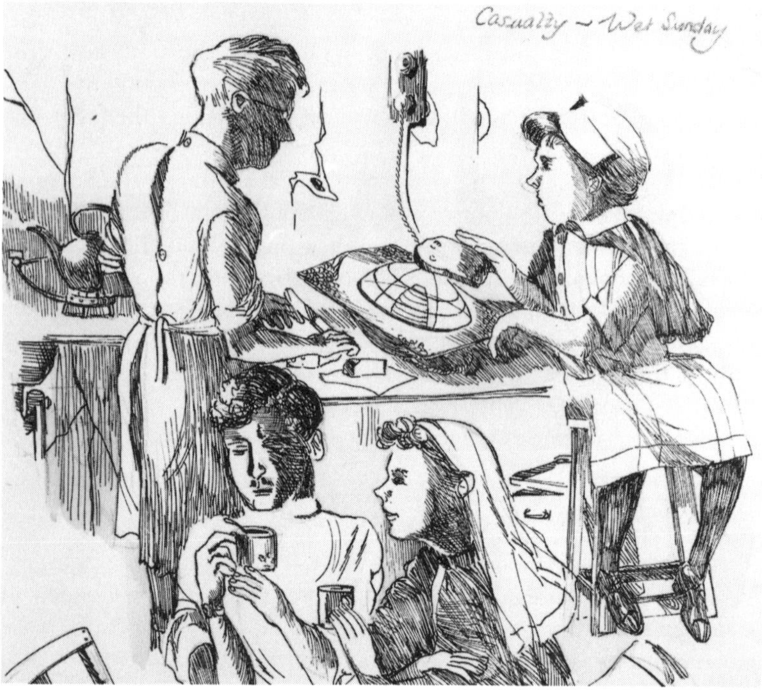

Titled 'Casualty—Wet Sunday', this is one of a number of sketches of nursing life at the Brisbane Hospital from 1942 to 1945 which were drawn by Mrs Rosemary Opala (nee Fielding) during her student days at the hospital. She completed her training in 1945. The nurse is making toast over one of the heaters and the kettle is boiling on a gas ring. (Fryer Library, University of Queensland. Rosemary Opala Collection. F3000.)

> Most times when my shift supposedly ended at 4 pm at the Children's I would find the pan-room over-flowing with nappies to be sorted and temporarily cleaned by the junior on duty only, and the room to be cleaned and spotless before the next shift. That could take at least another hour.[100]

These conditions were acknowledged publicly. The *Cairns Post* commented:

> Nursing is an arduous profession, but it carries with it great responsibilities, irregular and long hours, and a certain amount of danger from infection. The reason why so many girls go in for it is because, generally speaking, they are idealists, who wish to serve unfortunate people who are suffering in health. Because of this idealism they are likely to be made use of, for they are loth to fight for their rights

> like other classes of the community . . . Certainly something has been done in the last generation to improve nurses' conditions, which in the dim past could only be described as utterly unfair and cruel, especially during training. But they still do not get justice, in spite of the fact that every fair-minded person desires that they should.[101]

Miss C.E. Nell Grant wrote in the *ANJ* that it was not surprising that young women were not taking up nursing. This would not happen 'while girls can obtain employment in more lucrative professions where they are not required to do night duty nor work so strenuously, and have week-ends and public holidays off'.[102] A few lone voices suggested that the remedy lay in actually giving better conditions to nurses. In Federal Parliament Senator McLeay commented on the situation in November 1944:

> Why is the shortage of nurses so acute? One reason is that whilst the Government apparently is prepared to go to any length to improve working conditions in munitions factories, it is not willing to take similar action to improve the conditions of nurses who spend many years in training and engage in laborious work for many hours each day. The Government eventually will be forced to direct women to this important work, and to ensure that the remuneration of nurses shall be more comparable with that of women working in munitions factories and in other attractive avenues of employment. I make these suggestions because the position is becoming alarming.[103]

Nell Grant was more specific in her suggestions, suggesting eight-hour rosters for nurses.[104]

The situation was most serious in country areas, leading in some cases to the unprecedented step of nurses threatening and even taking strike action. Manpower authorities became involved and tried to recruit enough nursing and domestic staff to meet the needs. However they did not have much success for conditions remained poor, and women were discouraged by the fact that once they accepted work in a hospital they were forced to remain there by the wartime regulations. As a consequence the Manpower Directorate resorted to their powers of prosecuting women who did not obey these orders. In April 1944 the *Queensland Times* reported that 'man-power officials continue to direct women to hospitals where required, and to prosecute those who could not give good reasons for not obeying directions'. The Brisbane Summons Court fined Gertrude B. 5 pounds and 2 pounds 8 shillings costs in default three weeks imprisonment, for not reporting for work to the Goodna Mental Hospital on 7 April. Thelma B. was also fined,

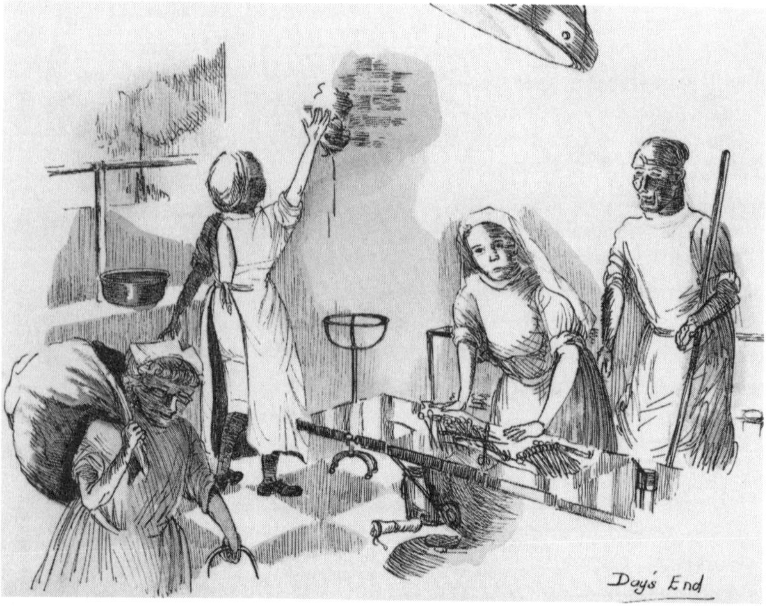

'Day's End' shows a nurse cleaning the walls of an operating theatre, another removing soiled linen, one sorting the instruments at the completion of the operation and a wardsman mopping the floor. This is one of the sketches of life at the Brisbane Hospital during the Second World War drawn by Mrs Rosemary Opala. (Fryer Library, University of Queensland. Rosemary Opala Collection. F3000.)

the magistrate saying that she had treated the direction order 'with some contempt'.[105]

The situation became so serious in some institutions that hospital workers took industrial action. Reekie discusses the 'persistent theme of female resistance to exploitation in the workplace' and found that in Western Australia 'women themselves initiated and carried through industrial action, often without the support of . . . male union executives'.[106] This was true of nurses' strikes in Queensland. They were not only initiated without the help of female or male union executive members, but in some instances were carried out totally without their knowledge or support.

In Queensland, nurses' strikes in 1944 and 1945 resulted from low staffing levels and poor working and living conditions as the nurses endeavoured to pressure the authorities into providing more staff. The situation became so bad at the Goodna Mental Hospital that female nurses, members of the Hospital Employees' Federation (HEF), went on strike. This had followed a deputation to the Manpower authorities in March 1944 and unsuccessful attempts by them to obtain an additional 50 nurses. The *Queensland Times* described the situation:

> To attend to the patients in 12 wards, only 14 nurses were stated to be on duty yesterday, while on Thursday only nine nurses were available for this work. Usually two or three nurses are fully occupied in each ward. In an effort to maintain efficiency, many of the nurses have been working 12 hour shifts.[107]

Mr F.E. Walsh, Deputy Director-General of Manpower in Queensland, reported that 'owing to staff shortages, the nurses employed had been carrying on under great strain and now felt that they could not continue this much longer'. Seventy women were needed immediately and the demand was so urgent that women were to be released from other protected undertakings for this work.[108] However additional nurses were not forthcoming and the female nurses went on strike on 13 April. This industrial action did not have the approval of their union and Mr L. Flower, HEF State Secretary, spoke against direct action, saying that union policy believed in other methods to solve difficulties. But, Flower said, 'the overwhelming vote of the women showed their feelings, and when it came to questions of danger to health, a strike was permissible'.[109]

There was great difficulty in getting additional staff for mental hospital work. Five women who reported for duty 'left almost immediately'.[110] By 18 April, with the nurses still on strike and the male nursing staff of 170 threatening to join them if the situation could not be alleviated, 55 additional workers including 25 Army nurses and four volunteers were obtained to begin work at the hospital. Walsh threatened to prosecute women who disobeyed direction orders without a satisfactory excuse.[111] The strike lasted five days.

In the same month, staff at the Willowburn Mental Hospital at Toowoomba threatened to strike. Manpower authorities attempted to direct women from non-essential employment to the hospital and 'combed' the retail stores for additional help,[112] but hospital staff decided that unless 47 additional employees were found within a week, strike action would be taken. Women were hastily directed to this work.[113] Shortages of nurses persisted and in March 1945, 61 nurses at Willowburn Mental Hospital, who cared for more than 600 patients, stopped work, requesting 21 additional nurses.[114] Manpower authorities responded by directing young women on the Darling Downs to this work.[115]

Industrial action was not confined to mental hospitals. Trainee nurses at Cairns Hospital went on strike over poor conditions and lack of staff. They complained of the 'excessive hours, overdue holidays, food conditions, lack of cutlery and ward utensils and no lounge in which to entertain friends' as well as an acute shortage of staff. The hospital needed an additional nineteen trainee nurses and six domestic staff.[116] A deputation of trainees explained to the local paper that they gave their food ration books to the hospital and that they were not receiving their share of food. One nurse stated that 'I do not know whether our rationed food goes into the wards or not . . . but I do know we don't get our proper issue. People outside get their fair share of such things as butter and meat, but we do not'. The deputation to the paper 'made it clear that they had no "grudge" against the matron, sub-matron or doctor'. The chairman of the hospital board appealed to the trainees to remain at work, but they refused.[117]

On 2 August 1944, 30 trainees went on strike for the day. After a lengthy conference with board members and the president and secretary of the local Trades and Labour Council, they resumed work on the condition that their demands were met within a week.[118] Manpower authorities combed the local area for young women to become trainee nurses and appealed to 'parents, employees and other persons likely in any way to influence any eligible young women, to do nothing to prejudice their taking up this urgent and essential hospital work'.[119] The local president of the Country Women's Association asked her members to help in recruiting nurses:

> We know that one does need to be of the necessary temperament to be a success; but there are many girls most suited for this profession, good, healthy Australians filled with the milk of human kindness. Will you try to convince your friends with growing girls that one of them at least might consider nursing as a career? The noblest of any![120]

The acute nursing shortage that persisted meant that two hospital wards remained closed.[121] One hundred young women were interviewed by Manpower staff but only three volunteered as nursing trainees and four were appointed as domestics. Eighteen direction orders were therefore issued by the Manpower authorities, sixteen for nursing trainees and two for domestic staff.[122] The attempts to direct women to work at Cairns Hospital mirrored the problems experienced earlier at Goodna. Only eight out of sixteen women directed to work at the hospital in August even turned up and a further four women had medical certificates stating that they were unfit for the work. Four women started work, but this number was offset by two nurses wanting to leave work because they were getting married. The hospital board asked the Army to release women to help ease the situation. However, despite all these efforts and the dire step of industrial action by the trainee nurses, there was a net gain of only eight nurses by the end of August 1944.[123]

Other hospitals and health services were also affected by the nurse shortage. Country towns supported nurses who were attempting to preserve health services in their communities. The position at Eidsvold Hospital was acute, with only a matron and two junior first year assistants, and district residents assisted the nurse with serious cases. The maternal and child welfare centres at Barcaldine, Longreach and Aramac, operated by one nurse, were closed indefinitely from 20 April 1944.[124] The Collinsville District Hospital in north Queensland also experienced difficulties. The coal miners in this town and nearby Scottville threatened to strike in sympathy with the overworked nurses, as they were 'determined to exert pressure on the authorities to see that the hospitals are adequately manned'.[125] In April 1944, when Manpower authorities suggested that the Gin Gin and Mt Perry Hospitals in central Queensland should be closed, the local shires protested vehemently.[126]

As with the Collinsville Hospital, nurses and trainees at the Cairns District Hospital were probably members of the ATNA but the ATNA was not involved in or notified of the strike of trainees in Cairns. Even after the strike it was the local TLC that the Cairns nurses approached about their working conditions. The ATNA Council, concerned at competition from the Cairns TLC, wrote to it stating that 'the Australian Trained Nurses' Association, Queensland Branch, is the Union of Nurses in Queensland and it would be appreciated if Nurses approaching their Union with complaints be advised to refer their difficulties to their own union where they will receive immediate consideration'. The council also sent application forms and information about the ATNA to the nurses and suggested that groups should be formed in each hospital to enable nurses to discuss their problems locally and refer them to the council for consideration.[127] Matron Henry of Charters Towers Hospital complained that nurses were being influenced by TLC delegates who had held meetings on the hospital premises. The nurses were very dissatisfied with their working conditions, the lack of amenities and the shortage of staff. Once again the ATNA wrote to the TLC requesting that any nurses approaching it be advised to refer their difficulties 'to their own Union, where they would receive immediate consideration'.[128]

By 1945 some hospitals were reporting their difficulties to the ATNA. The Atherton Hospitals Board asked why there was such difficulty getting trained staff. The ATNA Council replied that nurses would apply for positions at a hospital if the best possible accommodation and recreation facilities were provided. Concessions for travelling to and from home on annual leave would be an inducement for a nurse to accept a position in a country hospital, the council believed.[129] The Tully Hospital Secretary wanted to know if the ATNA could do something to improve the salaries and working conditions for nurses as the hospital board believed that it was an opportune time to do this, but the council felt that substantial increases had already been obtained.[130]

Most available labour had been recruited into the workforce by 1944, and the problem of finding enough women to work in hospitals was not solved. The severe difficulties faced by nurses as a result were not addressed by the ATNA Council. The Second World War so exacerbated poor working conditions that nurses in several hospitals spontaneously threatened or took strike action, something that would have been unthinkable prior to the war. Women 'felt so strongly about injustices suffered in the workplace that they dared defy a community consensus that there be no strikes in wartime. Women's militancy thus challenged the image presented in the media of the contented, patriotic female war worker'.[131] Such actions were all the more extraordinary when taken by the traditional carers of the community, nurses, who had absorbed the tradition of sacrifice to high degree.

Structure of ATNA

The character of the ATNA began to change during the war. Previously the only way a nurse could participate effectively in the organisation was to become a councillor but during the war various groups of nurses began requesting voices of their own. Groups with common problems joined together to seek solutions, with or without the assistance of the ATNA Council in Queensland. A trainee association was formed and district associations commenced. Nurses themselves initiated these changes and the ATNA Council had little choice but to accept these moves. The council, seeing itself as a professional organisation safeguarding the standards of nurses, did not agree that there was a need to develop a system of local representation which would widen the input of members and therefore did not initiate any such system. What was new, was that these nurses asked for a formal place within the organisa-

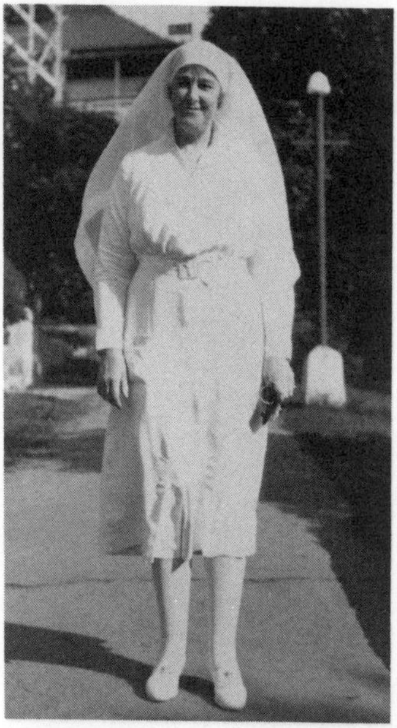

Miss Christense Sorensen was Matron of the Brisbane Hospital from 1928 to 1951, councillor of the ATNA from 1923 to 1943 and vice-president from 1943 to 1950. This photograph, taken in the early 1940s, shows Miss Sorensen on the path between the hospital and the nurses' home, a path known to the nurses as 'Cardiac Hill'. They would walk this path several times a shift as they went to their meals in the nurses' home. (Courtesy of the Royal Brisbane Hospital Graduate Nurses' Archive.)

tion where they could meet and discuss common needs, outside the council but with the assistance of this body when needed.

The increased role of women in the community during the war, a role much wider than that centred on the home, led women to participate more in the life of the community and to take decisions of their own. The participation in local community life and the responsibilities that women bore in wartime may have encouraged ordinary ATNA members to seek greater participation in the affairs of their association. Union membership increased from 32.8 per cent of the female workforce in 1939 to 51.9 per cent in 1945, while the rate of male membership increased 3.3 per cent in the same period.[132]

Late in 1941, following discussions with ATNA Councillors,[133] trainees at the Brisbane General Hospital and Brisbane Women's Hospital formed the Queensland Trainee Nurses' Association (which soon changed its name to the Student Nurses' Association of Queensland). They requested affiliation with the ATNA, and executive members of the Student Nurses' Association, who had to be associate members of the ATNA, were co-opted to council when they wanted to raise any matters. The trainees 'were congratulated upon their enterprise in forming an organisation, which the A.T.N.A. would endeavour to assist in every possible way'.[134]

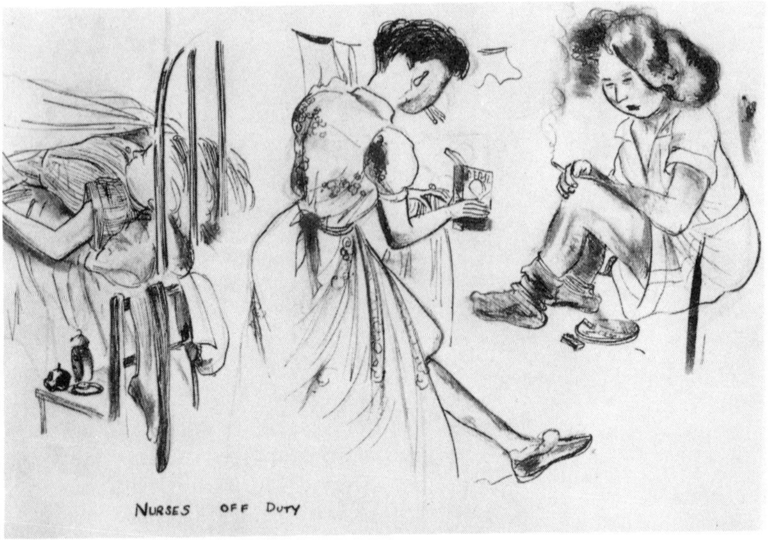

'Nurses Off Duty', a drawing by Mrs Rosemary Opala, depicts Brisbane Hospital nurses in their time off duty during the Second World War. The nurses shown are relaxing, smoking, doing their washing with the washing powder Persil and reading in bed with the alarm clock close at hand. (Fryer Library, University of Queensland. Rosemary Opala Collection. F3000.)

In mid-1942 they requested action from the council, asking that the award be changed so that a board and lodging allowance was paid to trainees while on annual leave. The council was 'most sympathetic' but decided that 'owing to the war situation the time was not opportune to take any action'. The trainees also wanted a reduction in train fares when going on annual leave. The council reported that they had tried several times to get reduced train fares for trainees and once again an approach to the Railways Commissioner was unsuccessful.[135]

The trainees' association, centred on the largest hospitals in the state and concerned primarily with nursing conditions, filled a gap for trainees in dealing with local problems. As the ATNA had no system of local representation via sub-branches or regional union representatives, the student group was the first mechanism established to handle these problems. It is interesting to speculate that these moves were first made by trainees, those not yet fully socialised into the unquestioning acceptance of poor conditions. Yet trainee nurses were an essential part of the hospital system, as one article in the *ANJ* commented:

> Hospitals are staffed to such a large extent by the student nurse. This has often placed far too great a burden upon her both physically and mentally. The hospital is dependent upon her, and she is made to feel responsible for all routine nursing duties, the tidiness of the ward, the cleanliness of the annexes and their equipment, and, in her senior years, for carrying out dressings and treatments; for no one else is available to do these things.[136]

The ATNA Council felt that:

> hospital authorities should remember that, for the student nurse employed in a hospital a long distance from her home, the hospital was the only home she had, and must become the centre of her social life when she was off duty. With the multiplicity of occupations open to them these days, girls were unlikely to be attracted to an occupation where this aspect was so neglected.[137]

In December 1943, the Queensland Student Nurses' Association asked the ATNA, as its 'parent body', to take over the organisation of the association throughout training schools in Queensland. A constitution was adopted in mid-1944 and Misses Winifred Payne and Frances Dunbar were appointed to represent the Student Nurses' Association on the council. A questionnaire was sent to matrons of training schools inquiring about the facilities for nurses, asking if there was a local student nurses' group and urging the formation of such a group in each training school.[138] The students themselves had formed their own associations, initiated the moves to become part of the ATNA and to gain representation at training schools throughout the state, thereby commencing the decentralisation of the union's structure with local decision-making bodies.

Moves for the greater representation of qualified nurses in country areas also came from the nurses themselves. The question of country representation was considered at the 1943 annual meeting when Miss C.E. Nell Grant, Matron of the Base Hospital, Longreach, proposed that country members should have direct representation on the council. Her idea, however, was a hospitals' association, not a nurses' association. She suggested a Western and Northern Hospital Association, with headquarters in Rockhampton or Townsville, which would submit ideas to the controlling council in Brisbane and send a representative to the annual meeting. Although the ATNA annual meeting 'considered that the idea is a good one',[139] nothing resulted. Positions on the ATNA Council were filled with matrons and nurses in senior positions and students and ordinary nurses still lacked the power to influence decisions easily.

The following year an approach for country representation came from Rockhampton, where nurses wanted to establish a branch of the ATNA and a Student Nurses' Association. Miss Eunice Paten visited Rockhampton to address a meeting of nurses about the objectives of the ATNA and subsequently 37 nurses attended the inaugural meeting of the Rockhampton Group on 1 August 1944. Interested nurses from country hospitals in the surrounding district were invited to participate and the council was 'very pleased with the result'.[140] The Rockhampton Group brought some of their problems to the ATNA, including the issue of the appointment of members of hospital boards who were not nurses or doctors. However, the ATNA Council was upset when an independent deputation of three Rockhampton nurses met with the Minister, Mr Thomas Foley, in February 1945. Yet the deputation's visit had some success as other matters were discussed with Foley and by this means the Rockhampton Group achieved a reduction in the period of night duty from three to two months.[141]

The Rockhampton Group continued to meet, held a street stall and bridge party to raise money, and conducted a club room for the benefit of the nurses and country visitors. By mid-1945 the council congratulated the Rockhampton nurses on 'the splendid and enthusiastic way in which the Group is functioning and the success of the monthly meetings'.[142]

Nurses who worked in medical practitioners' surgeries formed a group which approached the ATNA about an increase in wages. At the 1945 annual meeting Miss Kennedy asked that their salary be increased to 5 pounds 9 shillings per week, the same as industrial nurses. The meeting recommended this to the council for its consideration but the council, as usual wanting to check that a salary rise was acceptable to the employer, wrote to the BMA requesting that it discuss this matter with a view to voluntarily raising the salaries. The BMA replied that it was in favour of adequate salaries being paid but could not force doctors to pay this wage.[143] A conference of ATNA Councillors and representatives of nurses from doctors' surgeries and private nurses was held and Miss Kennedy again requested that the ATNA approach the Arbitration Court to gain the wage increase. She presented an itemised account of average living expenses which the current salary of 4 pounds 4 shillings was insufficient to meet. It was resolved that Miss Kennedy should gather evidence from nurses to support their case, and then present this to the council for its approval, with a view to making an application to the court for an increase in salary in 1946.[144] Once again any moves for salary increases had to be seriously vetted first and checked with potential or actual employers.

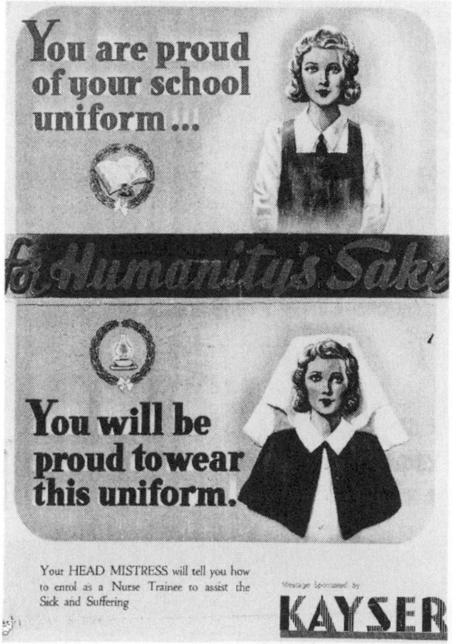

This poster was produced towards the end of the Second World War in an attempt to encourage young women to enter nursing. (Australian Archives (Vic.): CRS B551, Directorate of Man Power, Central Office, Correspondence Files 1942–46, item no. 1943/72/4727/1.)

Nurses at the Women's Hospital in Brisbane united to fight accommodation problems and even threatened industrial action. They claimed that the proposed nurses' quarters on the hospital roof would be cramped, restricting the privacy, ventilation and recreation facilities of the nurses, and noisy labour ward patients and crying babies would keep staff awake. The nurses were 'quite determined to strike should the government decide to go ahead with the building'.[145] Through the pages of the *Courier-Mail* one nurse protested that the Premier should not assume that:

> because we have not complained, there are no disadvantages in the accommodation on the fifth floor.
>
> The lifts are frequently out of order, and we have to use the stairs. The noise made by the lift dynamo is constantly heard. The noise made by the maids on the fourth floor, washing up in stainless steel sinks at frequent intervals between 6 a.m. and 8 p.m. has to be heard to be believed.
>
> The matron and sisters have frequently had to get out of bed and ask fourth floor nurses to remove babies from the nursery, because they could not sleep for their crying . . . This crying can be heard at times both day and night, and is sometimes most persistent.

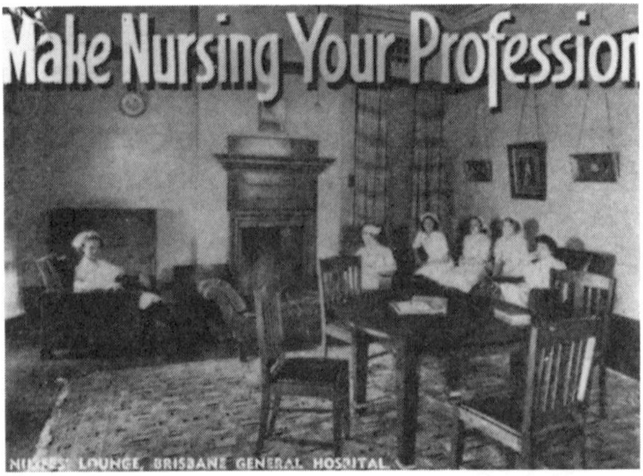

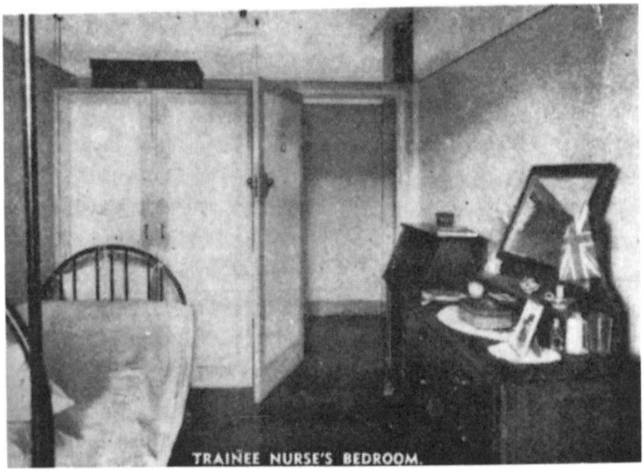

These photographs illustrated a pamphlet which urged young women to train as nurses. With headlines such as 'Basis of a Noble Career', 'High Position amongst the Professions' and 'Women's Hearts Must Surely Hear the Call', it stated that 'total war modifies every aspect of life and this has been most noticeable in the nursing profession, and has resulted in a shortage of nurses so acute that, in order to remedy the position, it is necessary to make an appeal to young women to make nursing their war-time work and the basis of their future career'. It talked about training: 'Florence Nightingale might well be described as the Apostle of Modern Nursing, and her insistency that probationers should be taught the principles underlying their work . . . is the guiding principle governing present-day training for the nursing profession. In Queensland, this training is thorough and wonderfully efficient.' The two illustrations depicted the comfortable life of nurses in the nurses' home at the Brisbane Hospital. (Australian Archives (Vic.): CRS B551, Directorate of Man Power, Central Office, Correspondence Files 1942–46, item no. 1943/72/4727/1.)

> We think the general public will agree that when the labour ward on the fourth floor is opened, more noise will be heard by the unfortunate nurses who will be living in the proposed roof quarters. . . . We do not want to live within the hospital.[146]

The nurses received support from many quarters[147] including the president of the League of Women Voters, Queensland, a non-party organisation, who suggested that the male decision-makers spend a night 'under prevailing conditions'. She concluded that 'the profession of nursing requires self-sacrifice, unknown in any other vocation, and nurses' housing should be equal to the contribution made by nurses to the welfare of the community'.[148] Although the ATNA Council requested a meeting of nurses at the Women's Hospital, and wrote to the hospital board requesting a conference to discuss the situation,[149] no further mention is made of the issue. The feelings of the nurses had run high and public support had been favourable. The ATNA, as usual, took a conservative line in its recommendations to its members.

Thus the push to deal with the difficulties in local working conditions and for increased wages once again came from the nurses directly involved. They fought issues themselves, took matters concerning them to annual meetings where they could have their say or established formal groups and then approached the ATNA. The student nurse associations grew out of a need for this category of nurses to tackle the problems encountered in hospitals. Not yet 'survivors' nor fully inculcated into the system where complaints about worsening conditions were frowned on, the students in some hospitals banded together to do something about their poor working conditions. The council responded by accepting groups when they were a *fait accompli* but did not actually facilitate the formation of more groups. The council guarded its territory very carefully and did not set up a structure or tangibly encourage local groups which could deal with the local problems of great significance to the individual nurse.

Although the council did not initiate moves to widen its representative base, it did alter its constitution to reduce significantly the influence of male medical practitioners who had held the position of president in the association since its inception. The annual meeting in July 1944 approved changes which gave medical practitioners a role 'only in a consultative and advisory capacity'.[150] Medical practitioners had played a vital role in determining the goals and activities of the ATNA in Queensland during its first 40 years. Holding some of the most senior medical posts in the state, their concerns as executive members of the association had revolved around the training and registration of nurses and they had been loath to request improved working conditions. Their involvement reflected the origins of the ATNA as a professional association and its continuing emphasis on activities related to this.

In 1944, Eunice Paten became the first president of the ATNA in Queensland who was a woman and a nurse. The war thus enabled the nurses to decrease their reliance on the men who often had the power and position to issue orders to them. The dramatic events of the Second World War, which brought rapid and extensive changes in the position of women, affected both nursing and the ATNA. Demand for labour during the war provided women with more employment options and, although most women still worked in traditional occupations, nursing suffered by comparison with other higher-paying jobs. However the ATNA reacted to changing circumstances reluctantly and did not initiate change. In particular, the extreme nursing shortage did not meet with a concerted effort from either the government or the nursing association to redress the causes of the decline in numbers. At the end of the war, problems associated with nurses' pay and conditions remained and would have to be tackled in the immediate post-war period.

CHAPTER 9

ATNA industrial activity, 1945 to 1950

' . . . over all these long years your Council had done its best, so far as possible, to keep that aspect [trade unionism] in the background.'[1]

Following the severe restrictions on labour during the war years, the post-war period was a time of industrial unrest and turmoil for many sectors of the community. The battle to achieve a shorter working week and a significant rise in the male basic wage lasted nearly five years. The industrial disputes which arose became very bitter and frequently polarised the community. Yet these events had little direct impact on the activities of the ATNA. It focused its concerns, as always, on the perceived needs of the nursing profession and did not see itself as part of the wider trade union movement. Although in this period there is the first statement in the minutes of the association that they are an industrial organisation, this is an isolated occurrence. The predominant view was that espoused by Miss Eunice Paten, president of the ATNA, who proudly avowed at a general meeting of members in 1947 that 'I have never liked Trade Unionism as applied to the profession of Nursing. The A.T.N.A. (Q) was forced . . . [to become] a Union and over all these long years your Council had done its best, so far as possible, to keep that aspect in the background and yet improve Nurses' conditions and salaries'.[2]

Unfortunately these two aspects were mutually exclusive, and the ATNA did not develop the industrial knowledge and expertise required to maintain and improve nurses' salaries and conditions because of its view that it was not truly an industrial organisation or trade union. Thus the attitudes and values of the ATNA in previous decades held sway after the war. The isolated strikes and threatened industrial action of the war were forgotten and the nurses' perception that they should not withdraw their labour was not challenged. The organisation continued to mirror the hierarchical structure of the hospitals and ignored the cries of its members. The philosophy which espoused the view that

'I have never liked trade unionism' determined the industrial fate of the union.

The post-war period was characterised by continuing shortages of nurses accompanied by complaints about poor working conditions and low pay. The unpopularity of the Manpower Regulations meant that they were repealed quickly, most by October 1945. Labour shortages meant that restrictions on the engagement of labour lasted longer, with the regulations dealing with the engagement of women between the ages of 18 and 45 being the last to go on 30 April 1946.[3] Restrictions on wage rises also lasted for several years. Once again the ATNA did not lead the way in seeking satisfactory working conditions, but reacted reluctantly to the strong pressures on it. Pressure from nurses themselves, community organisations and even government bodies were ultimately too hard to resist and the ATNA was forced to respond. The industrial cases that resulted slowly brought changes, however the ATNA exhibited such an extraordinary degree of ineptitude in these cases that successful award variations were delayed and nurses had to wait longer than necessary to gain improved working conditions.

The ATNA's inability to handle industrial cases was a result of the lack of training or experience of any of its office bearers in the preparation or advocacy of such cases, an area which was becoming increasingly specialised. The organisation did not appoint anyone with this experience. At the root of the problem lay their philosophical beliefs about the purpose of the ATNA, especially the overriding attitude that it was not an industrial organisation. Ultimately it was advice from government sources that helped it overcome its problems. The State Government, as the major employer of nurses, at times during the post-war period supported better pay and working conditions and was a significant outside pressure on the ATNA. Changes to the health-care system enhanced its importance as an employer. In 1945, the federal *Hospital Benefits Act* instituted a system of subsidy for each occupied bed in a public hospital, provided that free beds were offered in public wards. The subsidy came into effect on 1 January 1946 and formally abolished the voluntary hospital system in Queensland. Free treatment was extended to cover outpatients in this state.[4]

At the end of the war the traditional gender division of jobs was re-asserted. It had, of course, been made clear throughout the war, both by governments and individuals, that non-traditional jobs for women would not last into peacetime. As Mr E.C. McGrath, federal secretary of the Printing Industry Employees' Union, predicted:

> a belief which any woman may hold that she will be able to retain her industrial position is likely to bring unfortunate disillusionment to her. Gilded castles are being built for women which must inevitably crash to the ground, and our women will be justifiably wrathful on finding they have been misled by well-meaning but misguided champions.[5]

Asked what was women's appropriate place in society, McGrath referred to Queen Elizabeth's statement that after the war women 'would be called upon as homemakers to play a great part in rebuilding family life'.[6] The Re-establishment and Employment Bill of 1945 gave service personnel automatic preference for post-war employment and reinstatement in their pre-enlistment positions. Thus many women were forced out of jobs where they had learnt new skills and earnt more money. As well 'the predominantly male trade unions were determined that women would be pushed out of "male" industries'.[7]

The expectations of women were not uniform. Despite the strength of community feeling that women's place was in the home, surveys during the war showed that 'women did want to continue working, and many in the industry that they had worked at during the war'.[8] A Post-War Reconstruction Department report found that 69 per cent of servicewomen wanted paid employment after the war and 30 per cent wanted training. It 'was suggested that women wanted their own pay packets, the excitement of a job, and were determined to avoid the poorly paid areas of traditional women's work'.[9] On the other hand:

> many women were simply tired. They had worked long and often monotonous hours, been unable to change jobs, done the second shift of domestic work when they got home, borne the brunt of inadequate child-care and of food, clothing and petrol rationing, and often helped out with voluntary war work as well. If a newly returned husband was able to support them . . . there were many women who were only too glad to have their work-load lightened.[10]

Many women became pregnant, resulting in the 'baby boom' from 1946 to the early 1950s and emphasis on the nuclear family. Women's place at home caring for husband and children encouraged them to forgo paid employment.[11] For example, concern was expressed about the preservation of the 'feminine' qualities of women in the Australian Army Medical Women's Service. An education service was established for women in the services, 'the underlying principle of which was to stimulate and develop the natural feminine instincts which Service life could suppress. Cooking, dressmaking, baby care, handicrafts and gardening were some of the subjects taught'.[12] The prevailing ideology was one in which women should return to their homes with 'the obligation to nurse the returned soldiers'.[13]

The major industrial issue in the post-war years was the push by unions for an improvement in working conditions for 'the long hours of war production, overtime stresses, the strain of working in deteriorating conditions, and heavier taxation levels had by 1945 driven living standards to their lowest point in the War period'.[14] At the ACTU Congress that year the trade unions requested social and economic reforms and raised four main industrial issues: a 40-hour week, a substantial increase in the basic wage, an end to wage pegging and progress towards equal pay for women.[15] Wages were pegged by wartime regulations at their 1941 levels. The government foresaw that there would be a great deal of pressure to change this and 'the line pursued by the government was to delay and deflect industrial labour's array of demands in every conceivable way'.[16] The unions did not gain the increase of one pound in the basic (minimum adult male) wage which they were requesting until October 1950 when 'the Arbitration Court gave judgment in what was effectively the same case as it had commenced hearing in August 1940'.[17]

The battle for the 40-hour week was drawn out and it was not until 1 January 1948 that this was introduced in federal awards after a massive case involving 158 days of sitting, 8875 pages of transcript and 500 exhibits.[18] The Labor Government in New South Wales had already legislated for this change which came into effect in state awards on 1 July 1947 [19] and in October, Queensland legislated for this to commence on 1 January 1948.[20] The post-war years were industrially turbulent and in 1945, 1946 and 1947 almost five and a half million working days were lost due to strikes:[21]

> it was not simply that workers expected a real increase in their wages; they believed they were entitled to a 40 hour week as well. The sense of sacrifices made during the war, and the pent-up frustrations produced by wartime regulations, meant that they were prepared to take industrial action to win their objectives.[22]

But 'the picture for women was even worse, with wartime expectations that the female basic wage would at least be standardised at 75 per cent of the male rate—if not lifted to equality with it—being quite disappointed'.[23] Following the war a multiplicity of wage rates for women remained, from the low pre-war rate of 54 per cent of the male wage to the occasional 100 per cent. The government amended the Female Minimum Rates Regulations to provide for 75 per cent of the corresponding male award rate but the validity of this action was challenged in the High Court by employers' organisations and the issue was not resolved until the 1949–1950 Basic Wage Case.[24]

The ATNA remained aloof from the industrial happenings of the wider trade union movement; there is no mention of the industrial events of this period in their minutes or journal and the organisation resolutely continued to see itself as separate from the trade union movement. However, its members ultimately benefited from the gains that were made in reduced hours and increased wages.

Following the war there were still few acceptable jobs for women, especially ones which provided an education and offered status and upward mobility in society. Nursing fulfilled these conditions and accepted young women who had not completed secondary school. Given their limited opportunities, these women were unlikely to bring radical views to their union and would act as a conservative influence on the association. Thus, although there were a few complaints about pay and working conditions from members, there was no groundswell of opinion within the union. When fifteen trainees wrote to the *Courier-Mail* in 1946 complaining about their pay and working conditions, a trainee from the Brisbane Women's Hospital replied: 'There is more in nursing than "money" and "hours"; it is the most satisfying and thrilling work that any woman could undertake. I think you will find that, although a few "nitwits" are trying to pour water on old Florence, the lamp still burns.'[25]

However nurses were questioning the poor working conditions more vocally than ever before. One 'Disillusioned Trainee' from the Brisbane General Hospital blamed the officers of the ATNA for this situation:

> Though many members of the A.T.N.A. apparently desire to improve the lot of nurses, the A.T.N.A. does little in practice because it is dominated by matrons and senior sisters. In the hospitals, they act as the representatives of the Hospital Board. They are still the Board's representatives, in practice, on the A.T.N.A. Council when it takes action on behalf of trainees and younger members of the trained staff to improve living conditions.
>
> In addition, although trainee nurses are covered by the nurses' award, they have no say on the A.T.N.A. Council. It is difficult to imagine that there will be any improvement until the nurses themselves have a say in their own affairs.[26]

It was rare to see such insight publicly stated. A few weeks later 'Six Fed-Up Nurses', again from the Brisbane General Hospital, publicly aired their feelings in the daily newspaper:

> Do hospital matrons think they will receive a better staff while the conditions stay as they are?
>
> They will never have ample staff until there is more action and less talk. How do they expect young girls to leave their homes to begin nursing with the rate of pay they are receiving as well as the poor meals?[27]

At the time when trade unions were fighting hard to gain a 40-hour week, a group of trainee nurses from hospitals in the Brisbane area met with Mr Foley, Secretary for Health and Home Affairs, and requested a 44-hour week, along with a higher salary and improvements in living conditions. Foley pointed out that, although he would do all in his power to improve living conditions, the other matters had to be dealt with through the Industrial Court by changing the award. He went further and suggested to the trainees that they would need to approach the ATNA about these matters.[28] Deputations of Rockhampton nurses to the Department of Health and Home Affairs and the hospital board resulted in many improvements in working conditions.[29]

Thus groups of nurses thought that their most successful avenue for change was to lobby the minister and hospital boards directly and not work through their union. This action shows the nurses' view of the ATNA's usefulness to them when dealing with issues of better working conditions. It reflects how the ATNA officials were out of touch with the needs of nurses and trainees and the belief on the part of nurses lower down in the hospital order that changes in some conditions could be achieved more easily through direct negotiation with their employer.

For the first time there was widespread public acknowledgement by groups of nurses of how bad conditions were and these young nurses were prepared to go outside the nurses' organisation in an attempt to achieve their goals. The council of the ATNA was still operating in the world of charitable or community organisations. Its solution was to suggest that better publicity would overcome legitimate criticism of working conditions in a society which now offered women more prospects and better conditions at work.

There was a considerable amount of public pressure on the ATNA to re-evaluate nurses' working conditions and they were approached by organisations as diverse as the ALP and the United Graziers Association, as well as hospital boards. The Barcaldine Branch of the ALP sent the ATNA suggestions for improvements in nursing conditions. The United Graziers Association asked if the ATNA was taking any steps to improve nurses' wages and conditions, especially in country areas, and offered its support for this. It suggested that the new award should include increased salaries, six weeks annual leave and free rail passes each year for nurses working in country areas.[30] The Queensland Dairymen's Association wrote to the ATNA complaining that there was insufficient inducement for young women of the required education or standing to enter the nursing profession. They assured the ATNA of their whole-hearted support in any attempt to improve the pay and conditions of nurses.[31] Approaches to the ATNA also came from Trades and Labour Councils. The Women's Auxiliary of the Ipswich TLC approached the Minister for Health and Home Affairs about the provision of free text books for pupil nurses. The Minister replied that this was an industrial matter that should go to the Industrial Court. He suggested this to the ATNA, but no moves along these lines were made.[32] The Townsville TLC assured the ATNA of their support in any attempt to achieve wage rises.[33]

Conditions for nurses were presumably so bad and the difficulties of gaining and retaining staff in rural areas so great that several country hospitals asked the ATNA to initiate proceedings for improved conditions in the award. The Ayr Hospital Board in north Queensland offered their support in any approach to the Industrial Court for increased salaries and better conditions.[34] The Townsville Hospitals Board asked the ATNA Council to include a salary increase for the sister-in-charge and her assistant in the Maternity Block.[35] The Longreach Hospitals Board, in western Queensland, approached the Department of Health with a recommendation that the Western Parity Allowance be increased to 15 shillings a week.[36] Thus a strange situation emerged whereby employers requested the trade union to improve conditions in the award, even though this would add to the expense of running a hospital.

As well as offers of support the ATNA faced criticism of nursing conditions[37] and the inadequacy of its own actions. The council viewed these negative remarks as harmful and in December 1945 several executive members met with Mr R.G. Robinson, Under-Secretary of the Department of Health and Home Affairs, to consider improvements in nursing conditions. The result of the meeting was that a proposal was made that the 'destructive criticism of nursing affairs' be offset by a film and articles in local papers on nursing conditions.[38] The film, *A Noble Profession*, 'sought to communicate the message that a nurse "is not just a slave to nursing but that the nursing career helps to develop the individual characteristics each young lady may possess" '. It was designed to promote the benefits of a nursing career, but 'the professional element in nursing was . . . trivialised. One student began with the expected sense of vocation, one wanted to marry a doctor, one wanted to accumulate material for a novel and one wanted secure employment'.[39]

While community organisations and even employers were pressing for award changes to working conditions, nurses themselves took what action they could and bypassed the ATNA in seeking better conditions. The council had not yet separated its interests from those of the employing hospital boards and still saw itself as working with employers in the interests of nursing while numbers of its practitioners and community groups were complaining of the poor conditions.

Shortages of nurses

The cessation of fighting in August 1945 did not bring with it an increase in the number of nurses. In fact, the return to peacetime conditions exacerbated the dearth of trained nurses and trainees. Shortages of nursing staff were obvious and acknowledged by all sectors of the industry. The Queensland Government reported in 1946 that the position was the same in every state and that 'although it is expected that the position might ease to some extent so far as trainees are concerned, there appears to be little hope that there will be sufficient trained nurses to completely staff all public hospitals in Queensland for some time to come'.[40] In the three years from October 1943 to March 1946 the shortage of nurses in public hospitals had grown from 154 to 538 (including 307 trainees), an increase of 350 per cent.[41] The situation further deteriorated and in October 1948 the shortage of nurses was approximately 739.[42] Free treatment in public hospitals meant a growing number of hospital patients exacerbated the problem. An increase of almost 10 per cent in the number of in-patients was met with a decrease of 6 per cent in nursing staff.[43]

The staffing position in country hospitals was usually worse than in Brisbane. Townsville Public Hospital did not have enough trained staff to allow each ward to have a sister in charge.[44] Nurses were working up to 30 hours overtime a fortnight and annual leave could not be taken at the proper time. The hospital appealed over the radio for volunteers to relieve the critical staff shortage. Unless assistance could be obtained it was feared that three wards would have to be closed and the hospital would function solely on an emergency basis.[45]

The situation was so serious in many country hospitals that the *Courier-Mail* called it 'the most acute shortage of nurses in Australia's history'. While staff worked 'heroically' and waited, 'hoping that relief will come', 'districts which fostered local hospitals from the earliest days face[d] the prospect of having sick and injured transported long distances by air and road for treatment'.[46] The Cloncurry Hospital in the north-west of the state lost the matron and two sisters in early October 1945, leaving two sisters and six trainees to staff the 50-bed hospital.[47] Serious cases were sent to Mt Isa, 190 kilometres away, or Julia Creek, 130 kilometres away.[48] Towards the end of 1945 other regional hospitals were worried. Longreach had lost staff following the relaxation of the manpower restrictions with the result that it had half its normal complement of nurses and no matron.[49] In December 1946 the hospitals at Miles and Surat closed because of staff shortages.[50] By late 1948 another hospital had closed and 95 of the 113 public hospitals in the state were short of staff.[51] The situation in private hospitals was also grave. From 30 September 1939 to 25 March 1947, 86 private hospitals with a capacity of 689 beds closed.[52]

The state-wide staffing difficulties meant that 'matrons, sisters and trainees in hospitals in various parts of the State must assume added duties and responsibilities and undertake more arduous work than previously'.[53] Judges W.J. Riordan and T.E. Dwyer, hearing the nurses' cases in the Queensland Industrial Court in 1946 and 1947, felt that 'this shortage of nursing staff and the closure of hospitals has thrown abnormal work upon the nursing staffs who remain, as in addition to her normal work each nurse has now to attend to a greater number of patients than previously'.[54]

At a time of full employment, nursing suffered by comparison with other jobs. Overcoming the desperate shortage meant trying to recruit staff from an already depleted pool. By October 1945 the Manpower Regulations no longer allowed the direction of nurses, one of the major reasons for the continuing shortage according to the ATNA.[55] Despite some cries that servicewomen should take up nursing, many returned to 'home duties'.[56]

The reason why so many gave up nursing, Miss Joan Burgess, secretary of the ATNA in Queensland, believed, was the combination of poor salary and working conditions and lack of amenities in hospitals.[57] Justice Riordan felt that the shortage of nurses was caused by more general factors:

> During the war a number of women and girls who would have gone into training for nurses joined the Army and recruiting stopped for that period. That happened in many callings and even in rural industries. Boys who were taken from farms into the Services have not gone back to the farms to any great extent. The result is that labour in rural districts is scarce. The same thing applies in this case. There was the loss of all that time in training nurses.[58]

The conclusions drawn by Industrial Court judges were grim because 'unless greater numbers are attracted to the nursing profession there is a grave doubt as to the ability of the authorities to maintain health services to the public to the desired degree'.[59]

The continuing shortage of domestic staff placed added burdens on nurses. A report on ANF activities presented to the International Council of Nurses in May 1947 enumerated reasons for the shortages:

> living conditions undoubtedly need improvement, but the tendency to require nurses to perform other than nursing duties which was necessary during the war period still continues and appears to be the main cause of the trouble. Domestics whether for hospital or civilian service are practically unprocurable and until the status and conditions of this class of worker are bettered it is doubtful whether the position will be improved.[60]

The crux of the problem was identified by all sectors of the community as the poor conditions and low salaries. Miss Burgess felt that:

> if the living conditions in hospitals were made more attractive there would be more nurses. The hospital is a nurse's home. As many amenities as the authorities and the local community can manage should be put there.
>
> Nurses do not want coddling, but they do want reasonable treatment.[61]

Others saw the difficulties as more complicated. A 'Special Correspondent', writing in the *Courier-Mail* in November 1945, did not attempt a solution of this 'complex problem' but offered some suggestions to keep the hospitals open:

> The Florence Nightingale tradition has suffered in the material world of our time. Most young women now regard nursing as they would any other profession, in terms of salary and conditions—and matrimonial opportunity.
>
> They find themselves no longer obliged to stay in places they do not like.
>
> There is too much drudgery in nursing for girls who can get easier employment.
>
> In country hospitals life is dull, amenities are few.
>
> The public has not taken enough interest in the hospital staffs that serve it.
>
> In distant places particularly communities might follow the example of a generous few and give nurses a happier social life.[62]

In some cases nurses' quarters were inadequate and unsuitable for the climate. Trained nurses were 'requested to share small bedrooms, the quarters contain insufficient wash basins and no separate provision is made for the matron'.[63] Miss Burgess added that:

> the rooms are insufficiently ventilated, are small and meagrely furnished. In some country hospitals nurses have been accommodated on the verandah which is closed in with bags. The food often is inadequate, badly cooked and unpalatable. Nurses have refused their meals and the greater part of their salary has been spent in providing themselves with meals outside the hospital.[64]

The Roma Hospital Board advised the Department of Health and Home Affairs that it would be impossible adequately to staff hospitals in the west 'for years to come' unless amenities comparable to those found on the coast were available.[65] The ANF Conference in February 1946 resolved to urge all hospital boards to provide nurses and trainees with comfortable single rooms with adequate lighting and heating, facilities for bathing, laundry, writing and a recreation room. Where new accommodation was built it should include a visitors' reception room, a library and a pantry.[66]

The Queensland Government initially argued that its top priority was the provision of public housing, that its housing construction programme absorbed all available manpower and that it was 'impracticable for many hospital boards' to provide such accommodation.[67] However between the case in the Queensland Industrial Court in September 1946 and its continuation in April 1947, hospital boards in the state were instructed to provide all possible amenities for nurses as an expression of the government's appreciation of their loyalty and service.[68] According to Mr A. Jones, Secretary for Health and Home Affairs, the government was bound to provide better accommodation for nurses because 'the average nurse comes from a respectable family and it cannot be expected that she will be induced to take up a given class of employment if suitable accommodation is not provided'.[69]

Private employers were less happy about improving the standard of nurses' accommodation. Their advocate, Mr P.J. Self, argued that the accommodation claims were too expensive.[70] Canon Massey, speaking on behalf of St Martin's Hospital and the Church of England, felt they were 'too elaborate'. Two foot six inch wide beds provided 'ample and sufficient comfort'. Three foot wide beds as asked for would mean the added expense of buying new beds.[71] Massey defended the few rooms with two beds in them on the grounds that:

> numbers of beginners are lonely and need companionship, particularly in the solitude of a bedroom. By sharing rooms, in some cases a great number of employees have been retained in their employment

> when otherwise they would have left to return to their homes. Lasting friendships have also been formed in these circumstances, and that is surely to the advantage not only of the nurses themselves, but of the hospital itself and becomes reflected in the efficiency of the hospital.[72]

Other suggestions for alleviating the shortage came from the public. A letter to the *Courier-Mail* stated that:

> it does not seem fair that so many hospitals have to close down for need of help, especially in the country, where they are badly needed. There is much talk of demobilisation of the women's forces; is there any reason why they cannot be directed to the hospitals? Many of them have nursing and cooking experience.[73]

This suggestion brought an angry response:

> How can 'Wellwisher' . . . have the temerity to write such eyewash about demobilised servicewomen being 'directed' to work in hospitals? Does 'Wellwisher' think that girls who know what it is like to wash up greasy cooking dishes, dixies, &c., do guard every night, rough it in the semi-jungle, live on 4/4 or 6/ per day, have only 24 hours off a week, and be on duty for 24 hours a day, want to be 'directed' to do something along the same lines?
>
> Wake up, 'Wellwisher.' I suppose that you are one of those people who think the life of a servicewoman was easy. We did it out of a sense of duty, and didn't complain until we saw such a letter as yours.[74]

If better conditions were beyond the resources of government, perhaps altruism could be tried instead, as one writer to the women's pages of the *Courier-Mail* suggested:

> I should like to see the women of Brisbane who generously opened their homes to lads of the services during the war to do so again—this time to the trainees of the hospitals, whose homes are not in the city. These girls are just as much in need of the touch of home as the lads to whom everyone gave generously.
>
> They do not need elaborate entertainment, but a home in which to spend off-duty hours away from the hospital atmosphere, somewhere to wash their hair in tank water and relax in homely surroundings. Such a gesture might do much to help overcome the shortage of nurses. After all we need the nurses, so it is up to us.[75]

The images and language of military organisation, developed during the war years, were applied to the nursing crisis in a way that would not have fitted other occupations. The selflessness and poor conditions under which nurses laboured made the comparison with service life possible and reflected the military origins of the profession.

Male nurses and medical orderlies were used in an effort to alleviate the shortage of female nurses.[76] While some parliamentarians were in favour of this,[77] Mr Alf Muller, Member for Fassifern, did not agree: 'Because of their natures, men are not as suitable as nurses as women are'.[78] Other steps were taken to alleviate the shortage of nurses. At the Brisbane Women's Hospital nursing aids, young women of sixteen years, were employed to help the obstetrics trainees. Women without nursing training were accepted for an obstetrics training course of eighteen months which could be followed by a six months' course in maternal and child welfare. Nurses willing to undertake part-time and relieving duties were also employed by the board.[79] The age of entry to training was reduced from eighteen to seventeen. Mr Nicklin applauded this move saying that 'there is keen competition for girls leaving school. In the commercial world there are many attractive vacancies. Many businesses are paying above award wages to obtain the services of these girls'.[80] The minimum age of 21 for registration as a nurse was removed so that those qualifying could be registered immediately.[81] In October 1946, Mr Foley summed up the situation:

> I think I can say without fear of contradiction that the nurses who have been carrying on have given a very efficient service to patients despite the disabilities under which they have been working. Of course, we have paid a tremendous amount in overtime, and that cannot continue without having some effect upon the health of the staff as a whole.[82]

The broken shifts, overtime, poor accommodation and low salaries that nurses endured continued to compare unfavourably with the more attractive salaries and conditions offered in other occupations. The Industrial Court believed that 'the rates of remuneration prescribed by this award do not make adequate recompense for the duties called for and do not provide a sufficient inducement to trainees to undertake the necessary course of training to qualify for the profession'.[83] Statements by Mr Foley that the shortage was not due to poor remuneration[84] provoked an angry response in a letter to the *Courier-Mail* asking what he knew of nurses' conditions:

> There have been so many improvements and facilities made available for factory workers, wharf labourers, coal miners, and shop assistants, nobody, however, has troubled to think that nurses would like a few improvements and facilities as well.

> This nursing shortage is frequently discussed, yet nothing is ever done about it. Not until it is realised that nurses are human beings who need vitamins and good food, understanding, recreational facilities, and decent pay as well as other workers will there be any desire for girls and women to become nurses.[85]

Changing the award, 1946 and 1947

One solution that was obvious to the majority of the parties involved in the 'nursing crisis' was that improved conditions, including increased wages, were needed. Although committees during the war had pointed to the low pay and poor working conditions as a major cause of the dire nursing shortage it took until February 1946 for the Queensland Branch of the ATNA to decide to approach the Industrial Court for an award variation.[86] The catalyst for change in this period was the continuing, desperate shortage of nurses, exacerbated by a chronic shortage of hospitals at the end of the war.[87] The arguments put forward for wage rises for nurses in Queensland in 1946 relied heavily on the question of shortages. Miss Burgess, who presented the case for the ATNA, stressed that:

> owing to the falling off in applications for training in hospitals, mainly brought about by war conditions and more attractive positions offering in other occupations, e.g. higher salaries, greater recreation periods and better working and living conditions, the nursing situation is acute and some inducement must be made to girls to undertake nursing as a career and ensure the completion of their training.

When asked for further details she said that 'on several occasions . . . members of our association have resigned to take up other occupations. For instance, Army nurses are opening florists' shops with their deferred pay in preference to going back to nursing'.[88]

As nursing was an occupation that had existed for women long before the start of the Second World War, it had not benefited from any changes that occurred for 'new' female occupations or those for which male rates were paid. Nurses' wages were low because men were not employed as general nurses. Under the terms used for remedying an anomaly, the wages could not be raised very far because there was no male comparison and rates were always low. Since salaries for all nurses were depressed, comparison with other nurses' salaries could not lift them far out of this rut. Their salaries therefore remained low when compared with other workers, even other female workers.

While nurses suffered under the pressures of shortages, unable to secure salary increases, another set of regulations was gazetted that assisted some women workers. On 30 August 1945, the National Security (Female Minimum Rates) Regulations were amended so that 'any female employed in any occupation within a vital industry' was to be paid no less than 75 per cent of the corresponding minimum male rate.[89] The industries designated as vital included 'the occupations of the domestic staffs of hospitals, asylums and institutions of a like nature'.[90] A severe shortage of both domestic staff and nurses in hospitals was acknowledged, yet only the domestic staff were included in this regulation. Admittedly there was no comparable male rate for nurses yet neither was there for some of the classifications of domestic staff in hospitals, as a number of jobs were performed exclusively by women or men. This change upset the relativities between female staff in hospital employment.

Nurses' wages remained depressed as they could not be compared with other workers. They had not been subject to any ruling of the WEB or the adjustment of wages upward by regulation, but were bound by the application of the concept of anomaly. The slight improvement in their wages after the war only occurred when the staffing position of hospitals was so acute that the employers themselves approached the courts for increases or agreed that these increases were necessary and urgent.[91] Private employers, however, did not advocate wage increases and emphasised the qualities of self-sacrifice and dedication without reward. The fact that nursing was a unique female occupation in which service and sacrifice were essential components controlled the wage-fixing outcomes.

The case began in September 1946 but was not concluded until February the following year. Reduced hours were gained in 1946, however increased wages had to wait until 1947. Neither the ATNA nor Miss Burgess understood the complex National Security Regulations with which the court had to comply in order to grant wage increases. Although the Industrial Court believed that award rates of pay should be altered,[92] it could not legally do this until the requirements of the national regulations were met. Only with help from government sources and suggestions from the Industrial Court was the ATNA able to apply for and gain increases for nurses in 1947, who therefore waited longer than necessary for these changes.

To achieve increased wages the ATNA had to prove an anomaly existed in relation to the claim for a wage increase, yet it had no idea how to do this within the precise terms of the complex wartime regulations. The State Industrial Court had to undertake a preliminary examination of the case and, if there was sufficient evidence which met the precise terms of the regulations, a case could be submitted to the Chief Judge of the Commonwealth Court of Conciliation and Arbitration. If the Chief Judge agreed he could make an order authorising the State Industrial Court to hear and determine the case.[93] Changes in wages could be achieved if there was a change of circumstances in the employment or in comparable employment since the introduction of the regulations in 1942.[94] Increased workloads due to staff shortages were not deemed sufficient evidence.

The question of what an anomaly was and how it was judged was crucial to the assessment of nurses' wages. When the ATNA attempted to gain wage increases in 1946 the inadequacy of its evidence meant that the case was unsuccessful. The outcome hinged on what was legally considered to be an anomaly and this was judged very narrowly. An anomaly in nurses' wages existed only when there was a discrepancy among the rates paid to nurses, not a discrepancy among the wages paid to comparable groups of workers, such as other female occupations or hospital workers. Like was compared with like, so that an anomaly would be accepted when nurses' wages, as determined by one industrial authority, fell behind those determined by another authority. The ATNA did not understand how to prove this.

Lack of knowledge of relevant legislation and industrial relations practices and an unwillingness to seek advice meant that the ATNA in Queensland did not succeed in its claim for increased wages in 1946. The association put together a very rudimentary case for the hearing in September 1946. When dealing with claims for increases in nurses' salaries Miss Burgess steadfastly gave the reason that 'the anomaly is that owing to the change of circumstances the present rate is inadequate' or that 'the anomaly is the inadequacy of the present rates'.[95]

The members of the bench tried to help her by asking for further information. After hearing her response several times, Justice Ferry said 'you will have to show something more than that if you wish this Court to give you any assistance in getting an increase in the rates of pay'. He outlined the regulations, and said that 'the facts contained in your statement would not be sufficient for us to send to the Chief Judge of the Federal Court'. Ferry then asked if there was any change in the conditions of employment, to which Miss Burgess replied ineffectually, 'I think the duties of these employees have increased. The sick population has increased'. But no further evidence was brought by the ATNA to support this argument even though Ferry responded that if they could show these things, 'it would be something'. After more evidence from the ATNA Ferry again tried to assist the nurses, suggesting that it would help their case if they could show that nurses were leaving to take up other employment. When Miss Burgess answered 'yes' Ferry wearily replied, 'if you could do that, it might help'.[96]

The judges tried to point the union case in the right direction, but to no avail. The ATNA claimed an increase in salaries and when pressed for a reason said that it was because of the increased cost of living. But the Bench reminded the union that wages were still pegged by the Commonwealth Government and there had to be changed circumstances. Miss Burgess said that there had been increases in Western Australia, New South Wales and Victoria. Riordan replied that:

> the circumstances of your particular work have to change or we have to find that there is an anomaly. We cannot do that by saying the wages have changed in other States. They must have had changed circumstances there for the wages to increase. If they have changed here we will be only too pleased to recommend an increase for you.

Ferry advised them that the reasons given in other cases might assist them.[97] Miss Burgess did not address herself to the legal requirements necessary to achieve an increase, merely saying that 'if Queensland wishes to retain a high standard in the nursing profession, the Queensland rates should be made to compare favourably with those of the other States'. She concluded:

> the added duties for nurses, plus the shortage of nurses, throw extra responsibility on the existing staff. Nurses are carrying much greater responsibility than at the time of the last hearing. They cannot be given extra time off or extra leave and the only fair and equitable way of recompensing them for the additional duties is to grant them extra money. A critical stage is being reached in hospital staffs in Queensland, which, if not arrested early might result in calamity. The wages and nursing conditions must therefore be such as will attract enough of the right type of girl for this highly important national service.[98]

The ATNA's past history of rarely filing claims for better conditions was recalled. Riordan stated that 'the public generally have been led to believe that the nurses in Queensland . . . were in a very bad way. Probably they did not know that the nurses themselves appeared to be content inasmuch as they have not approached the Court for an increase'. Miss Burgess replied with the telling statement that 'the nurses themselves have requested us time and time again to approach the Court for increases in salary and better working conditions'. Riordan pointed out that they could have been in court a year earlier. Although that had been their intention, Miss Burgess replied, it had taken nearly a year to prepare the claim.[99]

Miss Burgess, representing the ATNA, believed in the justice of her case, and neither the public employers nor the judges of the Industrial Court doubted this. What the ATNA did not realise was that the rectitude of its case was not enough to gain wage increases, and the stringent legality of wartime regulations had also to be addressed. At the conclusion of the case in 1946, the members of the Industrial Court of Queensland submitted their opinion and reasons to the Chief Judge of the Commonwealth Court of Conciliation and Arbitration under Regulation 18 (3) of the National Security (Economic Organization) Regulations:

> the rates of remuneration prescribed by this award are anomalous in that they do not provide adequate recompense, when other awards are taken into consideration, for the skill, training and work required of nurses and that the existing staff shortages and consequent extra work provide *prima facie* evidence of changes in the circumstances of employment.[100]

Details used to reinforce this opinion were the acute shortage of nursing labour; the extra work this put on the remaining staff; rates of pay which did not adequately recompense staff or provide sufficient inducement for trainees to commence in the profession; the need for more highly specialised knowledge; loss of relativity between nurses' wages and those of domestic staff; the large number of nurses from the forces refusing to resume civilian nursing. Unless greater numbers were attracted into the profession there was 'grave doubt' that health services could be carried on 'to the desired degree'.[101]

In November 1946 however, Justice Drake-Brockman replied that he could not agree that the information given provided *prima facie* evidence that there were any changed circumstances which called for compensation or that the rates of pay were anomalous. If further and better evidence was made available, he would be prepared to reconsider the matter at any time.[102] The ATNA was aghast at this decision, although the lack of success in this case plainly derived from the union's poor preparation and its lack of industrial sophistication. A special council meeting of thirteen members decided to send a telegram to the Prime Minister protesting this decision with a letter stressing the fact that nurses in repatriation hospitals received a higher salary. The ATNA argued that the difference in the rates of pay between nurses under

Commonwealth and state awards was clearly an anomaly, this time using the term correctly.[103]

By December the union had submitted another claim for a variation of their award to the Industrial Court.[104] In February 1947 the council meeting decided that someone conversant with court procedure should present the case to the Industrial Court and Mr Robinson, Under Secretary, suggested that Mr H. Harvey, President of the Trades and Labour Council, might be able to assist the ATNA. The council approached him for advice on the arguments submitted by the opposing parties at the previous hearing and decided to accept his advice on award matters. The claim was filed immediately.[105]

Harvey presented a carefully researched submission giving precise details of the shortages in public hospitals and in April 1947 judges Riordan and Dwyer wrote to the Commonwealth Court saying that the ATNA had applied to the court to re-open the case on the grounds that they had further and better evidence. This evidence included precise details of the nursing shortage and its effects on the delivery of health care and the inadequacy of the pay. The court was of the opinion that there was *prima facie* evidence that alterations to the rates of pay should be made because of the shortage of nurses and the anomalous position which had come about because nurses in the Repatriation Department earnt more.[106] A few days later Judge Drake-Brockman replied that the Queensland Court could hear and determine the matter.[107]

In April 1947 wage increases of 17.5 per cent to 18.5 per cent were granted. The ATNA considered that Harvey had been 'to a great extent instrumental in gaining such gratifying increases'.[108] This was ironic because the ATNA steadfastly avoided thinking about itself as a trade union and it certainly could never have conceived of joining the Trades and Labour Council. Yet it had accepted the help of its chief officer when, even more remarkably, this had been suggested by a representative of the employers.

ATNA philosophy

In relation to wage increases, the ATNA still asked for increases in terms of the necessities of life and did not compare the work and remuneration of nurses with other occupations involving extensive training and responsibility. They did not compare themselves with other hospital workers in terms of the relativities that had traditionally existed. It is ironic that some of this evidence was used by the employers in support of their call for wage increases for nurses. The rationale for increased wages once again included nurses' inability to save for their old age. The ANF conference in early 1946 noted that:

> the salary of the average trained nurse in a hospital post, with the present high cost of living, is totally inadequate . . . In many instances it is little more than that paid to an unqualified person, and certainly not comparable with the mental and physical strain imposed on the trained nurse, nor does she have an opportunity to save for her future.[109]

The need for better conditions to attract more nursing recruits was also emphasised by Miss Burgess in the 1946 case as this would be 'a bigger inducement for girls to take up nursing and so relieve the situation . . . They commence training at present and due to long hours and lack of amenities they give up at the end of 12 months'.[110] In these views the ATNA was supported by public sympathies. Parliamentarians frequently spoke of the hardships of the nurse's life and complained about their low salaries.[111] Mr Tom Aikens, Member for Mundingburra, felt that trainees had a difficult life:

> Twenty-five bob a week and tucker and she does not get the same freedom of movement as the girl who works in industry. She is more or less under the rigid discipline of the matron . . . She must be in the hospital by a certain hour every night. If she wants to go out and spend an evening with her friends she must get permission. She must attend various lectures and lessons two or three times a week . . .
>
> After she has served for four years, after she has studied for four years and passed her first general nursing examination, she has to go to a hospital registered as a midwifery training centre and start all over again at a few shillings a week for another six or nine months in order to qualify for her midwifery certificate. So that for five years, that girl who starts at 18 years of age has to work for scandalously low wages . . . You cannot expect a girl to serve an apprenticeship of five years for the noblest profession any woman can follow and then at the end of it get not £2 14s. a week and tucker.[112]

Nurses were among the last groups in the community to receive a reduction in their hours of work, for the ATNA did not approach the Industrial Court about this until 1946. Nurses still worked a 96-hour fortnight. However, cases in 1946 and 1947 brought nurses into line with other workers by reducing their hours first to 88 and then to 80 hours per fortnight, a direct result of the general trade union push for a 40-hour week. When nurses finally received a reduction in their working hours, it was once again calculated over the period of a fortnight to give the employer more flexibility in arranging the nursing work of the hospital.

The initial reduction in hours to 88 per fortnight came years after this had been achieved by the majority of workers in Queensland. The way had been open for nurses to have a 44-hour week since the introduction of the *Industrial Conciliation and Arbitration Act* in 1932, which stipulated a 44-hour week.[113] The move by the ATNA to gain the shorter working week was prompted by a report to the council in March 1946 of a meeting of Brisbane and Ipswich trainee nurses with the Minister for Health and Home Affairs, Mr Foley, at which they requested a 44-hour week, higher salary and improved living conditions. Foley advised them to see the ATNA about these matters.[114]

When the ATNA applied for a reduction in hours in 1946, the past attitudes of the union returned to haunt it. At the court hearing in December that year the judge pointed out that 'on one occasion when application was made here for a 44-hour week, the nurses opposed it'. Miss Burgess could only reply that 'it was different in those times'.[115] The government gave evidence that 1013 Queensland hospital nurses were already working a 44-hour week, excluding overtime. The 1605 staff at all other country hospitals were on a 48-hour week. Nurses in Victoria, Western Australia and Tasmania worked a 44-hour week.[116] Justice Riordan said that there was no reason why nurses should not get a 44-hour week: 'The only reason you have not had it in the past is because you did not want it, generally speaking, but there is no reason why you should be asked to work longer hours.'[117] Thus on 23 December 1946, fourteen years after the enactment of legislation making such an application possible, the court granted nurses an 88-hour fortnight to bring them into line with other workers.

In October 1947, the Queensland Government legislated for a 40-hour week to commence from 1 January 1948 and the ATNA Council applied for an 80-hour fortnight.[118] There was no objection to the claim from the government or private hospitals although Mr D. Fraser, advocate for the Crown and hospital boards, pointed out that, because of the shortage of nurses, the staff would have to work longer than the 40 hours and overtime rates be paid.[119] From 1 January 1948, nurses joined much of the workforce with a shorter week[120] but because of staff shortages hospitals could not find the extra nurses needed and staff were paid four hours overtime on top of their pay for a 40-hour week.[121] Thus there was no immediate solution to the long hours actually worked. As nurses at the Ipswich Hospital commented:

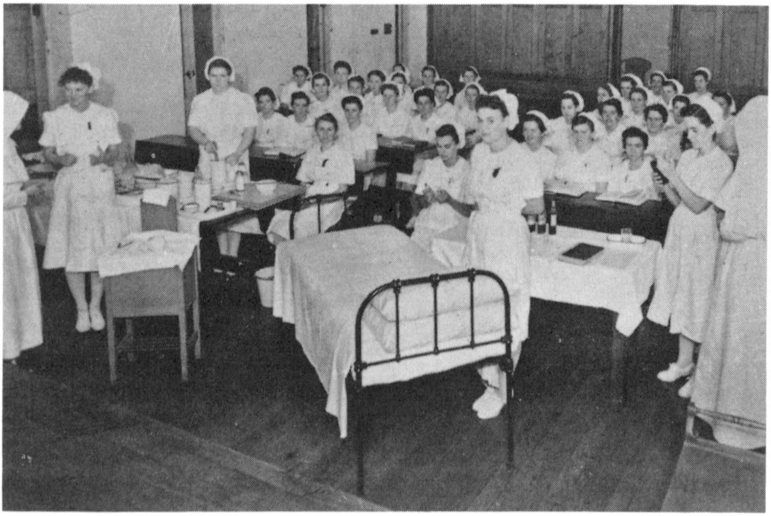

A practical demonstration in the nurses' study at the Mater Misericordiae Hospital, Brisbane, during off-duty hours, 1947. It shows bedmaking, preparing or measuring medicines, testing the temperature with a bath thermometer and preparing a treatment, possibly an eye bath. (Collection: John Oxley Library, Brisbane.)

> Whatever reduction in working hours per week we may be granted by the Court, the same work has to be done in the ward, actually in less time, and nurses will be working just as long unless staffs are increased.
>
> Whilst an increase in pay is appreciated by trainees, the extra overtime paid when a shorter week is worked will not in any way solve the problem of how to shorten nurses' working hours. The change will be in theory only and not in practice.[122]

This reduction in hours did not apply to matrons, who had to wait longer to have their hours regulated. In April 1948 the ATNA requested that matrons be given an 80-hour fortnight, with not more than twelve hours to be worked consecutively in any day.[123] The problem was that matrons in small hospitals were earning less than the sisters on their staff who were paid overtime. Also, country hospitals with less than nine beds, one-third of the total number of public hospitals in the state, had 'acute' staffing problems and great difficulty obtaining matrons. The matron was 'very often' the only trained nurse and 'not having a sufficient staff of Sisters means that the Matrons are called upon to work very long hours and are virtually on call almost continuously'.

The ATNA emphasised the important work of the matron: 'There is no doubt . . . that the Matron sets the tone for the whole hospital. If young nurses are to be inspired by a sense of service, consideration for their patients and a devotion to duty, it is the Matron by her precept and example who will be required to lead them in these matters.' The ATNA added that 'unless this position is given its correct status (and this is a very important point) as well as at least adequate remuneration and reasonable working hours, the right type of women will not apply for these positions and the whole structure of nursing will suffer'.[124] These difficulties were recognised by Cabinet which decided to increase the matrons' salaries from January 1948[125] and following a conference between the ATNA and the government, agreement was reached, with the hours of matrons remaining unspecified by the award. The wages were increased by 10 to 25 per cent, depending on the size of the hospital.[126]

More controversial than the reduction in hours was the ATNA request that nurses work unbroken eight-hour shifts, a condition that had first been requested by the QNA in 1921. Nurses wanted straight shifts and had asked the ATNA to pursue this. Broken shifts were 'quite customary' and for instance, frequently worked on two or three days a week at the Brisbane General and Ipswich Hospitals.[127] When working these shifts a nurse might 'not retire until 11 p.m. or even later, yet the nurse is expected to obtain sufficient rest following an arduous day's work and again be on duty at 6 a.m. the following day to face another day which may be heavier than the previous one'.[128] The ATNA's case was based on the need for shorter hours because of the hard work nurses performed:

> The work of a nurse is of a strenuous and tiring nature, requiring steady concentration and a keen and alert mind. To carry out her duties efficiently and thoroughly a nurse must be well rested and physically capable of executing her duties to the best of her ability.
>
> It is a well-known fact that the health of the majority of our nurses, as a result of the stress and overwork during the war years has been seriously undermined—mainly because of the long hours of duty they have had to perform.[129]

With the amount of overtime being worked, a nurse could be working twelve to fourteen hours a day.[130]

The uniqueness of nursing as an occupation was still emphasised in 1950. Many nurses and certainly the ATNA Council thought of nurses as different from other workers. This is evident in the view towards penalty rates for weekend work. Although nurses in repatriation hospitals under the federal award received these rates, a general meeting of ATNA members in Queensland in 1949 voted unanimousy that the ATNA should not apply for weekend penalty rates. Miss Paten's view was that 'the nurse who took up nursing whole-heartedly, knew that she would have to make many sacrifices of which working at the week-end was one'. Although Miss Kennedy, who had spoken for higher wages for nurses working outside hospitals, agreed in principal, she added that 'it must be realised that the nurses of to-day live on the same economic plane as other people'. But in the ensuing debate she agreed that overtime payments would be sufficient.[131]

Views of employers

At the initial hearing of the case in September 1946 the major employer, the State Government, opposed the increases proposed by the union[132] but the position of the government had changed considerably by the second hearing in April 1947 and it fully supported wage increases for nurses. Because of staff shortages the government saw it as 'imperative that the rates of remuneration of nurses, sisters and matrons should be such as will attract and retain the services of efficient and trained persons in the nursing staffs of the public hospitals of Queensland'.[133] Thus the severity of the staffing problem had overcome objections to the increased cost of running the state's hospitals.

Increases in nurses' wages in southern states disturbed the relativities which had existed between Queensland and the other states, and this, the government advocate Mr Fraser submitted, constituted an anomaly. Nurses in New South Wales had had their rates of pay increased from December 1946; in South Australia and Tasmania from January 1947; and in Victoria from 27 February 1947. Added to this, the higher wages of sisters in the Repatriation Department were 'a most prominent local anomaly'. These points, and the shortage of staff which had led to greater responsibility on the part of nurses, meant an increase should be granted.[134] Mr Fraser concluded the case for the public employers saying that although the government did not support 'the large and disproportionate increases sought by the Union', higher wages were necessary: 'It is in the national interests that increases in the remuneration of the nursing staffs of public hospitals be granted so as to attract and retain nursing staffs and thus remedy the staff shortages which threaten the efficient functioning of this important national service'.[135]

In addition the increased wages of domestic staff employed in public hospitals had severely disturbed the relativities in the wages of hospital employees. When domestic staff in hospitals had been granted 75 per cent of the male rate of pay in September 1945, their wages had risen from 3 pounds 13 shillings to 4 pounds 4 shillings and 9 pence.[136] This compared with a weekly salary of 3 pounds 8 shillings for a first year sister, grade II.[137] As one newspaper article commented, 'the final indignity to the trained nurse is the fact that when wages of women in industry were raised to 75 per cent of the male rate, a nursing assistant, with no experience, was paid more than the qualified girl with years of training'.[138]

The private hospitals were not as keen to accept wage rises. Mr P.J. Self, who appeared in the Industrial Court for the Private Hospitals' Association, Queensland Employers' Association and Chamber of Manufacturers, expressed the view that nurses' wages compared more than favourably with those of 'girls' in other callings. He stated that these hospitals did 'not find any evidence of discontent among . . . employees regarding their wages or conditions . . . we believe that their conditions would be more congenial than those in larger institutions'.[139] Self reported that 'private hospital proprietors agree that their nursing staffs are entitled to the best wages and conditions that can be offered, but do not consider that any substantial increases are justified in all the circumstances'.[140]

Naturally, the employers assessed the cost of the ATNA claim and decided that 'the main bone of contention in regard to this claim is its exorbitant nature'.[141] The private employers expressed concern that the increased wages would impose hardship on their hospitals and result in the closure of some of them.[142] For example, Self produced a letter from St Vincent's Private Hospital, Bundaberg, saying that if the claims were granted and fees were pegged then in desperation the hospital would close down. The letter continued:

> The A.T.N. Association ought to try and run a private hospital in these drought-stricken parts.
>
> It would not be an increase they would be asking for but a decrease in wages. You have no idea what the country is like here; farmers who crushed 2,000 to 3,000 tons a year [of sugar cane] will only crush 200 tons . . .
>
> How we are going to pay such a high increase in wages I do not know. I am afraid there will be very few Private Hospitals left if the Award and conditions come into force. My Banking Account shows £12 profit from February to June 30th. Puzzle it out and see if it will

allow an increase of £1 a week to trained nurses and all the other impossible conditions.

I am doing the work of 3 people so as to try and carry on; but I will not do it under the new Award. I will definitely close down.[143]

In the 1946 case Canon R.V. Massey, representing the Proprietors of St Martin's Hospital and the Church of England, Brisbane, did not oppose the proposed wage rates, saying that 'we admit at once that nurses are in every respect worthy of and deserve the increased remuneration proposed'.[144] But in the case the following April he opposed the addition of basic wage increases, which had been granted since the first claim had been lodged. He felt that an increase in salaries would not lead to an influx of nurses:

nursing is a vocation. People are called to it or not called to it. A good nurse cannot be bought with money. She will find her way there in spite of remuneration because with her that is a secondary consideration. On the other hand, attractive salaries would not attract other women and girls who are not keen to undertake the work. It is distasteful to them. If they did go into the nursing profession for what they could get out of it then the standard of nursing would be lowered and the patients, who are the people to be considered, would suffer.[145]

At the same time Massey said:

I think it is only a fair thing that an expression of gratitude should be given to the nurses for their work, but that such an increase must be subject to private hospitals being able to pay the extra expense. I do not say that they should not receive an adequate wage. We are all in favour of that. The people I represent want the nurses to be adequately paid, but we feel there must be a limit.[146]

Self claimed that benevolent institutions should not come under the award. He put forward the view that:

a trained certificated nurse is not essential to them. That is proved by the fact that in many of the homes no trained nurse is employed. However, when they get a woman who is prepared to devote her life to the work, because she is a trained nurse she must come under the award, while other places are allowed to go scot free. You get these charitably-minded women who are prepared to work the ends of their fingers off to help the old people in the homes, but if you ask them to add another £100 a year to the matron's salary they will possibly relax their efforts.[147]

Miss Burgess strenuously objected to this argument saying that if a nurse wanted to, she could donate a part of her salary to the benevolent institution for 'there is nothing to stop her from doing that if she receives extra and comes under our award'. She added:

> a nurse has to provide for her old age just the same as any other employee and she cannot do that on a mere pittance. If electricians and plumbers were employed in these places, they would undoubtedly come under an award, so why not nurses?[148]

There was still a very strong element, Canon Massey believed, of 'religious' dedication needed. He appealed to the perceived spirit of the profession in opposing a reduction in hours:

> Though it is recognised that any reduction of the existing hours of 96 a fortnight may seem to be warranted, if only for the purpose of more closely approximating the accustomed hours of work for employees generally, it would be wrong to lose sight of the fact that nursing is a profession with public service as its highest ideal.[149]

Thus the arguments were strongly made by the private employers that money would not attract the right sort of recruit. This view was held uniquely for nurses and never applied to male professions such as medicine which did not have to rely on the ethos of public obligation to gain status in the community.

The private hospitals opposed any reduction in hours. However, if hours were reduced they wanted twelve months notice of any change as well as the ability to work a fortnightly roster.[150] Massey vehemently opposed eight-hour shifts. The economic cost of the straight eight-hour shifts for St Martin's Hospital, he claimed, would be the employment of an additional eleven trainees and three sisters with one more nurse for the extra week's holiday in the union claim, at an extra cost of 1404 pounds a year. As well the additional staff would require a new building to accommodate them.[151] Massey believed that it was necessary for the majority of staff to work between the hours of 6 am and 10 am when duties such as sponging, dressing and breakfasts were given and the operating theatre was busiest. After 10 am large numbers of nurses were not required and it would be 'economically dangerous for any private hospital to retain on duty such of these employees whose services are no longer needed'. The remainder of the staff thus worked the rest of their hours later in the day. This was justified on the grounds that:

> nurses for the most part live on the premises and receive their days off for their own purposes, surely this practice dispels any suggestion that the broken hours involve a hardship . . . We submit it is

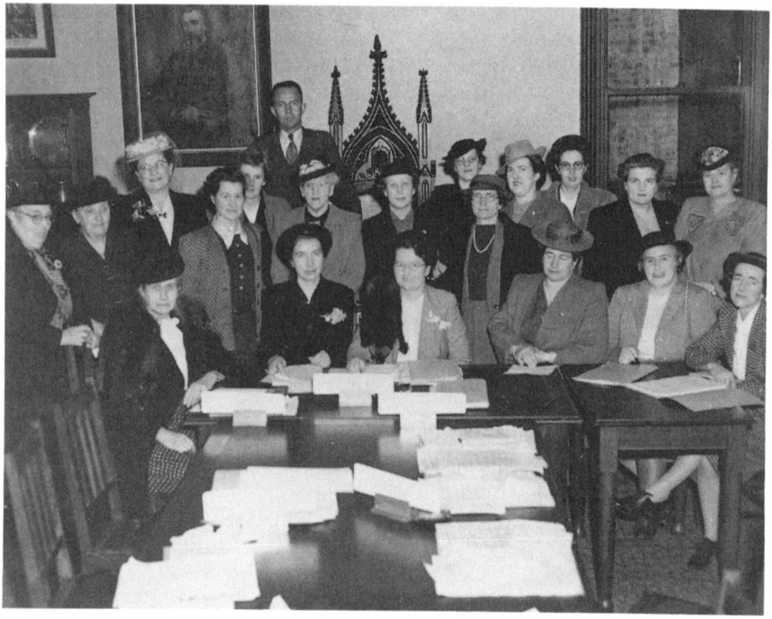

ATNA national council meeting, Melbourne, 1947. Miss Eunice Paten is standing second from the left. (Courtesy of ANF Federal Office, Melbourne.)

> indisputable that a nurse's efficiency and freshness are better preserved by broken time than by a continuous effort.[152]

Canon Massey asserted that he spoke 'from the point of view of patients'. From this perspective he believed that 'work on an unbroken shift as proposed means that nurses must to some extent at least get out of touch with their patients being off work 16 hours continuously in each day'.[153]

Canon Massey reiterated that the most valuable aspect of nursing was the life of dedication which nurses were expected to lead. Even though improved working hours might attract the required new staff 'the very essence of a profession, namely that the public interest is always uppermost, should not be cast aside by such a decrease in working hours as may impair the efficiency of the hospital'.[154] That is, nurses should be motivated by the public good: anything less than this was a threat to their professionalism. These views were reiterated by others in the community. Thomas Foley extolled the virtues of the nurse, saying that 'the old spirit that has existed from the days of the original nurse, Florence Nightingale, exists amongst our nurses still'.[155] But there was a new element in the claims of the ATNA. For the first time it compared the payment of nurses with those of other workers.

The ATNA in 1950

The ideals which had created the new female occupation of nursing in the nineteenth century were still evident in the 1940s. There were signs of change. Miss Joan Burgess compared nurses to other workers in the Industrial Court. Miss Abbott felt that the ATNA should 'attend to the material needs' of its members.[156] Miss Beatrice Roberts, secretary of the ATNA in New South Wales ('a purely ethical body') and Mr A.L. Hart, secretary of the New South Wales Nurses' Association (the industrial union) wrote to the *ANJ*:

> It may be that some nurses will dislike becoming members of a union, but where any body of people, whatever their walk in life, combine they immediately form a union, the only difference is that when an organization registers with the Court it becomes an industrial union . . . If nurses themselves do not register as an industrial union they will find their affairs controlled by people who know nothing about nurses or nursing, and as we cannot ever contemplate such a course of events taking place we suggest to all nurses to come closer together and not be as they are today pulling against each other.[157]

Yet Miss Paten was correct in saying that the Queensland Council of the ATNA had kept the industrial activities of the association 'in the background'.[158]

For the ATNA in Queensland, like most unions, the post-war years were dominated by industrial cases to gain wage increases and shorter hours. Dire shortages of nurses persisted after the war, exacerbating nurses' poor working conditions and gaining community support for improvements in wages and conditions. Long hours and restrictive labour legislation during the war had made these urgent demands for most unions. Where the ATNA differed from most other unions was that pressure from outside sources such as community organisations and even employers, had to be exerted before it would pursue such industrial activities. Even then its lack of industrial knowledge and ability meant that nurses' conditions did not improve as quickly as they could have done. An inability to understand what was required to meet the post-war industrial regulations meant that increases in wages were delayed. The ATNA Council displayed great reluctance to improve conditions and, in the most extreme case, the ATNA took fourteen years longer than necessary to gain a reduction in nurses' working hours from 96 to 88 a fortnight. This reticence to improve working conditions can be traced to the ATNA's belief that a nurse's life should be one of service and sacrifice, coupled with identification with the needs of the employer for a cheap workforce. The council's lack of acknowledgement of itself as an industrial organisation meant that it did not see this area of its work as legitimate and hence did not recognise the need to develop industrial expertise.

In 1950, the focus and activities of the Queensland Branch of the ATNA remained in Brisbane. Decision making was still the exclusive province of the council which was dominated by the leaders of the nursing profession with Miss Bardsley, Matron and Superintendent of Nurses, Child Welfare Service, as president and Miss Christense Sorenson, Matron of the Brisbane General Hospital, as vice-president.[159] The involvement of student nurses and nurses from other parts of the state was limited in the 1940s. Although prepared to enforce the preference clause to ensure membership, the ATNA viewed itself primarily as a professional organisation, forced by circumstances to take on the additional role of trade union. The *ANJ*, commenting on the moves to form a national organisation with an industrial focus, reflected this dichotomy: 'It is said that nursing is no longer a profession, and nurses are interested in material benefits only, but we assure you nothing in life is achieved with satisfaction if the only interest is the clock and the pay envelope, and we defy anyone to say that these are the only interests of nurses today'.[160]

CHAPTER 10

Conclusion

From the mid-nineteenth century to the end of the twentieth century the occupation of nursing in Australia changed dramatically and was part of the revolution in the delivery of health care in western industrialised countries. Nursing has been shaped by being a predominantly female occupation for most of these 150 years—a female occupation in a world where the public sphere of paid work, administration and decision making have been dominated by men.

Elements of service and sacrifice were prominent features in shaping nurses' attitudes to their conditions of work and the goals of their associations. While nurses attempted to lay claim to professional status by appealing to elements of sacrifice and selfless service, these attributes had to be measured in some way which set them apart from other workers, many of whom also worked long hours in harsh conditions. So the long hours, heavy work and the dangers present in contact with contagious diseases were not sufficient in themselves to show extreme dedication. However, when coupled with a low level of remuneration, nurses' work could be seen as unique, in the minds of both nurses and the public. Sacrifice and selflessness was demanded if one was to be classified as a true nurse and not a mere worker whose main motivation was money.

The ATNA as well as employers emphasised that the work of nursing itself provided intrinsic rewards: nurses did not work for money alone. These views determined that industrial issues would not be pursued vigorously by the ATNA. The ATNA in Queensland was first and foremost, by its own definition, a professional organisation, concerned with the standards of practice and training of nurses. The ATNA in Australia was very successful in attaining the goals of a professional organisation in a relatively short time. Within a decade of its establishment, State registration of nurses was attained in 1912. State certification was the ultimate seal of approval on the new occupation of nursing and the government accepted the ATNA views about training and certification of nurses as legitimate.

As aspiring professionals, nurses saw themselves as different from manual workers who engaged in bargaining with employers over wages and conditions, and even went on strike. The nursing associations, formed in order to promote the status of the trained nurse, could not be part of the trade union movement, whose prime motivation was the improvement of wages and working conditions. The ATNA in Queensland was different from other unions, even those of other professional workers, because of this emphasis on the individual sacrifice of the nurse. In the period to 1950 it was always external pressure that forced the ATNA Council to become involved in issues concerning wages and working conditions.

Established in Brisbane, the Queensland Branch did not believe that it was important to develop strong representative links with nurses in country areas so that the views of the ordinary nurse could be heard. In the period to 1950 nurses outside the capital city, student nurses and indeed staff nurses and private nurses generally, had little opportunity to influence the decisions of the association. However following the Second World War the structure of the Queensland Branch of the ATNA became a little more complex and a little more open to the ideas of its general membership. Sub-committees of council were formed in 1947, including one dealing with union matters and another handling education issues.[1] In 1949 the council wrote to the larger towns suggesting the formation of regional groups and student nurses' groups[2] but it was not until the 1950s that students began to participate actively in the association.

In the late 1940s the council was concerned by the lack of interest in the association and Miss Joan Abbott, first tutor sister at Brisbane Hospital in 1930,[3] visited all Queensland Hospitals to publicise the activities of the association.[4] Hospital authorities, particularly matrons, she reported, were pleased to see a representative of the ATNA, the first ever in most parts of the state. Responses from hospitals varied but most did not speak favourably of the ATNA's actions. Some believed that the ATNA was 'not in as much evidence as it could be' and 'repeatedly' asked 'what does the A.T.N.A. do for its members?' Others felt that the association was 'too Brisbane minded' and did not know anything about conditions in distant parts of Queensland. Another comment, 'mainly from the men', expressed the view that 'as soon as the A.T.N.A. behaves like any other Industrial Union the better'. Miss Abbott concluded that although nursing was a profession, the association had accepted a role as an industrial union as well and now had to behave as both:

> We must attend to the material needs of our members and we must also pay attention to the Ethical aspect and the educational requirements of a profession. At the same time as we find ourselves compelled to enforce the Preference Clause—we must find ourselves stressing the status of the profession.[5]

Miss Abbott's trip had revealed that the role of the ATNA had diminished. In response to this the council decided to enforce the preference clause, an unusual tactic for the ATNA to choose as it was so anti-union in its beliefs and preference clauses were associated with negative overtones of compulsory union membership and lack of choice.[6] But at a time when 'hospitals could not fill their staff establishments, let alone worry about offering employment to members of the ATNA before employing non members',[7] little could be achieved by this means.

By 1950 the ATNA still was not comfortable with its industrial role, although there was a gradually expanding awareness that nurses' working conditions should be perceived in a way similar to those of other workers. Justifications that better conditions were needed because it would result in improved patient care or that nurses could not save for their old age on their current salaries were no longer the sole reasons used to argue for upgraded conditions. However the council still saw itself as working with employers in the interests of nurses while groups of nurses and a wide variety of community organisations complained of poor conditions. The lack of acceptance of an industrial role meant that the lead in protesting against nurses' conditions did not come from the council and executive of their trade union, but from the public and some groups of nurses themselves.

In the decades since 1950 substantial changes have taken place in the occupation of nursing, including the transfer of nurse education courses from hospitals to universities. Changes in the 1940s stimulated discussions about nurse education. 'As a result of rapid advances in medical science', Miss Muriel Doherty, convener of the national subcommittee on Post-Graduate Nursing Education, exhorted, 'our profession requires overhauling and reorganizing in order to keep pace with progress and provide the community with an adequate and efficient nursing service'.[8] The Queensland Council of the ATNA was particularly concerned with the training of tutor sisters and felt that in many cases the number of trainees who failed their examinations was caused by the lack of trained teachers: 'Nursing appears to be the only profession in which teachers are not first of all instructed in teaching methods.'[9] The establishment of a College of Nursing in Queensland was discussed but did not eventuate[10] but a College of Nursing, Australia, was established in Melbourne with the specific role of offering post-graduate courses. It conducted its first courses in 1950 with Queensland nurses attending courses for tutor sisters[11] and from that time played an important part in the revision and development of nurse education.

Nurses' associations always maintained connections with each other and operated on a national basis when necessary, particularly during the Second World War. The ANF had been established in 1923 at a conference of the ATNA and RVTNA and the Queensland Branch of the ATNA, one of the state branches of the federation, paid capitation fees to the ANF and sent representatives to federal conferences. Concerned principally with training matters and professional recognition, its Federal Council discussed national matters and affiliated with the International Council of Nurses in 1937.[12] The federation continued as an organisation which co-ordinated national issues concerning the profession while the major work of the associations continued to be done within the state branches.

Although there had always been strong links between the ATNA branches, following the war there were calls for a national organisation of nurses. The debate about nationalisation of health services and a call for uniform control of nursing throughout Australia[13] encouraged discussion about the possibility of establishing one organisation to represent all nurses. The ANF feared that nurses' activities might be controlled by committees not made up of nurses and Miss R. Kirkcaldie, ANF president, 'stressed the need for nurses to control their own profession, and UNITY had to be their watchword'.[14] Moves to form a national association were started in 1946 by the Trained Nurses' Guild (formed in Victoria in 1921[15] and not a very active organisation). It approached the ANF concerning the amalgamation of the two associations.[16] The Queensland Branch decided that one nursing organisation for Australia was desirable and was prepared to take complicated administrative steps to enable this to occur.[17] However discussions between nursing organisations broke down at the 1948 conference principally over the admission of assistants in nursing to the new association. With the defeat of the federal Labor Government in 1949 plans for a national health service ceased and the forces propelling the disparate nursing organisation towards unity lessened and negotiations ended.[18] Decades of attempts to unite the state nursing associations followed and in 1989 the Queensland Nurses' Union forged new links with other nurses' trade unions through a process known as harmonisation, and has become an important member of the Australian Nursing Federation.

The nature of nursing and its role within health care has changed dramatically in the past one hundred years as nurses have defined a separate and independent role for themselves within the health-care system. This is exemplified in Virginia Henderson's widely accepted definition:

> The unique function of the nurse is to assist the individual, sick or well, in the performance of those activities contributing to health or its recovery (or to peaceful death) that he [*sic*] would perform unaided if he had the necessary strength, will or knowledge . . . This aspect of her [*sic*] work, this part of her function, she initiates and controls; of this she is master. In addition she helps the patient to carry out the therapeutic plan as initiated by the physician.[19]

In recent decades, nurses' views of industrial activity and even strike action have changed and nurses have fought long campaigns and taken prolonged industrial action in an effort to advance their claims.[20] These claims have included wage increases, better conditions, revised career structures and quality of patient care. No longer do nurses' unions stand outside the mainstream of the trade union movement in Australia as they are now members of local Trades and Labour Councils and the national federation, the Australian Council of Trade Unions. But it is only within the last decade that these changes have taken place, part of the trend also occurring in North America and Great Britain for nurses to identify themselves with other workers.[21]

However the ideals which had created the new female occupation of nursing in the nineteenth century were still evident even in 1950. Miss C.E. Grant, in an article titled 'The A.T.N.A. and What It Stands For', urged nurses to:

> Hold high the lamp which is your heritage from the woman whose name stands out like a beacon in the nursing world—Florence Nightingale. Emulating her we shall see to it that the standard of nursing is not lowered . . .
>
> May the present generation bring forth another Florence Nightingale to cause the nursing profession to rise like a phoenix from the ashes.[22]

Although parliamentarians could still call nursing 'the noblest profession',[23] many sectors of the community and many nurses themselves were beginning to assess the occupation of nursing and its working conditions in a way akin to other occupations. The ATNA would slowly respond to these pressures but in the period to 1950 'trade unionism' remained firmly 'in the background' in the activities of the nurses' union.

Endnotes

Introduction

1 Minutes of Council Meeting, ATNA Qld, 14 Aug. 1933.
2 For example, case 165 of 1946, transcript, 11 Apr. 1947, pp. 25–26, Queensland Industrial Commission (QIC).
3 See Stephen Deery, 'Union Aims and Methods' in *Australian Unions: An Industrial Relations Perspective*, eds Bill Ford & David Plowman, 2nd edn, Macmillan, Melbourne, 1989, pp. 74–103.
4 Allan Flanders, *Management and Unions*, Faber & Faber, London, 1970, p. 43.
5 Deery, 'Union Aims and Methods', p. 101.
6 Ann Game & Rosemary Pringle, *Gender at Work*, George Allen & Unwin, Sydney, 1983, p. 14.
7 Olga Maranjian Church, 'Historiography in Nursing Research', *Western Journal of Nursing Research*, vol. 9, no. 2, May 1987, p. 278.
8 ibid. p. 275.
9 Leslie Hardy & Anne Marie Rafferty, 'Nursing and History', *Nursing Times*, vol. 78, no. 37, 15 Sep. 1982, p. 1564.
10 M. Adelaide Nutting & Lavinia L. Dock, *A History of Nursing: The Evolution of Nursing Systems from the Earliest Times to the Foundation of the First English and American Training Schools for Nurses*, vols 1 & 2; Lavinia L. Dock, ed., *A History of Nursing: From the Earliest Times to the Present Day with Special Reference to the Work of the Past Thirty Years*, vols 3 & 4, G.P. Putnam's Sons, New York, 1907–1912.
11 Janet Wilson James, 'Writing and Rewriting Nursing History: A Review Essay', *Bulletin of the History of Medicine*, no. 58, Winter 1984, p. 571.
12 For example, Lumby discusses the history of nursing from animals to Florence Nightingale, relying heavily on Donahue, which in turn relies on early nursing texts such as Dock and Nutting and does not use recent scholarship. (Judy Lumby, *Nursing: Reflecting on an Evolving*

Practice, Deakin University Press, Geelong, 1991, pp. 2–6; M. Patricia Donahue, *Nursing: The Finest Art: An Illustrated History*, C.V. Mosby, St Louis, 1985.) Lumby's rendition of nursing history bears out James' argument that history theses done within nursing schools in the USA have ignored recent historical scholarship: 'The writers seem to be unaware of current social history and . . . the history of women'. (James, 'Writing and Rewriting Nursing History', p. 574.)

13 James, 'Writing and Rewriting Nursing History', p. 570.

14 Agnes E. Pavey, *The Story of the Growth of Nursing as an Art, a Vocation, and a Profession*, 5th edn, Faber & Faber, London, 1959. For example, Richard H. Shryock, *The History of Nursing: An Interpretation of the Social and Medical Factors Involved*, W.B. Saunders, Philadelphia, 1959; Charles Marie Frank, *Foundations of Nursing*, 2nd edn, W.B. Saunders, Philadelphia, 1959.

15 Vern L. Bullough & Bonnie Bullough, *The Emergence of Modern Nursing*, 2nd edn, Macmillan, Toronto, 1969; J.M. Mellish, *A Basic History of Nursing*, 2nd edn, Butterworths, Durban, 1990.

16 Eva Gamarnikow, 'Sexual division of labour: the case of nursing' in *Feminism and Materialism: Women and Modes of Production*, eds Annette Kuhn & AnnMarie Wolpe, Routledge & Kegan Paul, London, 1978.

17 Dock, *A History of Nursing*, vol. 3, p. vii.

18 ibid. vol. 4, p. 180.

19 Nutting & Dock, *A History of Nursing*, vol. 1, p. 3.

20 Jocalyn Lawler, *Behind the Screens: Nursing, Somology, and the Problem of the Body*, Churchill Livingstone, Melbourne, 1991, p. vi. Original italics.

21 Isabel Stewart, 'The science and art of nursing', *Nursing Education Bulletin*, vol. 2, no. 1, Winter 1929, p. 1, quoted in Donahue, *Nursing: The Finest Art*, p. 467.

22 Donahue, *Nursing: The Finest Art*, p. 11.

23 Shryock, *The History of Nursing*, p. 318.

24 Celia Davies, ed., *Rewriting Nursing History*, Croom Helm, London, 1980; Ellen Condliffe Lagemann, ed., *Nursing History: New Perspectives, New Possibilities*, Teachers College, New York, 1983; Christopher Maggs, ed., *Nursing History: The State of the Art*, Croom Helm, London, 1987.

25 Barbara Melosh, *'The Physician's Hand': Work Culture and Conflict in American Nursing*, Temple University Press, Philadelphia, 1982, p. 7.

26 Susan M. Reverby, *Ordered to Care: The Dilemma of American Nursing, 1850–1945*, Cambridge University Press, Cambridge, 1987, p. 1.

27 Christopher Maggs, *The Origins of General Nursing*, Croom Helm, London, 1983.

28 For example, Victoria Hobbs, *But Westward Look: Nursing in Western Australia 1829–1979*, University of Western Australia Press, Perth, 1980; Richard Trembath & Donna Hellier, *All Care and Responsibility:*

A History of Nursing in Victoria 1850–1934, Florence Nightingale Committee, Melbourne, 1987; Helen Gregory, *A Tradition of Care: A History of Nursing at the Royal Brisbane Hospital*, Boolarong, Brisbane, 1988.

29 Mary Dickenson, *An Unsentimental Union: The NSW Nurses Association 1931–1992*, Hale & Iremonger, Sydney, 1993, p. 57.

30 John Tyrer, *History of the Brisbane Hospital and its Affiliates*, Boolarong, Brisbane, 1993, pp. 145–148.

31 L. McGuire, 'Surgical History of the Royal Brisbane Hospital', *Proceedings of the Division of Surgery Royal Brisbane Hospital*, 1985, p. 12.

32 F. E. Hare, *The Cold-bath Treatment of Typhoid Fever*, Macmillan, London, 1898, p. 30.

33 Tyrer, *History of the Brisbane Hospital*, p. 262.

34 McGuire, 'Surgical History of the Royal Brisbane Hospital', p. 14; L. McGuire, 'Surgical History of the Royal Brisbane Hospital—1931–1967', *Proceedings of the Division of Surgery Royal Brisbane Hospital*, 1987, pp. 13–14.

35 Dickenson, *An Unsentimental Union*, p. 57.

36 Sheila Bunting & Jacquelyn C. Campbell, 'Feminism and nursing: Historical perspectives', *Advances in Nursing Science*, vol. 12, no. 4, Jul. 1990, pp. 11–24; Mercia Bush, 'Nursing as a Feminist Issue', *The Lamp*, Apr. 1981, pp. 25–29.

37 Bunting & Campbell, 'Feminism and nursing', pp. 19–20.

38 Minutes of Extraordinary General Meeting, ATNA Qld, 22 Oct. 1947.

39 John Davis, *Florence Nightingale, or the Heroine of the East*, Arthur Hall, Virtue, London, 1856, p. 3.

Chapter 1

1 Evidence of Walter Balls-Headley, Medical Society of Victoria, question 2451, Minutes of Evidence, Royal Commission on Charitable Institutions, *Victorian Parliamentary Papers (VPP)*, 1892.

2 Brian Abel-Smith, *A History of the Nursing Profession*, Heinemann, London, 1960, p. 4.

3 Katrina Alford, *Production or Reproduction? An economic history of women in Australia, 1788–1850*, Oxford University Press, Melbourne, 1984, p. 183.

4 K.S. Inglis, *Hospital and Community: A History of the Royal Melbourne Hospital*, Melbourne University Press, Melbourne, 1958, p. 95.

5 Alford, *Production or Reproduction?*, p. 209.

6 ibid. p. 184.

7 Minutes of Evidence, Select Committee on the Hospitals of the Colony, *Queensland Parliamentary Papers (QPP)*, 1866, pp. 1620, 1624.

8 ibid. pp. 1629–1630.

9 ibid. pp. 1625, 1650, 1660.
10 Trembath & Hellier, *All Care and Responsibility*, pp. 9–10.
11 Minutes of Evidence, Select Committee on the Hospitals of the Colony, *QPP*, 1866, pp. 1621,1631.
12 M.P. Susman, 'Lucy Osburn and Her Five Nightingale Nurses', *Medical Journal of Australia (MJA)*, 1 May 1965, pp. 633–642.
13 Gregory, *A Tradition of Care*, pp. 13–16.
14 Ronald Lawson, *Brisbane in the 1890s: A Study of an Australian Urban Society*, University of Queensland Press, Brisbane, 1973, p. 149.
15 Brian Dickey, *No Charity There: A Short History of Social Welfare in Australia*, Nelson, Melbourne, 1980, pp. 72–73.
16 Brian Dickey, 'Health and State in Australia, 1788–1977', *Journal of Australian Studies*, vol. 2, Nov. 1977, p. 53.
17 Jacqueline Bell, 'Queensland's Public Hospital System: Some Aspects of Finance and Control' in *Social Policy in Australia: Some Perspectives 1901–1975*, ed. Jill Roe, Cassell, Sydney, 1976, p. 285.
18 Ronald Lawson, *Brisbane in the 1890s*, p. 149.
19 Dickey, 'Health and State in Australia, 1788–1977', p. 55.
20 Dickey, *No Charity There*, p. 69.
21 Quoted in Abel-Smith, *A History of the Nursing Profession*, p. 18.
22 Patricia Branca, *Silent Sisterhood: Middle Class Women in the Victorian Home*, Croom Helm, London, 1975, p. 7.
23 Abel-Smith, *A History of the Nursing Profession*, p. 17.
24 Katrina Alford & Michelle McLean, *Partners or Parasites of Men? Women's Economic Status in Australia, Britain and Canada, 1850–1900*, Working Paper in Economic History no. 66, Australian National University, Canberra, 1986, pp. 8–9, 44.
25 Proportion of females to each 100 males. (The Australian figures do not include the Aboriginal population.)

	1871	**1880**
England and Wales	105.38	105.47
Queensland	66.87	67.47
New South Wales	81.05	78.90
Victoria	82.42	83.44
South Australia	93.72	91.40

(Registrar-General's Report—Vital Statistics, *Queensland Votes and Proceedings*, vol. 1, 1881, p. 688.)

26 Census of Queensland, 1891, *Queensland Votes and Proceedings*, vol. 3, 1892, pp. 1051,1155. Comparative figures cannot be obtained for Queensland as the census in 1881 did not give a separate category for nurses. (Census of Queensland, 1881, *Queensland Votes and Proceedings*, vol. 1, 1882, p. 1080.)
27 Trembath & Hellier, *All Care and Responsibility*, p. 14. Trembath and Hellier warn that the figures indicate trends only.

28 For example, evidence of Isabella Rathie, questions 7261–7265, Minutes of Evidence, Royal Commission on Charitable Institutions, *VPP*, 1892.
29 Trembath & Hellier, *All Care and Responsibility*, p. 14.
30 Quoted in Trembath & Hellier, *All Care and Responsibility*, p. 13.
31 Quoted in Inglis, *Hospital and Community*, p. 96.
32 Quoted in Ann M. Mitchell, *The Hospital South of the Yarra: A history of Alfred Hospital, Melbourne from foundation to the nineteen-forties*, Alfred Hospital, Melbourne, 1977, p. 79.
33 'Training School for Nurses', *Australian Medical Journal*, 15 Nov. 1889, p. 507.
34 ibid.
35 Inglis, *Hospital and Community*, p. 96.
36 Gregory, *A Tradition of Care*, pp. 16–23.
37 Ross Patrick, *The Royal Women's Hospital, Brisbane—The First Fifty Years*, Boolarong, Brisbane, 1988, pp. 15,17.
38 Gregory, *A Tradition of Care*, p. 21.
39 Inglis, *Hospital and Community*, p. 97.
40 Minutes of Evidence, Royal Commission on Charitable Institutions, *VPP*, 1892.
41 Answer by respondents, Hospitals & Awards, 21/1332, COL/367, Queensland State Archives (QSA).
42 Evidence of Walter Balls-Headley, question 2451, Minutes of Evidence, Royal Commission on Charitable Institutions, *VPP*, 1892.
43 Evidence of Rev. Mervyn Whitton, question 19517, ibid.
44 Evidence of Robert Duncan, question 20497, ibid.
45 Evidence of William Avison, question 12488, ibid.
46 Evidence of James Webb, questions 17098, 17136, ibid.
47 Maggs, *The Origins of General Nursing*, p. 26.
48 Evidence of Mary Muffitt, questions 6496, 6497, and Alice Martelli, question 6529, Minutes of Evidence, Royal Commission on Charitable Institutions, *VPP*, 1892.
49 Evidence of Henrietta Strong, questions 6335–6337, 6345, ibid.
50 Evidence of Hubert Miller, question 18401, ibid.
51 Evidence of Harloe Fleming, question 21551, ibid.
52 Evidence of Leonard Robinson, questions 18061, 18062, 18065, ibid.
53 Evidence of Ralph Stevenson, questions 20085–20086, ibid.
54 Evidence of John Klein, questions 12035–12038, ibid.
55 Report of the Royal Commission on Charitable Institutions, p. xix, *VPP*, 1892, p. xix.
56 Minutes of Evidence, Royal Commission on Charitable Institutions, *VPP*, 1892.
57 Gregory, *A Tradition of Care*, p. 31.
58 Evidence of Robert Norman, questions 1864, 1901, Minutes of Evidence, Royal Commission on Charitable Institutions, *VPP*, 1892.

59 Evidence of Isabella Rathie, question 7198, ibid.
60 Evidence of Robert Norman, question 1864, and Isabella Rathie, question 7198, ibid.
61 M. Voysey, *Nursing: Hints to Probationers on Practical Work*, Scientific Press, London, 1905, p. 4 quoted in Maggs, *The Origins of General Nursing*, pp. 23–24.
62 Mitchell, *The Hospital South of the Yarra*, pp. 78–79.
63 ibid. p. 80.
64 Gregory, *A Tradition of Care*, p. 30.
65 Martha Vicinus, *Independent Women: Work and Community for Single Women 1850–1920*, Virago, London, 1985, p. 97.
66 Abel-Smith, *A History of the Nursing Profession*, p. 23.
67 Maggs, *The Origins of General Nursing*, p. 12.
68 Evidence of Archibald Colquhoun, question 11615, Minutes of Evidence, Royal Commission on Charitable Institutions, *VPP*, 1892.
69 Evidence of Elizabeth Finlay, question 7172, and Isabella Rathie, question 7209, ibid.
70 Evidence of Henrietta Strong, question 6310, ibid.
71 Evidence of Dorothy Smith, questions 6235–6238, ibid.
72 Evidence of Catherine Caffyn, question 7416, ibid.
73 Evidence of Thomas Fitzgerald, question 3118, ibid.
74 Evidence of Alice Martelli, questions 6543, 6558, ibid.
75 Details of this evidence from Trembath & Hellier, *All Care and Responsibility*, pp. 34–35.
76 Gregory, *A Tradition of Care*, p. 29.
77 Evidence of Margaret Watson, questions 16723, 16726, 16744, Minutes of Evidence, Royal Commission on Charitable Institutions, *VPP*, 1892.
78 Lawson, *Brisbane in the 1890s*, p. 66.
79 Eddie Clarke, *Female Teachers in Queensland State Schools: A History 1860–1983*, Department of Education, Brisbane, 1985, p. 7.
80 Evidence of Archibald Colquhoun, questions 11586, 11587 and Dorothy Smith, questions 6216, 6239, Minutes of Evidence, Royal Commission on Charitable Institutions, *VPP*, 1892.
81 Evidence of James Barrett, question 2723, ibid.
82 Evidence of Thomas Fitzgerald, questions 3121–3123, ibid.
83 Evidence of Thomas Rowan, question 3215, ibid.
84 Evidence of Henrietta Strong, questions 6316–6321, ibid.
85 Evidence of Isabella Rathie, questions 7246, 7250, ibid.
86 Evidence of Alice Martelli, questions 6526, 6539 ibid.
87 Anne Marie Lynzaat, 'Respectability and the outworker: Victorian Factory Acts 1885–1903' in *In pursuit of justice: Australian women and the law 1788–1979*, eds Judy Mackinolty & Heather Radi, Hale & Iremonger, Sydney, 1979, p. 86.

88 Details of this debate from Trembath & Hellier, *All Care and Responsibility*, pp. 36–38.
89 *Victorian Parliamentary Debates*, vol. LXXIX, 1895–1896, p. 4326.
90 *Factories and Shops Act of 1900* (Qld).
91 Reverby, *Ordered to Care*, p. 127.
92 ibid. p. 128.
93 Gregory, *A Tradition of Care*, pp. 31–32.
94 For example, Bendigo Hospital, question 11610, Minutes of Evidence, Royal Commission on Charitable Institutions, *VPP*, 1892.
95 Trembath & Hellier, *All Care and Responsibility*, p. 36.
96 Patrick, *The Royal Women's Hospital, Brisbane*, p. 17.
97 *Factories and Shops Act of 1900* (Qld), Section 45.
98 Evidence of Archibald Colquhoun, question 11595, Minutes of Evidence, Royal Commission on Charitable Institutions, *VPP*, 1892.
99 Evidence of Sarah Bishop, questions 7303–7308 and Dorothy Smith, questions 6221–6265, ibid.
100 Evidence of Hubert Miller, questions 18403, 18404, ibid.
101 Quoted in Gregory, *A Tradition of Care*, p. 33.
102 Evidence of Isabella Rathie, question 7198, Minutes of Evidence, Royal Commission on Charitable Institutions, *VPP*, 1892.
103 Evidence of Isabella Rathie, questions 7227–7239, ibid.
104 Inglis, *Hospital and Community*, p. 100.
105 Evidence of Marie Magill, questions 7361–7375, Minutes of Evidence, Royal Commission on Charitable Institutions, *VPP*, 1892.
106 Gregory, *A Tradition of Care*, p. 35.
107 ibid. p. 23.
108 Maggs, *The Origins of General Nursing*, p. 120.
109 ibid. p. 121 & Vicinus, *Independent Women*, p. 108.
110 Gregory, *A Tradition of Care*, p. 89.
111 H. O'Neill & E. Barnett, *Our Nurses and the Work They Have to Do*, Ward, Lock, London, 1888, pp. 14–15, quoted in Vicinus, *Independent Women*, p. 92.
112 Vicinus, *Independent Women*, p. 109.
113 Reverby, *Ordered to Care*, p. 54.
114 Maggs, *The Origins of General Nursing*, p. 119.
115 Vicinus, *Independent Women*, p. 101.
116 ibid. p. 111.
117 Reverby, *Ordered to Care*, p. 58.
118 ibid. p. 59.
119 Nancy A. Hewitt, 'Beyond the search for sisterhood: American women's history in the 1980s', *Social History*, vol. 10, no. 3, Oct. 1985, p. 315.
120 Reverby, *Ordered to Care*, p. 6.

121 John Rickard, *Class and Politics: New South Wales, Victoria and the Early Commonwealth, 1890–1910*, Australian National University Press, Canberra, 1976, pp. 308–309.
122 Lawson, *Brisbane in the 1890s*, p. 129.
123 Clarke, *Female Teachers in Queensland State Schools*, p. 6.
124 Noeline Kyle, *Her Natural Destiny: The Education of Women in New South Wales*, New South Wales University Press, Sydney, 1986, p. 137.
125 *Queensland Parliamentary Debates (QPD)*, vol. LXXXIII, 1899, p. 1363.
126 Maggs, *The Origins of General Nursing*, p. 25.
127 Evidence of John Taylor, question 10956, Minutes of Evidence, Royal Commission on Charitable Institutions, *VPP*, 1892.
128 Evidence of David Bennett, questions 10872–75, ibid.
129 Evidence of Mrs Edith Morris, question 6032, ibid.
130 Reverby, *Ordered to Care*, p. 3.
131 Quoted in Melbourne Hospital, Report of Sub-Committee of Enquiry on Trained Nurses, Jul. 1871, p. 14.
132 *Argus*, 1856, quoted in Trembath & Hellier, *All Care and Responsibility*, p. 10.
133 J. Frederick Watson, *The History of the Sydney Hospital from 1811 to 1911*, W.A. Gullick, Sydney, 1911, p. 134.

Chapter 2

1 Editorial, *Australasian Nurses' Journal (ANJ)*, Mar. 1903, p. 3.
2 Susan B. McGahey, 'The Nursing Organisations in the Australasian Commonwealth', *The Nursing Record and Hospital World*, 21 Dec. 1901, p. 494.
3 General Meeting of Nurses and Medical Men, Sydney, 26 May 1899 & Minutes of First Meeting of Proposed Nurses' Association, Sydney, nd.
4 Minutes of Committee Meeting of Proposed Nurses' Association, Sydney, 21 Jun. 1899.
5 'In Memoriam', *Una*, Jul. 1903, p. 24.
6 Australasian Trained Nurses' Association, *Report of Council 1900*, R.T. Kelly, Sydney, 1900, p. 7.
7 ibid. & Australasian Trained Nurses' Association, *Register of Members 1904*, Websdale, Shoosmith, Sydney, 1904, p. 73.
8 Australasian Trained Nurses' Association, *Report of Council 1900*, pp. 7–8.
9 Geoffrey Millerson, *The Qualifying Associations: A Study in Professionalization*, Routledge & Kegan Paul, London, 1964, pp. 28–30.
10 ibid. pp. 30–39.
11 Melosh, *'The Physician's Hand'*, p. 29.
12 Millerson, *The Qualifying Associations*, p. 256.

13 Australasian Trained Nurses' Association, *Report of Council 1900*, p. 6.
14 ibid. p. 9.
15 McGahey, 'The Nursing Organisations in the Australasian Commonwealth', p. 495.
16 Minutes of Council Meeting, ATNA NSW, 18 May 1900.
17 ibid. 25 Jun 1902.
18 Australasian Trained Nurses' Association, *Report of Council 1900*.
19 Samuel T. Knaggs, letter to editor, *Daily Telegraph*, 4 Aug. 1899.
20 Minutes of Special General Meeting, ATNA NSW, 22 Feb. 1901.
21 Minutes of Council Meeting, ATNA NSW, 17 Apr. 1903.
22 Editorial, *ANJ*, Mar. 1903, pp. 2–3.
23 Minutes of Council Meeting, ATNA NSW, 24 Jan. 1900 & 31 Jan. 1901.
24 Hobbs, *But Westward Look*, p. 18.
25 The VTNA became the Royal Victorian Trained Nurses' Association (RVTNA) in 1904. (Trembath & Hellier, *All Care and Responsibility*, p. 53).
26 ibid. pp. 45–47.
27 A.M. Payne to Secretary, ATNA NSW, minutes of ATNA, Qld, 17 Nov. 1903.
28 A.M. Payne to Secretary, ATNA NSW, ibid. 4 Dec. 1903.
29 A.M. Payne to Secretary, ATNA NSW, ibid. 17 Nov. 1903.
30 'Trained Nurses' Association', *Brisbane Courier*, 26 Feb. 1904.
31 Minutes of Council Meeting, ATNA NSW, 18 Mar. 1904.
32 Minutes of General Meeting and Council Meeting, ATNA Qld, 27 Apr. 1904. The subscription fees were £1 1s for medical practitioners, 10s 6d for general nurses and 5s for midwifery nurses.
33 Minutes of General Meeting, ATNA Qld, 27 Apr. 1904.
34 Draft Rules to govern the establishment and working of State Branches of the ATNA, Minutes of ATNA Qld.
35 In 1922, 863 general nurses, 333 obstetric nurses and 20 mental nurses were members. ATNA Qld, (Annual Report for year ending 30 Apr. 1922.)
36 Minutes of Council Meeting, ATNA Qld, 18 Apr. 1907.
37 ibid, 21 Feb. 1907.
38 Executive positions of the Queensland Branch were president, two vice-presidents, treasurer, two secretaries and a council of 21. All positions were honorary. The council was made up of six medical practitioners representing general nurses, twelve general nurses, one medical practitioner representing midwifery nurses and two midwifery nurses. ('Trained Nurses' Association', *Brisbane Courier*, 26 Feb. 1904.)
39 Ross Patrick, 'Ernest Sandford Jackson', in *Australian Dictionary of Biography*, vol. 9, eds Bede Nairn & Geoffrey Searle, Melbourne University, Melbourne, 1979–1988, p. 457.
40 Gregory, *A Tradition of Care*, p. 63.

41 Minutes of General Meeting, ATNA Qld, 27 Apr. 1904 & Gregory, *A Tradition of Care*, p. 165.
42 Minutes of Council Meeting, ATNA Qld, 19 Jan. 1912 & Minutes of Annual General Meeting, ATNA Qld, 1 Jun. 1912.
43 Dr Jackson, 'Notes on the Objects of a Trained Nurses' Association', *ANJ*, Jan. 1905, pp. 140–141.
44 Trembath & Hellier, *All Care and Responsibility*, p. 49.
45 Reverby, *Ordered to Care*, p. 121.
46 'The Special General Meeting', *ANJ*, May 1908, pp. 146–147.
47 'Matronships of Country Hospitals', editorial, *ANJ*, Apr. 1907, p. 99.
48 'The Conference', *ANJ*, Aug. 1909, pp. 291–292.
49 'Shorter Hours', editorial, *ANJ*, Jan. 1910, p. 2.
50 Jackson, 'Notes on the Objects of a Trained Nurses' Association', p. 141.

Chapter 3

1 Robert Scott, 'The Preliminary Training of Nurses', *Una*, Dec. 1904, p. 151.
2 'Preliminary Education', editorial, *ANJ*, Apr. 1909, p. 118.
3 'Circular to Training Schools', *ANJ*, Jan. 1906, p. 10.
4 Minutes of Council Meeting, ATNA Qld, 14 Oct. 1919.
5 'Preliminary Education', p. 118.
6 Robert Longhurst, *In the Footsteps of the Mercies: A History of Nursing at the Mater Misericordiae Public Hospitals, Brisbane*, Mater Misericordiae Public Hospitals, Brisbane, 1992, p. 71.
7 Rupert Goodman, *Secondary Education in Queensland, 1860–1960*, Australian National University Press, Canberra, 1968, pp. 178–179.
8 ibid. p. 181.
9 Kyle, *Her Natural Destiny*, p. 116.
10 *Census of the Commonwealth of Australia Taken for the Night Between the 2nd and 3rd April, 1911; Volume 1; Statistician's Report*, p. 182.
11 Stuart Macintyre, *The Oxford History of Australia, Volume 4: 1901–1942: The Succeeding Age*, Oxford University Press, Melbourne, 1986, p. 61.
12 Kyle, *Her Natural Destiny*, p. 116.
13 Coral Chambers, *Lessons for Ladies: A social history of girls' education in Australasia 1870–1900*, Hale & Iremonger, Sydney, 1986, pp. 90, 122, 127.
14 Paula Miller & Ian Davey, 'The Common Denominator: Schooling the People', in *Constructing a Culture: A People's History of Australia since 1788*, eds Verity Burgmann & Jenny Lee, McPhee Gribble, Melbourne, 1988, p. 25.

15 Kerreen M. Reiger, *The disenchantment of the home: Modernizing the Australian family 1880–1940*, Oxford University Press, Melbourne, 1985, p. 56.
16 Chambers, *Lessons for Ladies*, pp. 157–158.
17 Dr Scott was Resident Surgeon at Ballarat Hospital from 1886 to 1891 and subsequently held the posts of Honorary Physician, Surgeon and Chairman of the honorary medical staff until 1911. (Anthea Hyslop, *Sovereign Remedies: A history of Ballarat Base Hospital 1850s to 1980s*, Allen & Unwin, Sydney, 1989, pp. 143–144, 369.)
18 Robert Scott, 'The Preliminary Training of Nurses', p. 149.
19 'Country Hospitals', *ANJ*, Apr. 1904, p. 2.
20 'Probationers and Private Hospitals', *Una*, Jan. 1907, p. 1.
21 'Annual Meeting of the Queensland Branch', *ANJ*, Jul. 1907, p. 211.
22 Minutes of Council Meeting, ATNA Qld, 30 Jan. 1906. Details of staff from Bartz Schultz, *A Tapestry of Service: The Evolution of Nursing in Australia: Volume I; Foundation to Federation*, Churchill Livingstone, Melbourne, 1991, p. 374 & Tyrer, *History of the Brisbane Hospital*, p. 435.
23 'Circular to Training Schools', pp. 10–11.
24 'Graduation Hospitals', editorial, *ANJ*, Dec. 1905, p. 177.
25 Australasian Trained Nurses' Association, *Register of Members 1909*, Websdale, Shoosmith, Sydney, 1909, pp. 16–18.
26 Australasian Trained Nurses' Association, *Register of Members 1904*, pp. 14–15.
27 Australasian Trained Nurses' Association, *Register of Members 1902*, L. Bruck, Sydney, 1902, p. 11.
28 Australasian Trained Nurses' Association, *Register of Members 1909*, pp. 16–18.
29 'Graduation Hospitals', p. 178.
30 'Country Hospitals', p. 2.
31 ibid.
32 'The Private Hospital as a Training School for Nurses', *ANJ*, Mar. 1906, p. 67.
33 ibid. p. 68.
34 ibid. p. 69.
35 ibid.
36 Australasian Trained Nurses' Association, *Register of Members 1904*, pp. 14–15.
37 ibid.
38 Minutes of Council Meeting, ATNA NSW, 17 Apr. 1903.
39 Australasian Trained Nurses' Association, *Report of Council 1905*, p. 18.
40 Minutes of Council Meeting, ATNA NSW, 20 May 1904.
41 Minutes of Council Meeting, ATNA Qld, 20 May 1909.
42 ibid. 17 Aug. 1905.

43 'The Continuous Training of Probationers', editorial, *ANJ*, Nov. 1907, p. 325.
44 Minutes of Annual General Meeting, ATNA Qld, 18 Jun. 1910.
45 'The New Year', *ANJ*, Jan. 1905, p. 117.
46 Minutes of Council Meeting, ATNA NSW, 22 Jul. 1904.
47 ibid.
48 Circular to Training Schools, 1906, pp. 7–9.
49 Minutes of Council Meeting, ATNA Qld, 9 Aug. 1906.
50 Australasian Trained Nurses' Association, *Report of Council 1904*, pp. 16–18.
51 Minutes of Council Meeting, ATNA Qld, 20 Apr. 1911.
52 'Circular to Training Schools', p. 6.
53 ibid. p. 7.
54 Australasian Trained Nurses' Association, *Register of Members 1905*, Websdale, Shoosmith, Sydney, 1905, p. 21.
55 Reiger, *The disenchantment of the home*, p. 3.
56 Glennon, 'Housekeeping', *Una*, Jun. 1904, p. 51.
57 'Domestic Training of Nurses', *Una*, Jan. 1905, p. 1.
58 E. Glover, 'What are the Duties of a Nurse?', letter to editor, *Una*, Apr. 1905, p. 32.
59 Gregory, *A Tradition of Care*, p. 44.
60 Reverby, *Ordered to Care*, p. 60.
61 Editorial, *Una*, Apr. 1903, p. 1.
62 Scott, 'The Preliminary Training of Nurses', p. 149.
63 ibid.
64 *Argus*, 10 Jun. 1904, quoted in *Una*, Jul. 1904, p. 78.
65 Editorial, *Una*, Sep. 1904, p. 1.
66 E.M.G., 'A Plea for a Higher Standard of Education', *Una*, Feb. 1905, p. 188. (The writer is probably Miss E. Glover, member of the RVTNA Council.)
67 Felix Meyer, 'Nursing: Its Higher Aspects', *Una*, Jan. 1904, p. 71.
68 Madge A. Jones, 'Nurses and Political Influence', letter to editor, *Una*, Jun. 1904, p. 64.
69 E.M.G., 'A Plea for a Higher Standard of Education', p. 188.
70 ibid.
71 Scott, 'The Preliminary Training of Nurses', p. 151.
72 'The Social Position of the Nurse', editorial, *Una*, May 1905, p. 1.
73 ibid.
74 'Preliminary Education', editorial, *ANJ*, Apr. 1909, p. 118.
75 'The Qualification of Probationers', editorial, *Una*, Nov. 1904, p. 1.
76 ibid.
77 'The Nurse and the Doctor', editorial, *Una*, Apr. 1905, p. 1.
78 *Argus*, 10 Jun. 1904, quoted in *Una*, Jul. 1904, p. 78.
79 Edith E. Johnstone, 'What are the Duties of a Nurse?' letter to editor, *Una*, Mar. 1905, p. 5.

80 Scott, 'The Preliminary Training of Nurses', p. 151.
81 Reverby, *Ordered to Care*, p. 117.
82 MacLean, 'Lecture by Miss MacLean', *Una*, Jul. 1903, p. 34.
83 ibid.
84 S.D., 'Is the Eight Hour System for Hospital Nurses a Success?' *ANJ*, Jun. 1909, p. 194.
85 E. Glover, 'Nurses and Women's Suffrage', letter to editor, *Una*, Apr. 1903, p. 11.
86 Quoted in Reverby, *Ordered to Care*, p. 128.
87 Glover, 'Nurses and Women's Suffrage', p. 11.
88 Gregory, *A Tradition of Care*, p. 43.
89 Minutes of Annual General Meeting, ATNA Qld, 18 Jun. 1910.
90 Maggs, *The Origins of General Nursing*, p. 110.
91 Reverby, *Ordered to Care*, p. 70.
92 ibid.
93 Macintyre, *1901–1942: The Succeeding Age*, pp. 113–121.
94 'Discontent', editorial, *ANJ*, Nov. 1911, p. 361.
95 ibid.
96 Jenny Hughey, 'Equal pay and the Queensland Teachers' Union: the seventy year struggle by women teachers' in *Battlers and Bluestockings: Women's Place in Australian Education*, eds Sandra Taylor & Miriam Henry, Australian College of Education, Canberra, 1989, pp. 52–57.
97 Janice N. Brownfoot, 'Vida Jane Mary Goldstein', *Australian Dictionary of Biography*, vol. 9, pp. 43–45.
98 Vida Goldstein, 'Miss Goldstein and Hospital Nurses', letter to editor, *Una*, May 1904, p. 48.
99 Vida Goldstein, letter to *Argus*, reprinted in *Una*, Apr. 1904, p. 32.
100 Goldstein, 'Miss Goldstein and Hospital Nurses', p. 48.
101 'A Wellwisher', 'How to Ventilate Grievances', letter to editor, *Una*, Apr. 1904, p. 32.
102 Jones, 'Nurses and Political Influence', p. 64.
103 'Trained Nurse', 'Nurses and Women's Suffrage', letter to editor, *Una*, Jul. 1903, p. 40.
104 'A Faculty of Nursing', editorial, *ANJ*, May 1912, pp. 145–146.
105 Isla Blomfield, 'Some Defects in the Training of the Nurse'. *ANJ*, Aug. 1918, p. 380.
106 'Interested', 'College of Nursing', *ANJ*, Aug. 1918, p. 382.
107 Anne Summers, *Damned Whores and God's Police: The Colonization of Women in Australia*, Penguin, Melbourne, 1975, p. 329.
108 Quoted in Longhurst, *In the Footsteps of the Mercies*, pp. 71–72.
109 Maggs, *The Origins of General Nursing*, p. 197.
110 Cynthia Nolan, *A Bride for St Thomas*, Constable, London, 1970, p. 13.
111 Maggs, *The Origins of General Nursing*, p. 197.

112 'Nursing, Its Ideals and Realities, Before and After', *The Hospital*, 8 Feb. 1896, quoted in Anon., *Nursing in South Australia: First Hundred Years 1837–1937*, reprinted with supplements of 1939–1945 and 1989, Nurses' Memorial Foundation of SA Incorporated, Adelaide, 1989, p. 368.

Chapter 4

1 'State Registration of Nurses', *MJA*, 14 Nov. 1914, p. 475.
2 Registration was gained in South Australia in 1920, Western Australia in 1921, Victoria in 1923, New South Wales in 1924 and Tasmania in 1927.
3 Evan Willis, *Medical Dominance: The division of labour in Australian health care*, George Allen & Unwin, Sydney, 1983, p. 29.
4 L.L. Dock, 'The Progress of Registration', *Una*, Mar. 1906, pp. 9–10.
5 Melosh, *'The Physician's Hand'*, p. 15.
6 ibid. p. 16.
7 ibid. pp. 28–29.
8 'State Registration', *ANJ*, Dec. 1907, pp. 360–361 & 'A State Register for Nurses', *ANJ*, Dec. 1906, p. 388.
9 'State Registration', *ANJ*, Dec. 1907, pp. 359–360.
10 Minutes of council meeting, ATNA NSW, 18 Mar. 1904.
11 'The Progress of Registration', *Una*, Mar. 1906, p. 9.
12 'State Registration', *ANJ*, Jan. 1904, pp. 117–118.
13 'State Registration', *ANJ*, Dec. 1907, p. 360.
14 'Conference', *Una*, Apr. 1906, p. 24 & Willis, *Medical Dominance*, p. 107.
15 Willis, *Medical Dominance*, p. 94.
16 ibid. p. 106.
17 'Conference', *Una*, Apr. 1906, p. 24.
18 Neville Hicks, *'This Sin and Scandal': Australia's Population Debate 1891–1911*, Australian National University Press, Canberra, 1978, pp. 25–27.
19 'State Legislation in Regard to Private Hospitals', *ANJ*, Nov. 1906, pp. 351–352.
20 'Special General Meeting', *ANJ*, Jul. 1908, p. 224.
21 *Private Hospitals Act of 1908* (NSW).
22 'Private Hospitals Act', *ANJ*, Feb. 1909, p. 47.
23 'Nurses' Registration Bill', *ANJ*, Sep. 1915, p. 323.
24 *New South Wales Parliamentary Debates (NSWPD)*, vol. XXXIII, 1909, p. 855.
25 ibid. pp. 855–856.
26 'Nurses' Registration Bill', *ANJ*, Nov. 1909, p. 398.
27 'State Registration in New South Wales', *ANJ*, May 1908, p. 151.

28 'The Special General Meeting', editorial, *ANJ*, May 1908, p. 146.
29 'State Registration in New South Wales', pp. 151–152.
30 'Special General Meeting', *ANJ*, Jul. 1908, p. 226.
31 *NSWPD*, vol. XXXIII, 1909, pp. 857–858.
32 ibid. p. 858.
33 ibid. vol. XXXIX, 1910, p. 453.
34 ibid. p. 456.
35 ibid. vol. XXXIII, 1909, pp. 1022–1023.
36 ibid. pp. 1038–1039.
37 ibid. p. 1029.
38 'Nurses' Registration Bill, N.S.W.', *ANJ*, Sep. 1915, p. 322.
39 *NSWPD*, vol. XXXIX, 1910, p. 453 & vol. LI, 1913, p. 1416.
40 Sir Charles Mackellar died at the age of 81 in 1926. Ann M. Mitchell, 'Sir Charles Kinnaird Mackellar' in *Australian Dictionary of Biography*, vol. 10: 1891–1939, eds Bede Nairn & Geoffry Searle, Melbourne University Press, Melbourne, 1986, pp. 297–298.
41 'State Registration in Qld.', *ANJ*, Mar. 1912, p. 74.
42 J.B. McLean & E.L. Hunter, Honorary Secretaries Qld, to Dr Dansey, Honorary Secretary NSW, 29 Aug. 1911, *ANJ*, Sep. 1911, pp. 294–295.
43 *Health Act Amendment Act of 1911* (Qld).
44 'State Registration In Queensland', *ANJ*, Sep. 1911, p. 295.
45 ATNA, Qld, to Home Secretary, n.d., in 'State Registration In Queensland', *ANJ*, Sep. 1911, p. 295.
46 *QPD*, vol. CVIII, 1911–1912, pp. 519–520.
47 ATNA, Qld, to Home Secretary, n.d., in 'State Registration In Queensland', pp. 295–296.
48 *Health Act Amendment Act of 1911* (Qld).
49 ibid.
50 'Council Meetings: Queensland Branch', *ANJ*, Feb. 1912, p. 39.
51 'State Registration', editorial, *ANJ*, Sep., 1911, p. 289.
52 Minutes of Council Meeting, ATNA Qld, 18 Jul. 1912.
53 *QPD*, vol. CV111, 1911, pp. 727–728.
54 ibid. p. 725.
55 ibid. p. 532.
56 ibid. p. 725.
57 ibid. p. 734.
58 ibid. p. 729.
59 ibid. pp. 724–725.
60 'Trained Nurses—Deputation to Home Secretary', *Brisbane Courier*, 29 Aug. 1911.
61 Willis, *Medical Dominance*, p. 53.
62 *Health Act Amendment Act of 1911* (Qld).
63 'State Registration of Nurses', *MJA*, p. 475.

64 Zachary Cope, *Six Disciples of Florence Nightingale*, Pitman Medical, London, 1961, p. 17.
65 Report of Nurses' Registration Board, *QPP*, vol. 2, 1913, p. 42.
66 ibid. vol. 2, 1914, p. 27.
67 Minutes of Council Meeting, ATNA Qld, 10 Aug. 1916.
68 Report of Nurses' Registration Board, *QPP*, vol. 1, 1927, p. 710.
69 *Health Act Amendment Act of 1911* (Qld).
70 *QPD*, vol. CLXXIII, 1938, p. 954.
71 ibid. p. 1510.
72 *Nurses and Masseurs Registration Acts Amendment Act of 1938*, (Qld).
73 'Council Meetings: Queensland Branch', *ANJ*, Feb. 1912, p. 39.
74 Memo to Hospitals, 10 Dec. 1912, Minutes of Council Meeting, ATNA Qld.
75 Minutes of Council Meeting, ATNA Qld, 16 Jan. & 20 Feb. 1913.
76 *QPD*, vol. CXXV, 1916–1917, p. 2852.
77 Minutes of Council Meeting, ATNA Qld, 20 Mar. 1913.
78 'Volunteer!', *ANJ*, Oct. 1914, p. 329.
79 Marianne Barker, *Nightingales in the Mud: The Digger Sisters of the Great War 1914–1918*, Allen & Unwin, Sydney, 1989, p. 188.
80 'The Staffing of Military Hospitals: Conference with the P. M.O.'s', *ANJ*, Dec. 1915, p. 414.
81 ibid. p. 413 & minutes of Council Meetings, ATNA Qld, 18 Nov. & 9 Dec. 1915.
82 Minutes of Council Meeting, ATNA Qld, 9 Dec. 1915.
83 'The Staffing of Hospital Ships', editorial, *ANJ*, Jan. 1916, p. 1.
84 Minutes of Council Meeting, ATNA Qld, 13 Jan. 1916.
85 'The Staffing of Hospital Ships', p. 2.
86 Mary Dickenson, 'The Nursing Profession as a Pressure Group', *Australian Journal of Social Issues*, vol. 11, no. 2, May 1976, p. 90.
87 *Nurses and Masseurs Registration Act of 1928* (Qld).
88 Dickenson, 'The Nursing Profession as a Pressure Group', p. 91.
89 ibid. p. 90.
90 ibid. p. 98.
91 Fred E. Katz, 'Nurses' in *The Semi-Professions and Their Organization: Teachers, Nurses, Social Workers*, ed. Amitai Etzioni, Free Press, New York, 1969, pp. 71–72.
92 Andrew C. Twaddle & Richard M. Hessler, *A Sociology of Health*, C.V. Mosby, Saint Louis, 1977, p. 187.
93 Bryan S. Turner, *Medical Power and Social Knowledge*, Sage, London, 1987, p. 135.
94 Hospital Employees (Nursing Staff—Australian Capital Territory) Case, *Commonwealth Arbitration Reports (CAR)*, vol. 90, 1958, pp. 362–363.
95 'All at Sea', editorial, *ANJ*, Mar. 1973, p. 4.

96 Registered Nurses Professional Rates Case, decision D89/0211, 19 May 1989, Victorian Industrial Relations Commission.
97 See for instance Etzioni, *The Semi-Professions and Their Organization*; Twaddle & Hessler, A *Sociology of Health*; Millerson, *The Qualifying Associations*; Paul Boreham, Alec Pemberton & Paul Wilson, eds, *The Professions in Australia: A Critical Appraisal*, University of Queensland Press, Brisbane, 1976. This approach is discussed in Terence Johnson, *Professions and Power*, Macmillan, London, 1972, chapter 2.
98 Turner, *Medical Power and Social Knowledge*, pp. 134–135.
99 Johnson, *Professions and Power*, p. 10.
100 Millerson, *The Qualifying Associations*, pp. 4–5.
101 ibid. p. 4.
102 ibid. p. 10.
103 ibid. p. 9.
104 Katz, 'Nurses', pp. 75–76.
105 Twaddle & Hessler, A *Sociology of Health*, p. 188.
106 For a fuller discussion of this see Reverby, *Ordered to Care*, pp. 199–207.
107 Marie Francoise Colliere, 'Invisible care and invisible women as health-care providers', *International Journal of Nursing Studies*, vol. 23, no. 2, 1986, pp. 102–103.
108 See, for example, evidence given to the Royal Commission on Charitable Institutions, *VPP*, 1892 and Gregory, A *Tradition of Care*, p. 23.
109 Willis, *Medical Dominance*, p. 21.
110 ibid. p. 25.
111 Colliere, 'Invisible care and invisible women as health care-providers', p. 103.
112 Katz, 'Nurses', p. 58.
113 Reverby, *Ordered to Care*, p. 1.
114 Gregory, A *Tradition of Care*; Trembath & Hellier, *All Care and Responsibility*; Reverby, *Ordered to Care*.
115 Colliere, 'Invisible care and invisible women as health-care providers', p. 104.
116 Reverby, *Ordered to Care*, p. 4.
117 Johnson, *Professions and Power*, p. 22.
118 ibid. p. 18.
119 Twaddle & Hessler, A *Sociology of Health*, pp. 188–189.
120 Richard L. Simpson & Ida Harper Simpson, 'Women and Bureaucracy in the Semi-Professions' in *The Semi-Professions and Their Organization*, p. 197.
121 ibid. p. 198.
122 Australian Bureau of Statistics, *Labour Statistics Australia, 1993*, cat. no 6101.0, (Canberra: Australian Bureau of Statistics, 1994), p. 43.
123 Simpson & Simpson, 'Women and Bureaucracy in the Semi-Professions', pp. 234–235.

124 ibid. p. 235.
125 Melosh, '*The Physician's Hand*', p. 18.
126 ibid. p. 25.
127 Turner, *Medical Power and Social Knowledge*, p. 135.
128 ibid. p. 140.
129 Melosh, '*The Physician's Hand*', p. 19.
130 Willis, *Medical Dominance*, p. 30.
131 'Conference of the Councils of the A.T.N.A. with the Council of the R.V.T.N.A.', *Una*, Feb. 1913, p. 299.
132 Turner, *Medical Power and Social Knowledge*, p. 141.
133 Ross Patrick, *A History of Health and Medicine in Queensland 1824–1960*, University of Queensland Press, Brisbane, 1987, p. 86.
134 Articles discussing whether nursing is a profession abound. See, for example, Joan E. Lynaugh & Claire M. Fagin, 'Nursing Comes of Age', *Image*, vol. 20, no. 4, Winter 1988, pp. 184–190; E. Crowder, 'Historical Perspectives of Nursing's Professionalism', *Occupational Health Nursing*, vol. 33, no. 4, 1985, pp. 184–190; Margaret Parsons, 'The Profession in a Class by Itself', *Nursing Outlook*, vol. 34, no. 6, 1986, pp. 270–275.
135 Johnson, *Professions and Power*, p. 32.

Chapter 5

1 J.McLean, Medical Superintendent Brisbane Hospital, to Under Secretary, Home Secretary's Office, 28 Mar. 1921, 21/1868, COL/367, QSA.
2 Details of survey results from the file Hospitals & Awards, 21/1332, COL/367, QSA. Numbers of hospitals tallied for each section varies as not all hospitals answered all questions.
3 Social Statistics of Queensland 1920, *QPP*, vol. II, 1922, p. 262.
4 Replies of hospitals to Under Secretary, Home Secretary's Office, Mar. 1921, Hospitals & Awards, 21/1332, COL/367, QSA.
5 The matron or head of the nursing section of a hospital or the sole nurse (when only one was employed in a hospital) was paid anything between 100 pounds per annum at Mungindi Hospital to 250 pounds at Camooweal Hospital, both hospitals employing two nurses. The majority of matrons (52) received between 120 pounds and 150 pounds, with the matron of Brisbane General Hospital being paid 250 pounds to 300 pounds. Nurses designated as sister earnt from 80 pounds to 140 pounds, with an average salary of 103 pounds. The salary of staff nurses averaged 95 pounds, with wages varying from 52 pounds to 130 pounds. Staff nurses at the Brisbane General Hospital earnt 72 pounds and sisters were paid from 105 pounds to 145 pounds. Married couples, acting as matron and wardsman, staffed three hospi-

tals earning a joint salary of 400 pounds at Burketown, 250 pounds at Kynuna and 130 pounds at Eidsvold.

6 The value of board and lodging was variously estimated by the hospitals at between 16 shillings 6 pence and 2 pounds 10 shillings a week. No explanation was given of how the monetary value of this provision was calculated but the majority of hospitals placed a value of between 52 pounds and 78 pounds per year on board and lodging.

7 *Queensland Government Gazette* (QGG), vol. CXIII, no. 312, 16 Dec. 1919.

8 Reply of Hospital for Sick Children, Brisbane, 12 Mar. 1921, 21/2158, COL/367, QSA.

9 Minutes of Council Meeting, ATNA Qld, 20 Jul. 1920.

10 Minutes of Special General Meeting, ATNA Qld, 14 Sep. 1920.

11 Minutes of Council Meeting, ATNA Qld, 14 Dec. 1920.

12 ibid. 9 Nov. 1920.

13 ibid. 14 Dec. 1920.

14 ibid. 18 Jan. 1921.

15 ibid.

16 ibid. 19 Jul. 1921.

17 'An Appeal to Members of the A.T.N.A. Queensland Branch', *ANJ*, Nov. 1921, p. 380.

18 Application for Registration, ATNA, 8 Nov. 1921, file 96, Queensland Industrial Commission (QIC).

19 RANF Application to amend Registration in respect to callings, 4 Jan. 1971, file 96, QIC.

20 The only records of the activities of the QNA that have been obtained are those at the QIC. These contain membership numbers and the details of claims filed with the court. No other records are known to be extant.

21 Interview with Bartz Schultz, 12 Jun. 1995, Brisbane.

22 Denis Murphy, *Ken Laidlaw: A White Collar Union Leader*, Australian Bank Employees Union, Brisbane, 1979, pp. 8, 17, 67.

23 ibid. pp. 16–25.

24 ibid. pp. 63–64.

25 ibid. p. 23.

26 QNA Constitution and Rules, file 87, QIC.

27 ibid.

28 This Australian Nurses' Federation is not the same organisation as the Australian Nursing Federation formed in 1924. Information regarding the federal registration of the Australian Nurses' Federation in 1921 comes from copies of documents made in 1949 from the federal Industrial Registry's files and contained in the papers of the RANF, Melbourne. The original Industrial Registry file no longer exists.

29 Transcript of telephone conversation from ATNA Qld to Secretary, ATNA NSW, 7 Jun. 1949, RANF Melbourne. The transcript stated that, as far as they could ascertain, the registration was effected on 5 July 1949.
30 Mary B. Harper, secretary ATNA Qld, to E. Evans, General Secretary ANF, 7 Jun. 1949, RANF, Melbourne.
31 Copy of letter from K. Laidlaw, Secretary QNA to Industrial Registrar, Melbourne, 18 Aug. 1924, RANF, Melbourne.
32 Application for Registration of an Industrial Association (or Trade Union) of Employees by QNA, Industrial Registrar 10 Jan. 1921, file 87, QIC.
33 Membership included 77 out of approximately 125 nurses at the Brisbane General; 65 out of approximately 72 at the Children's Hospital; 35, approximately all, nurses at the Diamantina Hospital; ten out of fifteen nurses at Roma Hospital; two nurses at Townsville General Hospital. (QNA List of Members up till 31 Dec. 1921, Industrial Registrar 11 May 1922, file 87, QIC; Social Statistics 1920, *QPP*, vol. 2, 1922, p. 262.)
34 QNA List of Members up till 31 Dec. 1921 Industrial Registrar 11 May 1922, file 87, QIC and Gregory, *A Tradition of Care*, pp. 69–70, 165.
35 Superintendent, Diamantina Hospital to Under Secretary, Home Secretary's Office, 2 Mar. 1922, COL/367, QSA.
36 Trembath & Hellier, *All Care and Responsibility*, pp. 126–148.
37 K.H. Laidlaw, Honorary Secretary QNA, to Industrial Registrar, 5 Apr. 1933, file 87, QIC.
38 QNA List of Members for year ending 31 Dec. 1932, file 87, QIC.
39 QNA List of Members for year ending 31 Dec. 1933, file 87, QIC.
40 K.H. Laidlaw to Industrial Registrar, 26 Mar. 1936, file 87, QIC.
41 File 87, QIC.
42 Gillian Whitehouse & Kenneth Wiltshire, *The History of the Queensland Professional Officers' Association*, Royal Australian Institute of Public Administration, Brisbane, 1987, pp. 14, 49, 65.
43 Flanders, *Management and Unions*, p. 43.
44 Hobbs, *But Westward Look*, p. 237; Dickenson, *An Unsentimental Union*, p. 59; Trembath & Hellier, *All Care and Responsibility*, p. 172.
45 Whitehouse & Wiltshire, *The History of the Queensland Professional Officers' Association*, p. 27.
46 'Australasian Trained Nurses' Association Conference', *ANJ*, Aug. 1921, p. 258.
47 Claims of the QNA, COL/367, QSA.
48 J. McLean, ATNA President, 18 Mar. 1921, COL/367, QSA.
49 Minutes of Annual General Meeting, ATNA Qld, 21 Jun. 1921.
50 J. McLean, ATNA President, 18 Mar. 1921, COL/367, QSA.
51 ibid.

52 'Nurses and Hospitals', Editorial, *MJA*, 16 Jul. 1921, pp. 47–48.
53 Country Hospitals' Association, 11 Apr. 1921, Hospitals & Awards, 21/1332, COL/367, QSA.
54 Answer to application by Dr E. Humphrey, Townsville, 18 Mar. 1921, case 52 of 1921, QIC.
55 Answer by respondents, Stanthorpe Hospital Committee, 16 Mar. 1921, Hospitals & Awards, 21/1332, COL/367, QSA.
56 Answer by respondents, Gladstone Hospital, 10 Mar. 1921, Hospitals & Awards, COL/367, QSA.
57 Answer to application by Dr E. Humphrey, Townsville, 18 Mar. 1921, case 52 of 1921, QIC.
58 Hospitals & Awards, 21/1332, COL/367, QSA.
59 Answer by respondents, Gladstone Hospital, 10 Mar. 1921, Hospitals & Awards, 21/1332, COL/367, QSA.
60 Hughenden District Hospital to Under Secretary, Home Secretary's Office, 26 Mar. 1921, Hospitals and Awards, 21/1332, COL/367, QSA.
61 QGG, vol. CXVI, no. 290, 23 Jun. 1921.
62 J.B. McLean, Medical Superintendent, Brisbane Hospital, to Under Secretary, Home Secretary's Office, 28 Feb. 1921, 21/1868, COL/367, QSA.
63 J.B. McLean, Medical Superintendent, Brisbane Hospital, to Under Secretary, Home Secretary's Office, 17 Feb. 1921, 21/1539, COL/367, QSA.
64 Hospitals & Awards, 21/1332, QSA.
65 QGG, vol. CXVI, no. 290, 23 Jun. 1921. No transcript of nurses' cases in the 1920s exists at the QIC or in ATNA records.
66 Social Statistics 1921, *QPP*, vol. 2, 1923, pp. 711–712.
67 QGG, vol. CXVI, no. 290, 23 Jun. 1921.
68 QGG, vol. CXVIII, no. 197, 8 Jun. 1922.
69 ibid.
70 Social Statistics 1921, *QPP*, vol. 2, 1923, pp. 711–712.
71 Printing Trades Case, South Australia, 1918 in George Anderson, *Fixation of Wages in Australia*, Macmillan, Melbourne, 1929, pp. 389–398.
72 Harvester decision, *CAR*, vol. 2, 1907–1908, p. 3.
73 Fruit-pickers' case, *CAR*, vol. 6, 1912, p. 72.
74 Anderson, *Fixation of Wages in Australia*, p. 398.
75 Clothing Trades case, *CAR*, vol. 13, 1919, p. 691.
76 *Industrial Arbitration Act of 1916* (Qld), Section 9.
77 Answer by respondents, Stanthorpe Hospital Committee, 16 Mar. 1921, Hospitals & Awards, 21/1332, COL/367, QSA.
78 *Industrial Arbitration Act of 1916* (Qld), Section 8.
79 This question was examined in a case in which the QTU claimed equal pay for women teachers. Justice McCawley concluded that 'even if the work of the female is shown to be equally or more important,

or equally or more valuable, it is not established that the work is the "same work" '. He decided that the union case had not established that female and male teachers did the same work and equal pay was not granted. The court would have faced problems too great to bear if it had seriously entertained the idea that females contributed more than male teachers, for how could males have been paid less? (QGG, vol. CXIII, no. 296, 11 Dec. 1919.)

80 Margaret Power, 'Woman's Work Is Never Done—by Men: A Socio-Economic Model of Sex-Typing in Occupations', *Journal of Industrial Relations*, vol. 17, no. 3, Sep. 1975, pp. 227–229.

81 Anderson, *Fixation of Wages in Australia*, pp. 279–281.

82 QGG, vol. CXVI, no. 290, 23 Jun. 1921.

83 Minutes of Sub-committee Meeting, ATNA Qld, 14 Mar. 1921, COL/367, QSA.

84 Answer to QNA claim by Committees of Cloncurry, Hughenden, Richmond and Winton Public Hospitals, COL/367, QSA.

85 QGG, vol. CXVI, no. 290, 23 Jun. 1921.

86 *Factories and Shops Act of 1900* (Qld), Section 45.

87 Anderson, *Fixation of Wages in Australia*, p. 435.

88 Hospitals & Awards, 21/1332, COL/367, QSA.

89 QGG, vol. CXVI, no. 290, 23 Jun. 1921.

90 ibid.

91 Anderson, *Fixation of Wages in Australia*, p. 429.

92 A fourth year trainee's salary was 34 per cent of a wardsman's wage or 45 per cent after the value of board and lodging has been deducted from the male rate. Pantrymaids, housemaids, waitresses and generals received 29 per cent of the male salary, or 39 per cent after the value of board and lodging has been deducted from the male wage. Laundresses received 35 per cent of the salary of a laundryman, or 47 per cent if board and lodging is considered.

93 Details of QNA claim from Application for Award by Queensland Nurses' Association, COL/367, QSA. Answer and comments of ATNA from Meeting of ATNA Sub-committee, 14 Mar. 1921, observations on QNA claim, COL/367, QSA. Details of award from QGG, vol. CXVI, no. 290, 23 Jun. 1921.

94 Social Statistics 1921, *QPP*, vol. 2, 1923, pp. 711–712.

95 Anderson, *Fixation of Wages in Australia*, pp. 510–513. In Queensland, shop assistants worked 47 hours a week, clerks worked 44 hours a week in the central and southern divisions of the state and 40 hours in the northern division, and Queensland Public Service clerks and typists worked 36 3/4 hours each week. (QGG, vol. CXV, no. 69, 5 Aug. 1920; no. 103, 20 Aug. 1920; no. 320, 22 Dec. 1920.)

96 *Industrial Arbitration Act of 1916* (Qld), Section 10.

97 QGG, vol. CXVI, no. 290, 23 Jun. 1921.

98 The QNA claim was similar to other awards including the Clerks' Award, Queensland Public Service General Officers' Award and Teachers' Award. (QGG, vol. CXV, no. 164, 23 Sep. 1920; vol. CXVI, no. 104, 23 Mar. 1921; no. 187, 21 Apr. 1921.)

99 Meeting of ATNA Sub-committee, 14 Mar. 1921, observations on QNA claim, COL/367, QSA.

100 The QNA proposed that overtime should be paid at the rate of time-and-a-half for day work and double time for night work. This was opposed by the ATNA who emphasised that 'double time should never be paid'. Double time was paid in some other awards, with shop assistants receiving this rate for all overtime worked after 9.30 pm. (QGG, vol. CXV, no. 69, 5 Aug. 1920.)

101 *Industrial Arbitration Act of 1916* (Qld), Section 10.

102 QGG, vol. CXVI, no. 290, 23 Jun. 1921.

103 Other hospital workers received a maximum of three weeks sick leave each year while clerks received a maximum of twelve days paid sick leave each year, shop assistants one week and Queensland Public Servants one week on full pay and one week on half pay each year. (QGG, vol. CXIII, no. 312, 16 Dec. 1919; vol. CXV, no. 69, 5 Aug. 1920; no. 103, 20 Aug. 1920; no. 320, 22 Dec. 1920.)

104 'Editorial Notes', *ANJ*, Dec. 1919, p. 398.

105 Claims of the QNA, COL/367 QSA; Meeting of Sub-committee of ATNA, 14 Mar. 1921, observations of QNA claim, COL/367 QSA; QGG, vol. CXVI, no. 290, 23 Jun. 1921.

106 J.K. Galbraith, 'The Economics of the American Housewife', *The Atlantic*, Aug. 1973 quoted in Kathleen Taperell, Carol Fox & Margaret Roberts, *Sexism in Public Service: The employment of women in Australian Government Administration*, AGPS, Canberra, 1975, p. 17.

107 QGG, vol. CXVI, no. 290, 23 Jun. 1921.

108 ibid.

109 C. Chuter, Discussion of award clauses, COL/367, QSA.

110 *Industrial Arbitration Act Amendment Act of 1924* (Qld).

111 Affidavit, Dorothy Corlass & Kenneth H. Laidlaw, President & Secretary QNA, 6 Jul. 1925, case no 302 of 1925, QIC and affidavit and application of the Queensland Government Professional Officers' Association to be joined as a party, 25 Jul. 1925, case no 302 of 1925, QIC.

112 Minutes of Council Meeting, ATNA Qld, 15 Jul. 1925.

113 Reply of the Brisbane and South Coast District Hospitals Board, 25 Jul. 1925, case 302 of 1925, QIC.

114 'Concerning 44 hour week, for nurses in General Hospitals', COL/367, QSA.

115 QGG, vol. CXXV, no. 40, 8 Aug. 1925.

116 Glenda Law (nee Strachan), ' "I have never liked Trade Unionism": the Development of the Royal Australian Nursing Federation,

Queensland Branch, 1904–45' in *Women, Class and History: Feminist Perspectives on Australia 1788–1978*, ed. Elizabeth Windschuttle, Fontana, Melbourne, 1980, p. 204.

117 Trembath & Hellier, *All Care and Responsibility*, p. 73.

118 ibid.

119 ibid.

120 ibid.

121 Letter to editor, *New Idea*, 6 Apr. 1985, p. 101.

Chapter 6

1 Florence Chatfield, Royal Commission on Public Hospitals, *QPP*, vol. 1, 1930, p. 673.

2 Brian Costar, 'Was Queensland different?' in *The Wasted Years? Australia's Great Depression*, ed. Judy Mackinolty, George Allen & Unwin, Sydney, 1981, p. 162.

3 Ross Fitzgerald, *A History of Queensland from 1915 to the 1980s*, University of Queensland Press, Brisbane, 1984, p. 168.

4 Costar, 'Was Queensland different?', p. 159.

5 Brian Costar, 'Labor, Politics and Unemployment: Queensland during the Great Depression', PhD thesis, University of Queensland, 1981, p. xvi.

6 ibid. p. xvii.

7 L.J. Louis, *Trade Unions and the Depression: A Study of Victoria, 1930–1932*, Australian National University Press, Canberra, 1968, p. 142.

8 Costar, 'Labor, Politics and Unemployment', pp. 139, 151.

9 Judy Mackinolty, 'Woman's place . . . ' in *The Wasted Years?*, ed. Mackinolty, pp. 101–102.

10 Josephine Castle, *Nursing at the Wollongong Hospital 1926–1982*, University of Wollongong Press, Wollongong, 1984, p. 15.

11 Mackinolty, 'Woman's place . . . ', p. 102.

12 ibid. p. 110.

13 Margaret Power, 'Women and Economic Crises: the Great Depression and the Present Crisis' in *Women, Class and History*, ed. Windschuttle, p. 497.

14 ibid. p. 499.

15 Louis, *Trade Unions and the Depression*, p. 142.

16 Case 173 of 1930, transcript, 6 Oct. 1930, p. 2, QIC.

17 Application for New Award, case 173 of 1930, QIC.

18 Basic Wage and Wage Reduction Inquiry, CAR, vol. 30, 1931, p. 31.

19 Mark Bray & Malcolm Rimmer, *Delivering the Goods: A History of the Transport Workers' Union in New South Wales 1888–1986*, Allen & Unwin, Sydney, 1987, p. 133.

20 Costar, 'Labor, Politics and Unemployment', p. 55.
21 Whitehouse & Wiltshire, *The History of the Queensland Professional Officers' Association*, pp. 81, 83.
22 Andrew Spaull & Martin Sullivan, *A History of the Queensland Teachers' Union*, Allen & Unwin, Sydney, 1989, pp. 181–182.
23 Minutes of Council Meeting, ATNA Qld, 14 Oct. 1930.
24 Notice of Motion of Henry Bolton, 5 Sep. 1930, case 173 of 1930, and Notice of Motion and Affidavit of Henry Bolton, 2 Oct. 1930, case 188 of 1930, QIC.
25 Application for New Award, Case 173 of 1930, QIC.
26 Minutes of Council Meeting, ATNA Qld, 9 Sep. 1930.
27 Answer of ATNA, 17 Sep. 1930, case 173 of 1930, QIC.
28 Case 173 of 1930, transcript, 24 Oct. 1930, p. 1, QIC.
29 Case 173 of 1930. transcript, 6 Oct. 1930, p. 3, QIC.
30 QGG, vol. CXXXV, no. 159, 31 Oct. 1930.
31 ibid. no. 196, 1 Dec. 1930.
32 ibid. vol. CXXXVII, no. 29, 1 Jul. 1931.
33 Notice of Motion filed by Henry Bolton, 5 Sep. 1930, case 173 of 1930, QIC.
34 Bray & Rimmer, *Delivering the Goods*, pp. 131–132.
35 *Industrial Conciliation and Arbitration Act of 1929* (Qld).
36 Royal Commission on Public Hospitals, *QPP*, vol. 1, 1930, p. 649. Transcript of the evidence is not given in the report of the Royal Commission and there are no records of this in the Queensland State Archives.
37 ibid. p. 673.
38 ibid. pp. 673 & 674.
39 Case 173 of 1930, transcript, 6 Oct. 1930, p. 2, QIC.
40 Royal Commission on Public Hospitals, 1930, p. 674.
41 Tom Sheridan, *Mindful Militants: The Amalgamated Engineering Union in Australia 1920–1972*, Cambridge University Press, Cambridge, 1975, p. 111.
42 ibid.
43 'Question of Ethics', *ANJ*, May 1925, p. 229.
44 Letter to editor, *ANJ*, Jul. 1933, p. 152.
45 'The Accommodation for the Nursing Staff in Hospitals', *ANJ*, Nov. 1927, p. 338.
46 Case 173 of 1930, transcript, 6 Oct. 1930, pp. 1–2, QIC.
47 ibid. p. 3.
48 QGG, vol. CXXXV, no. 137, 11 Oct. 1930.
49 ibid.
50 Answer of ATNA, 17 Sep. 1930 & answer of QNA, 18 Sep. 1930, and transcript, 24 Oct. 1930, p. 3, case 173 of 1930, QIC.
51 QGG, vol. CXXXV, no. 159, 31 Oct. 1930.

52 Bradon Ellem, *In Women's Hands? A History of Clothing Trades Unionism in Australia*, New South Wales University Press, Sydney, 1989, p. 181.
53 Spaull & Sullivan, *A History of the Queensland Teachers' Union*, p. 187.
54 *Daily Mail*, 24 Feb. 1931, quoted in Gregory, *A Tradition of Care*, p. 75.
55 Case 173 of 1930, transcript, 6 Oct. 1930, p. 3, QIC.
56 ibid. 24 Oct. 1930, p. 4.
57 ibid. p. 3.
58 ibid. p. 4.
59 ibid.
60 ibid.
61 Minutes of Council Meeting, ATNA Qld, 17 Jan. 1928.
62 ibid., 14 Jul. 1931.
63 QGG, vol CXLVIII, no. 65, 1 Apr. 1937.
64 Notice of Motion filed by Myra Spooner, ATNA Secretary, 16 Feb. 1937, Case 36 of 1937, QIC.
65 Case 36 of 1937, transcript, 16 Apr. 1937, p. 3, QIC.
66 Ross Fitzgerald & Harold Thornton, *Labor in Queensland from the 1880s to 1988*, University of Queensland Press, Brisbane, 1989, pp. 113–114.
67 Case 36 of 1937, transcript, 16 Apr. 1937, p. 3, QIC.
68 ibid. p. 5.
69 Minutes of Council Meeting, ATNA Qld, 12 Jun. 1933.
70 ibid. 10 Jul. 1933.
71 ATNA claim, 16 Feb. 1937, case 36 of 1937, QIC & QGG, vol. CXLVIII, no. 105, 4 May 1937.
72 Case 36 of 1937, transcript, 16 Apr. 1937, pp. 7–9, QIC.
73 Minutes of Council Meeting, ATNA Qld, 11 May 1937.

Chapter 7

1 Minutes of Council Meeting, ATNA Qld, 14 Aug. 1928.
2 Reverby, *Ordered to Care*, pp. 180–183.
3 Fitzgerald & Thornton, *Labor in Queensland*, p. 110.
4 Reverby, *Ordered to Care*, p. 104.
5 ibid. p. 100.
6 Sister Lena, 'Difficulties and Dangers in Private House Nursing', *Una*, Oct. 1903, p. 49.
7 Reverby, *Ordered to Care*, p. 96.
8 Sister Lena, 'Difficulties and Dangers in Private House Nursing', p. 49.
9 ibid. p. 46.
10 Melosh, *'The Physician's Hand'*, p. 82.
11 Reverby, *Ordered to Care*, p. 96. (Original italics.)
12 Minutes of Meeting of Private Nurses, ATNA Qld, 24 Jan. 1922.

13 Melosh, '*The Physician's Hand*', pp. 79–87 & letters to *ANJ* and *Una*, 1903 to 1914.
14 Sister Lena, 'Difficulties and Dangers in Private House Nursing', p. 48.
15 Janet M. Geister, 'Hearsay and Facts in Private Duty', *American Journal of Nursing*, vol. 26, no. 7, Jul. 1926, pp. 517–518.
16 Amy Mercer Smith to Dr McLean, 24 Oct. 1904, ATNA minutes, Qld Branch.
17 Minutes of General Meeting, ATNA Qld, 16 Feb. 1905.
18 Minutes of Annual General Meeting, ATNA Qld, 16 May 1905.
19 Madge S. Jones, letter to editor, *Una*, Oct. 1903, p. 60.
20 R.D.K.L., 'Re Scale of Fees for Private Nursing', letter to editor, *Una*, Jul. 1904, p. 79.
21 'A Daughter of Erin', 'A Nurse's Grievance', letter to editor, *Una*, Jun. 1905, p. 64.
22 Minutes of Council Meetings, ATNA Qld, 11 Feb. 1915 & 10 Feb. 1920; minutes of Special Council Meeting, ATNA Qld, 2 Feb. 1920.
23 Wray Vamplew, ed., *Australians: Historical Statistics*, Fairfax, Syme & Weldon, Sydney, 1987, p. 161.
24 Reverby, *Ordered to Care*, pp. 102–103.
25 Melosh, '*The Physician's Hand*', pp. 88–90.
26 'Special General Meeting', *ANJ*, Jul. 1911, p. 228.
27 ibid. p. 229.
28 ibid. p. 231.
29 ibid.
30 ibid. p. 230.
31 'Sympathiser', 'What is to become of the Australian Nurse?: 1. A Rejoinder', *ANJ*, Jul. 1913, p. 232.
32 'Nurses' Fees: A Suggestion', *ANJ*, Aug. 1912, p. 269.
33 'Puck', 'What is to become of the Australian Nurse?', *ANJ*, Jun. 1913, p. 195.
34 'What is to become of the Australian Nurse?', editorial, *ANJ*, Aug. 1913, pp. 253–254.
35 'Nurses' Fees', editorial, *ANJ*, Nov. 1913, p. 362.
36 As well as letters to the *ANJ*, letters to *Una* in 1912 supported this.
37 'Organize', letter to editor, *Una*, Sep. 1912, p. 165.
38 'Oberon', 'Underpaid Nurses II', *ANJ*, Sep. 1913, p. 297.
39 'Nurse', letter to editor, *Una*, Mar. 1912, p. 9.
40 'Dress Basket', letter to editor, *Una*, May 1912, p. 61.
41 Editor's comment, *Una*, May 1912, p. 61.
42 'Oberon', 'Underpaid Nurses II', p. 297.
43 E. Ludowici, 'Increased fees', *ANJ*, Oct. 1913. p. 340.
44 Minutes of Council Meeting, ATNA Qld, 18 Jul. 1912.
45 ibid. 21 Nov. 1912.
46 The questions that the nurses had to answer in the ballot were very confused but almost half the nurses wanted an increase in fees and

many more wanted an increase in the charge for laundry. One hundred and forty-five wanted all fees to be raised by half a guinea; 82 wanted an increase of half a guinea on the two guinea fee only; 155 voted for an increase in laundry charges; 83 wanted no increase in fees. ('Nurses' Fees', *Una*, Nov. 1912, p. 218.)

47 'Special General Meeting', *ANJ*, Nov. 1913, p. 368.

48 ibid. p. 367.

49 ibid. p. 371.

50 'Nurses' Fees', editorial, *ANJ*, Nov. 1913, p. 362.

51 Two hundred and ninety-eight nurses voted in favour of an increase in fees and 220 voted against. As a result of this the council resolved that weekly fees would be increased by 5 shillings 6 pence with the extra charge of 2 shillings 6 pence for laundry abolished. ('Result of Ballot re Fees', *Una*, Jan. 1913, p. 264.)

52 J.B. McLean to editor, quoted in 'The Raising of Fees and the Referendum' editorial, *ANJ*, Dec. 1913, p. 398.

53 'Queensland Branch: Special General Meeting', *ANJ*, Jan. 1914, pp. 8–11.

54 Minutes of Council Meeting, ATNA Qld, 19 Feb. 1914.

55 Minutes of Special Council Meeting, ATNA Qld, 27 Feb. 1914.

56 Trembath & Hellier, *All Care and Responsibility*, p. 72.

57 Minutes of Council Meeting, ATNA Qld, 18 Jan. 1921.

58 ibid. 15 Feb. 1921.

59 'Australasian Trained Nurses' Association Conference', *ANJ*, Aug. 1921, p. 257.

60 Minutes of Council Meeting, ATNA Qld, 10 Jan. 1922.

61 Minutes of Meeting of Private Nurses, ATNA Qld, 24 Jan. 1922.

62 ibid. 7 Feb. 1922.

63 Minutes of Executive Meeting, ATNA Qld, 21 Mar. 1922.

64 Minutes of Council Meeting, ATNA Qld, 11 Jul. 1922.

65 'A.T.N.A. (Queensland Branch) Private Nurses' Claim now before the State Arbitration Court', *ANJ*, Oct. 1922, p. 382.

66 QGG, vol. CXIX, no. 224, 23 Dec. 1922.

67 ibid.

68 Minutes of Council Meeting, ATNA Qld, 12 Jun. 1928.

69 ibid. 10 Jul. 1928.

70 ibid. 14 Aug. 1928.

71 ibid. 11 Dec. 1928.

72 Minutes of Special General Meeting, ATNA Qld, 30 Jan. 1929.

73 Minutes of Council Meeting, ATNA Qld, 14 May 1929.

74 Melosh, '*The Physician's Hand*', p. 111.

75 Hobbs, *But Westward Look*, p. 82.

76 Bill Gammage & Peter Spearritt, eds, *Australians: 1938*, Fairfax, Syme & Weldon, Sydney, 1987, p. 154.

77 Minutes of Council Meeting, ATNA Qld, 14 Jul. 1931.

78 Minutes of Special General Meeting, ATNA Qld, 1 Sep. 1931.
79 The result of the ballot was 411 nurses in favour of reducing the charge to three guineas a week and 88 nurses in favour of retaining the 4 guinea fee, although only 512 ballot papers were returned out of 1308 issued. The fees were lowered but it was decided that there would be no change in the fees charged for broken time which would remain the same as the amounts on the 1929 scale of fees. (Minutes of Council Meeting, ATNA Qld, 10 Nov. 1931.)
80 Minutes of Special General Meeting, ATNA Qld, 13 Jul. 1937.
81 ibid. 14 Sep. 1937.
82 ibid. 12 Jul. 1938.
83 Fitzgerald & Thornton, *Labor in Queensland*, p. 116.
84 Minutes of Council Meeting, ATNA Qld, 14 Feb. 1939.
85 ibid. 9 May 1939.
86 ibid. 10 Feb. 1942.
87 Minutes of Meeting of Private Nurses, ATNA Qld, 24 Feb. 1942.
88 Minutes of Council Meeting, ATNA Qld, 14 Apr. 1942.
89 ibid. 14 Jul. 1942.
90 Minutes of Annual General Meeting, ATNA Qld, 25 Jul. 1942.
91 Minutes of Council Meeting, ATNA Qld, 15 Sep. 1942.
92 ibid. 15 Dec. 1942.

Chapter 8

1 Report of the Committee Appointed by the Minister for Defence, 4 Jun. 1945; Department of Defence III Correspondence File Multiple Number System (Class 301) (Classified); 'Medical Manpower Position in Relation to the Services & Civilian Needs—Statement by Medical Services Directors' 1943–1946: A816, item 11/301/552, Australian Archives, ACT.
2 Rupert Goodman, *Queensland Nurses: Boer War to Vietnam*, Boolarong, Brisbane, 1985, p. 207.
3 Minutes of Annual General Meeting, ATNA Qld, 24 Jul. 1940.
4 Minutes of Council Meeting, ATNA Qld, 12 Nov. 1940.
5 ibid. 10 Dec. 1940.
6 Paul Hasluck, *The Government and the People, 1939–1941*, Australian War Memorial, Canberra, 1952, pp. 403–405.
7 S.J. Butlin, *War Economy 1939–1942*, Australian War Memorial, Canberra, 1955, pp. 225–226.
8 Hasluck, *The Government and the People 1942–1945*, pp. 283–284.
9 Wallace C. Wurth, *Control of Manpower in Australia: a general Review of the Administration of the Man-Power Directorate February, 1942–September, 1944*, Government Printer, Sydney, c.1944, pp. 107–110.

10 S.J. Butlin & C.B. Schedvin, *War Economy 1942–1945*, Australian War Memorial, Canberra, 1977, pp. 29, 31.
11 Quoted in Megan McMurchy, Margot Oliver & Jeni Thornley, *For Love or Money: a pictorial history of women and work in Australia*, Penguin, Melbourne, 1983, p. 110.
12 Wurth, *Control of Manpower in Australia*, pp. 71, 81–88.
13 ibid. p. 86.
14 ibid. pp. 97, 99, 102–103.
15 ibid. p. 63.
16 Edna Ryan & Anne Conlon, *Gentle Invaders: Australian Women at Work*, 2nd edn, Penguin, Melbourne, 1989, pp. 137–138.
17 Hasluck, *The Government and the People 1942–1945*, p. 291.
18 Butlin & Schedvin, *War Economy 1942–1945*, pp. 349,368.
19 Kate Darian-Smith, *On the Home Front: Melbourne in Wartime 1939–1945*, Oxford, Melbourne, 1990, pp. 57–58.
20 Wurth, *Control of Manpower in Australia*, p. 390.
21 ibid. pp. 101–102, 111.
22 Marilyn Lake, 'The War over Women's Work' in *A Most Valuable Acquisition: A People's History of Australia since 1788*, eds Verity Burgmann & Jenny Lee, McPhee Gribble, Melbourne, 1988, p. 205.
23 Gail Reekie, 'Women's Responses to War Work in Western Australia 1942–1946', *Studies in Western Australian History*, no. 7, Dec. 1983, p. 52.
24 ibid. p. 55.
25 Darian-Smith, *On the Home Front*, p. 67.
26 Ryan & Conlon, *Gentle Invaders*, p. 136 & Darian-Smith, *On the Home Front*, p. 64.
27 McMurchy, Oliver & Thornley, *For Love or Money*, p. 111.
28 Helen Crisp, 'Women in Munitions', *Australian Quarterly*, vol. 13, no. 3, Sep. 1941, p. 72.
29 ibid. pp. 72–73.
30 Lake, 'The War over Women's Work', p. 209.
31 McMurchy, Oliver & Thornley, *For Love or Money*, p. 113.
32 Lake, 'The War over Women's Work', p. 209.
33 McMurchy, Oliver & Thornley, *For Love or Money*, p. 112.
34 Ryan & Conlon, *Gentle Invaders*, pp. 133–134.
35 Darian-Smith, *On the Home Front*, pp. 69–72 & Reekie, 'Women's Responses to War Work in Western Australia', pp. 51–53.
36 Darian-Smith, *On the Home Front*, pp. 69, 79.
37 Lake, 'The War over Women's Work', p. 209.
38 Wurth, *Control of Manpower in Australia*, p. 162.
39 Allan S. Walker, *Middle East and Far East*, Australian War Memorial, Canberra, 1953, pp. 21, 51–52.
40 Allan S. Walker, *Medical Services of the R.A.N. and R.A.A.F.*, Australian War Memorial, Canberra, 1961, p. 428.

41 Goodman, *Queensland Nurses*, pp. 121–129.

42 Walker, *Medical Services of the R.A.N. and R.A.A.F.*, p. 420.

43 ibid. pp. 170, 415–473.

44 Alice Jackson, 'Nurses share mateship of war in New Guinea', *The Australian Women's Weekly*, 4 Dec. 1943, p. 12; Harry Keys, 'A.I.F. Nurses Inspired Besieged Singapore', *The Australian Women's Weekly*, 21 Feb. 1942, p. 7; 'Nightingales of the 9th Division', *The Australian Women's Weekly*, 3 Apr. 1943, p. 14.

45 'Devoted nursing saves thousands of lives', *The Australian Women's Weekly*, 10 Jun. 1944, p. 22.

46 Private X, 'Blitz-Worn Angel', *The Australian Women's Weekly*, 3 Jul. 1943, p. 10.

47 Director-General of Health to Secretary, Department of Defence Co-ordination, 24 May 1940; Department of Defence III General Correspondence (Unclassified) Series 'O' Multiple Number System; 'Manpower Proposal for Reservation of Triple Certificated Nursing Sisters' 1940: A663, item 0130/3/103 P, Australian Archives, ACT.

48 Report of proceedings of conference held for the purpose of discussing difficulties experienced in hospital management owing to the shortage of nurses, 26 Sept. 1941. Department of Defence III General Correspondence (Unclassified) Series 'O' Multiple Number System: 'Control of Nurses' 1942–1943: A663, item 0130/1/731, Australian Archives, ACT.

49 After a search of Australian Archives, unfortunately it seems that the records of the Queensland MCC no longer exist and were possibly lost or destroyed before reaching the Archives.

50 Minutes of Council Meeting, ATNA Qld, 14 Oct. 1941.

51 Minutes of Annual General Meeting, ATNA Qld, 24 Jul. 1940.

52 Minutes of Council Meeting, ATNA Qld, 14 Oct. 1941.

53 Proceedings of meeting of CMCC, 6 Jun. 1942; Department of Health, Reports of the Central Medical Control Committee 1938–Feb. 1946; 'Central Medical Co-ordination Committee 6 June 1942': CP94/1, item bundle 24, Australian Archives, ACT.

54 Report of meeting of Nurses' Sub-committee of CMCC, Melbourne, 1 Aug. 1942; Department of Health, Reports of Central Medical Control Committee 1938–Feb. 1946: CP94/1, item bundle 30, Australian Archives, ACT.

55 Sir Alan Newton, Deputy Chairman CMCC to all Deputy Chairmen, 5 Aug. 1942; Department of Health Central Medical Co-ordination Committee General Correspondence 1939–1945, 'Nurses Co-ordination' 1942: CP432/2, item bundle 3, Australian Archives, ACT.

56 Control of the Nursing Profession, Memorandum by Dr J.H.L. Cumpston, Director-General of the Emergency Medical Service, 16 Oct. 1942; Department of Defence III, General Correspondence (Un-

classified) Series 'O' Multiple Number System 'Control of Nurses' 1942–1943: A663, item 0130/1/731, Australian Archives, ACT.

57 A.N. Kellett and E. Evans, President and General Secretary, ANF, to Prime Minister, 4 Sep. 1942; Department of Defence, ibid.

58 Minutes of Council Meeting, ATNA Qld, 15 Sep. 1942.

59 J. Bell, ANF to H.S. Ward, Secretary, CMCC, 9 Dec. 1942; Department of Defence III General Correspondence (Unclassified), Series 'O' Multiple Number System 'Control of Nurses' 1942–1943: A663, item 0130/1/731, Australian Archives, ACT.

60 Dr Cumpston to W.C. Wurth, 22 Jan. 1943; Department of Defence, ibid.

61 Wurth, *Control of Manpower in Australia*, p. 179 & Annual Report of Council, 1942–1943, ATNA Qld, p. 3.

62 Wurth, *Control of Manpower in Australia*, pp. 179–180.

63 ibid. p. 177.

64 ibid. p. 180.

65 W.C. Wurth to Deputy Director-General, 10 Apr. & 18 Aug. 1943; Department of Labour and National Service Correspondence: B550, Australian Archives, Victoria.

66 Wurth, *Control of Man Power in Australia*, p. 180.

67 W.C. Wurth, Director General Man Power to Deputy Directors General, 28 Jun. & 21 Sep. 1943; Department of Labour and National Service Correspondence: B550, Australian Archives, Victoria.

68 W.C. Wurth, Director General Man Power to all Deputy Directors General, 25 Jul. 1944; Department of Labour and National Service, ibid.

69 Deputy Director General of Man Power NSW to Director General of Man Power, 28 Sep. 1943; Department of Labour and National Service Correspondence File, 'Nursing', 1942–1943: SP 191/1, Item 33100 Pt 1, Australian Archives, NSW.

70 Circular No. 306, Office of the Deputy Director General of Man Power NSW, 30 Nov. 1943; Department of Labour and National Service, ibid.

71 Butlin & Schedvin, *War Economy 1942–1945*, p. 374.

72 W.C. Wurth, Director General Man Power to Secretary Department of Defence, 20 Jun. 1944; Department of Defence III General Correspondence (Unclassified) Series 'O' Multiple Number System ('Medical Manpower Services and Civilian Requirements') 1944: A663, item 0130/1/791, Australian Archives, ACT.

73 W.C. Wurth, Director General Man Power to all Deputy Directors General, 28 Jul. 1943; Department of Labour and National Service, Correspondence File, 'Nursing', 1942–1943: SP191/1, item 33100, Pt 1, Australian Archives, NSW.

74 W.C. Wurth, Director General Man Power to all Deputy Directors General, 6 Oct. 1943; Department of Labour and National Service Correspondence: B550, Australian Archives, Victoria.
75 Wurth, *Control of Manpower in Australia*, p. 181.
76 ibid. p. 177.
77 S.R. Burston, Major-General D.G.M.S., to Director-General of Man Power, 24 Jul. 1944; Department of Defence III Correspondence File Multiple Number System (Class 301) (Classified), 'Medical Manpower Position in Relation to the Services & Civilian Needs—Statement by Services Medical Directors' 1943–1946: A816, item 11/301/552, Australian Archives, ACT.
78 Report of Committee Appointed by the Minister for Defence, 4 Jun. 1945; Department of Defence, ibid.
79 Control of the Nursing Profession Memorandum by Dr J.H.L. Cumpston, Director-General of the Emergency Medical Service, 16 Oct. 1942; Department of Health Central Medical Co-ordination Committee, General Correspondence 1939–1945 'Nurses Co-ordination' 1942: CP432/2, item bundle 3, Australian Archives, ACT.
80 Peter Punch, *Guidebook to Australian Industrial Law*, 4th edn, CCH, Sydney, 1984, pp. 19–21.
81 Minutes of Special Council Meeting, ATNA Qld, 4 Nov. 1942 & Minutes of Council Meetings, ATNA Qld, 15 Dec. 1942 & 19 Jan. 1943.
82 Pritchard Marsland & Co, solicitors, to Secretary, ANF, 18 Dec. 1942. E83/20, Archives of Business and Labour, Australian National University.
83 Minutes of Council Meeting, ATNA Qld, 14 Nov. 1944.
84 Nurses (Queensland Public Hospitals) Award 1991, decision 19 Jun. 1991, print J7768, Australian Industrial Relations Commission.
85 The only exception to this was those few matrons in charge of 100 to 150 bed hospitals in Port Pirie, South Australia who earned less than their Queensland counterparts. (Department of Health, Central Medical Co-ordination Committee, General Correspondence 1939–1945 'Nurses Co-ordination' 1942: CP432/2, item bundle 3, Australian Archives, ACT.)
86 Minutes of Special Council Meeting, ATNA Qld, 27 Feb. 1940.
87 QGG, vol. CLXI, no. 71, 8 Sep. 1943.
88 ibid.
89 ibid.
90 QGG, vol. CLIV, no. 99, 20 May 1940; vol. CLXI, no. 27, 2 Aug. 1943 & no. 71, 8 Sep. 1943.
91 Calculated from weighted average nominal weekly rates. Commonwealth Bureau of Census and Statistics, *Labour Report 1947*, Commonwealth Bureau of Census and Statistics, Canberra, 1948, pp. 58 & 60.
92 QGG, vol. CLXI, no. 71, 8 Sep. 1943.

93 ibid. vol. CLXIII, no. 84, 4 Nov. 1944.
94 Minutes of Council Meeting, ATNA Qld, 10 Jul. 1945.
95 ibid. 10 May 1938.
96 Annual Report of Council, 1939–1940, ATNA Qld, p. 5.
97 Minutes of Annual General Meeting, ATNA Qld, 19 Jul. 1939.
98 Minutes of Council Meeting, ATNA Qld, 10 Feb. 1942.
99 ibid. 15 Sep. 1942.
100 Reminiscences of nurses Gloria Becker nee Moore & Gladys Thiele nee Lewis, Graduate Nurses Archive, Royal Brisbane Hospital.
101 'Melbourne Letter: Nurses' Salaries', *Cairns Post*, 7 Aug. 1944.
102 C.E. Nell Grant, 'Annual Meeting, Queensland', *ANJ*, Jun. 1945, p. 84.
103 *Commonwealth Parliamentary Debates*, vol. 180, 1944, p. 2429.
104 Grant, 'Annual Meeting, Queensland', p. 84.
105 'Two Women Fined', *Queensland Times*, 29 Apr. 1944.
106 Gail Reekie, 'Industrial Action by Women Workers in Western Australia during World War II', *Labour History*, no. 49, Nov. 1985, p. 81, 82.
107 'Nurses Threaten Strike', *Queensland Times*, 8 Apr. 1944.
108 'Urgent Need', *Queensland Times*, 11 Apr. 1944.
109 'Strike to-morrow', *Queensland Times*, 12 Apr. 1944.
110 'Strike Threat', *Queensland Times*, 13 Apr. 1944.
111 'Goodna Strike', *Queensland Times*, 17 Apr. & 19 Apr. 1944.
112 'Nurses Threaten to Strike', *Queensland Times*, 27 Apr. 1944.
113 'Strike Threatened', *Queensland Times*, 28 Apr. 1944.
114 'Nurses Stop Work To-Day', *Courier-Mail*, 21 Mar. 1945 & '243 Patients Unattended', *Courier-Mail*, 22 Mar. 1945.
115 'Girls Ordered to Willowburn', *Courier-Mail*, 23 Mar. 1945.
116 List of Strikes in Queensland for month of August, 1944; Department of Labour and National Service, Central Office; General Correspondence of the Secretariat, and Administrative an Industrial Relations Divisions, 1940–c.1950: MP574/1, item 420/1/18, Australian Archives, Victoria.
117 'Trainees' Threat', *Cairns Post*, 1 Aug. 1944.
118 'Trainees Strike', *Cairns Post*, 2 Aug. 1944.
119 'Securing Hospital Staff', *Cairns Post*, 3 Aug. 1944.
120 M. Christina Atherton to editor, *Cairns Post*, 8 Aug. 1944.
121 'Hospital Staff', *Cairns Post*, 8 Aug. 1944.
122 'Hospital Staff', *Cairns Post*, 10 Aug. 1944.
123 'Closing of Wards', *Cairns Post*, 29 Aug. 1944.
124 'Staff Shortages', *Queensland Times*, 21 Apr. 1944.
125 'Nurses Threaten to Strike', *Queensland Times*, 27 Apr. 1944.
126 'Closure of Hospitals', *Queensland Times*, 22 Apr. 1944.
127 Minutes of Council Meeting, ATNA Qld, 9 Jan. 1945.
128 ibid. 8 May 1945.

129 ibid. 9 Oct. 1945.
130 ibid. 8 May 1945.
131 Reekie, 'Industrial Action by Women Workers in Western Australia during World War II', p. 81.
132 Lynn Beaton, 'The importance of women's paid labour: Women at work in World War II' in *Worth Her Salt: Women at work in Australia*, eds Margaret Bevege, Margaret James & Carmel Shute, Hale & Iremonger, Sydney, 1982, p. 94.
133 Minutes of Council Meeting, ATNA Qld, 14 Oct. 1941.
134 ibid. 9 Dec. 1941. Student nurses were admitted to the ATNA as associate members in 1933.
135 ibid. 9 Jun. & 14 Jul. 1942.
136 Agnes Pavey, 'Post-War Reconstruction in Schools of Nursing', *ANJ*, May 1942, p. 75.
137 'Trained Nurses Plan Safeguard Move', *Courier-Mail*, 28 Jul. 1944.
138 Minutes of Council Meeting, ATNA Qld, 18 Jan., 16 May, 15 Aug., 10 Oct. 1944 & 10 Apr. 1945; minutes of Annual General Meeting, ATNA Qld, 27 Jul. 1944.
139 Minutes of Annual General Meeting, ATNA Qld, 24 Jul. 1943.
140 Minutes of Council Meeting, ATNA Qld, 20 Jun. & 15 Aug. 1944.
141 ibid. 13 Mar. & 12 Jun. 1945.
142 ibid. 12 Jun. & 10 Jul. 1945.
143 Minutes of Annual General Meeting, ATNA Qld, 18 Jul. 1945; minutes of Council Meeting, ATNA Qld, 14 Aug. & 11 Sep. 1945.
144 Report on Conference of Council Members and Representative Nurses from Doctor's Surgeries and Private Nurses, ATNA Qld, 9 Oct. 1945.
145 Minutes of Special Council Meeting, ATNA Qld, 26 Mar. 1945.
146 'Nurses Reject "Same Old Story" ', *Courier-Mail*, 1 May 1945.
147 'Opposes Nurses Living on Roof', *Courier-Mail*, 12 Mar. 1945 & A.Tipper, 'Housing Nurses on Roof Opposed', letter to editor, *Courier-Mail*, 16 Mar. 1945.
148 Lillian M. Troedson, 'Housing Nurses', letter to editor, *Courier-Mail*, 7 May 1945.
149 Minutes of Council Meeting, ATNA Qld, 8 May 1945 & minutes of Special Council Meeting, ATNA Qld, 26 Mar. 1945.
150 Minutes of Special Council Meeting, ATNA Qld, 8 Jun. 1944; minutes of Annual General Meeting, ATNA Qld, 27 Jul. 1944.

Chapter 9

1 Minutes of Extraordinary General Meeting, ATNA Qld, 22 Oct. 1947.
2 ibid.
3 Butlin & Schedvin, *War Economy 1942–1945*, p. 701.
4 Fitzgerald & Thornton, *Labor in Queensland*, pp. 115–116.

5 E.C. McGrath, 'The Future of Women In Industry', *Australian Quarterly*, vol. 15, no. 2, Jun. 1943, p. 39.
6 ibid. p. 45.
7 Carolyn Allport, 'Left off the Agenda: Women, Reconstruction and New Order Housing', *Labour History*, no. 46, May 1984, p. 18.
8 ibid. p. 19.
9 ibid.
10 McMurchy, Oliver & Thornley, *For Love or Money*, p. 114.
11 ibid. pp. 114, 128.
12 Walker, *Medical Services of the R.A.N. and R.A.A.F.*, p. 487.
13 Allport, 'Left off the Agenda', p. 19.
14 Jim Hagan, *The History of the A.C.T.U.*, Longman Cheshire, Melbourne, 1981, p. 188.
15 ibid. p. 118.
16 Tom Sheridan, 'Planners and the Australian Labour Market 1945–1949', *Labour History*, no. 53, Nov. 1987, p. 99.
17 Hagan, *The History of the A.C.T.U.*, p. 120.
18 Standard Hours Enquiry, *CAR*, vol. 59, 1947, p. 586.
19 *Industrial Arbitration (Forty Hours Week) Amendment Act of 1947* (NSW).
20 *Industrial Conciliation and Arbitration Acts Amendment Act of 1947* (Qld).
21 Hagan, *The History of the A.C.T.U.*, p. 122.
22 ibid. p. 204.
23 Tom Sheridan, 'The trade unions and postwar reconstruction' in *Better Dead Than Red: Australia's First Cold War: 1945–1959, vol. 2*, eds Ann Curthoys & John Merritt, Allen & Unwin, Sydney, 1986, p. 14.
24 Basic Wage Inquiry, *CAR*, vol. 68, 1950, p. 840.
25 'Another One' (Brisbane Women's Hospital), 'Nurse Says: "Lamp Still Burns" ', letter to editor, *Courier-Mail*, 1 Oct. 1946.
26 'Disillusioned Trainee' (Brisbane General Hospital), 'Nurses' Conditions', letter to editor, *Courier-Mail*, 3 Nov. 1945.
27 'Six Fed-Up Nurses' (General Hospital), 'Hospital Staffs', letter to editor, *Courier-Mail*, 26 Nov. 1945.
28 Minutes of Council Meeting, ATNA Queensland, 13 Mar. 1946. Hospitals represented were Brisbane, Mater, Turrawan, St Helen's, St Martin's (all in Brisbane) and Ipswich.
29 Minutes of Annual General Meeting, ATNA Qld, 30 Jul. 1946.
30 Minutes of Council Meeting, ATNA Qld, 13 Mar. & 8 Oct. 1946.
31 ibid. 14 May 1946.
32 ibid. 13 Aug. 1946.
33 ibid. 8 Oct. 1946.
34 ibid. 14 May 1946.
35 ibid. 13 Aug. 1946.
36 ibid. 13 Nov. 1946.

37 'Disillusioned Trainee', 'Nurses' Conditions'.
38 Minutes of Council Meeting, ATNA Queensland, 8 Jan. 1946.
39 Gregory, *A Tradition of Care*, p. 100. This film is not in the collections of the National Library or National Film and Sound Archive and could not be located elsewhere.
40 Case 165 of 1946, transcript, 13 Sep. 1946, p. 31, QIC.
41 ibid. 11 Apr. 1947, pp. 2–3.
42 *QPD*, vol. CLXIV, 1948, p. 1009.
43 The number of in-patients increased from 127 030 for the year ended June 1944 to 139 315 for the year ended June 1946 while at the same time the average number of nursing staff decreased from 2732 to 2564. (Case 165 of 1946, transcript, 11 Apr. 1947, p. 12, QIC.)
44 Case 165 of 1946, transcript, 11 Apr. 1947, p. 12, QIC.
45 'Hospital's Radio Call for Helpers', *Courier-Mail*, 16 Dec. 1946.
46 'Nurses' Conditions should be Improved', *Courier-Mail*, 1 Nov. 1945.
47 'Hospital Fear of Staff Cut', *Courier-Mail*, 10 Oct. 1945.
48 'Nurse Lack Forces Patients out of Cloncurry', *Courier-Mail*, 1 Oct. 1945.
49 'Hospital Fear of Staff Cut', *Courier-Mail*, 10 Oct. 1945.
50 'Staff Shortages Close Hospitals', *Courier-Mail*, 21 Dec. 1946.
51 *QPD*, vol. CXCIII, 1948, p. 861.
52 Case 165 of 1946, transcript, 11 Apr. 1947, p. 2, QIC.
53 ibid. p. 12.
54 Case 165 of 1946, Statement of Industrial Court, 14 Apr. 1947, p. 2, QIC.
55 Case 165 of 1946, transcript, 11 Apr. 1947, p. 3, QIC.
56 Of 4856 women discharged from the services from June to August 1945, almost half (2352) 'immediately took up home duties'. ('Army Girls Prefer Home', *Courier-Mail*, 20 Nov. 1945.)
57 Case 165 of 1946, transcript, 13 Sep. 1946, pp. 5–6, QIC.
58 ibid. 11 Apr. 1947, p. 29.
59 Case 165 of 1946, Statement of the Industrial Court of Queensland, 14 Apr. 1947, p. 2, QIC.
60 'ANF 1937–1947', report to International Council of Nurses meeting, May 1947, p. 2.
61 'Need for Amenities', *Courier-Mail*, 1 Nov. 1945.
62 ibid.
63 Case 165 of 1946, transcript, 13 Sep. 1946, p. 11, QIC.
64 ibid. p. 26.
65 'Shortage of Nurses Creates Serious Position', *Western Star*, 23 Nov. 1945.
66 'Australian Nursing Federation', *ANJ*, Feb.–Mar. 1946, p. 43.
67 Case 165 of 1946, transcript, 13 Sep. 1946, p. 47, QIC.
68 ibid. 11 Apr. 1947, p. 6.
69 *QPD*, vol. CLXIV, 1948, p. 1024.

70 Case 165 of 1946, transcript, 13 Sep. 1946, p. 68, QIC.
71 ibid. p. 55.
72 ibid. p. 56.
73 'Wellwisher', 'Girls For Hospitals', letter to editor, *Courier-Mail*, 9 Oct. 1945. The editor replied that this power of direction no longer existed.
74 A.W.A., 'Servicewomen Object', letter to editor, *Courier-Mail*, 12 Oct. 1945.
75 Mrs C.E. Smith, 'Plea For Nurses', letter to editor, *Courier-Mail*, 9 Dec. 1946.
76 *QPD*, vol. CLXXXVII, 1946, p. 2090.
77 ibid. vol. CLXXXVIII, 1946, p. 504.
78 ibid. p. 507.
79 ibid. p. 2090.
80 ibid. vol. CXCIV, 1948, p. 1067.
81 ibid. p. 1065.
82 ibid. vol. CLXXXVIII, 1946, p. 508.
83 Case 165 of 1946, Statement of Industrial Court, 14 Apr. 1947, p. 2, QIC.
84 *QPD*, vol. CLXXXVIII, 1946, p. 509 & ' "Poor Pay Not To Blame For Lack Of Nurses" ', *Courier-Mail*, 11 Dec. 1946.
85 B.M.C., 'Mr. Foley and Nursing', letter to editor, *Courier-Mail*, 17 Dec. 1946.
86 Minutes of Council Meeting, ATNA Qld, 12 Feb. 1946.
87 Butlin & Schedvin, *War Economy 1942–1945*, p. 790.
88 Case 165 of 1946, transcript, pp. 5, 7, 13 Sep. 1946, QIC.
89 National Security (Female Minimum Rates) Regulations, Statutory Rule no. 139, 1945.
90 *Commonwealth Gazette*, no. 170, 4 Sep. 1945.
91 Nursing Staffs in Repatriation Institutions Case, Determination 19 of 1946, *Commonwealth Public Service Arbitration Reports*, vol. 26, p. 111.
92 Case 165 of 1946, Statement of Industrial Court, 14 Apr. 1947, pp. 2–3, QIC.
93 National Security (Economic Organization) Regulations, Statutory Rule no. 11, 1945.
94 National Security (Economic Organization) Regulations, Statutory Rule no. 332, 1942.
95 Case 165 of 1946, transcript, 13 Sep. 1946, pp. 5–6, QIC.
96 ibid. pp. 6–7.
97 ibid. p. 16.
98 ibid. pp. 76–77.
99 ibid. p. 76.
100 Case 165 of 1946, Industrial Registrar to Chief Judge, Commonwealth Court of Conciliation and Arbitration, 26 Sep. 1946, QIC.
101 ibid.

102 Case 165 of 1946, Further Statement of Industrial Court and Approval of Senior Judge of Commonwealth Court, QIC.
103 Minutes of Special Council Meeting, ATNA Qld, 28 Nov. 1946.
104 ibid. 20 Dec. 1946.
105 ibid. 25 Feb. 1947.
106 Case 165 of 1946, Statement of Industrial Court, 14 Apr. 1947, QIC.
107 Case 165 of 1946, E. Drake Brockman, Judge, Commonwealth Court to Queensland Industrial Court, 18 Apr. 1947, QIC.
108 Minutes of 43rd Annual General Meeting, ATNA Qld, 29 Jul. 1947.
109 'Australian Nursing Federation', *ANJ*, Feb.–Mar. 1946, pp. 43–44.
110 Case 165 of 1946, transcript, 13 Sep. 1946, p. 22, QIC.
111 *QPD*, vol. CLXXXIII, 1944, p. 1867 & vol. CLXXXVIII, 1946, p. 507.
112 ibid. vol. CLXXXV, 1945, p. 916.
113 *Industrial Conciliation and Arbitration Act of 1932* (Qld), section 10.
114 Minutes of Council Meeting, ATNA Qld, 13 Mar. 1946.
115 Case 165 of 1946, transcript, 13 Sep. 1946, p. 21, QIC.
116 ibid. p. 41.
117 ibid. p. 23.
118 Minutes of Council Meeting, ATNA Qld, 11 Nov. 1947.
119 Case 804 of 1947, notice of motion, 27 Nov. 1947 & transcript, 18 Dec. 1947, QIC.
120 QGG, vol. CLXX, no. 5, 5 Jan. 1948.
121 Case 147 of 1948, transcript, 2 Dec. 1948, p. 1, QIC.
122 Case 165 of 1946, transcript, 13 Sep. 1946, pp. 21–22, QIC.
123 Case 147 of 1948, notice of motion, 23 Apr. 1948, QIC.
124 Case 147 of 1948, transcript, 2 Dec. 1948, pp. 2–3, 11, QIC.
125 ibid. p. 2.
126 QGG, vol. CLXXI, no. 148, 1 Nov. 1948 & no. 248, 25 Dec. 1948.
127 Case 165 of 1946, transcript, 13 Sep. 1946, pp. 22–23, QIC.
128 ibid. p. 21
129 ibid. p. 20.
130 ibid. p. 21.
131 Minutes of General Meeting, ATNA Qld, 29 Apr. 1949.
132 Case 165 of 1946, transcript, 13 Sep. 1946, pp. 32–35, QIC.
133 ibid. 11 Apr. 1947, p. 7.
134 ibid. p. 10.
135 ibid. pp. 22–23.
136 ibid. p. 14.
137 QGG, vol. CLXVIII, no. 30, 10 Feb. 1947.
138 Geraldine Turner, 'Tough Times For Nurses', *Herald*, 5 Feb. 1946.
139 Case 165 of 1946, transcript, 13 Sep. 1946, p. 64.
140 ibid. 11 Apr. 1947, p. 31.
141 ibid. p. 28.
142 ibid. 13 Sep. 1946, pp. 52, 61.

143 ibid. pp. 62–63.
144 ibid. p. 51.
145 ibid. 11 Apr. 1947, p. 26.
146 ibid. p. 25.
147 ibid. 13 Sep. 1946, p. 73.
148 ibid. p. 74.
149 ibid. p. 52.
150 ibid. p. 66.
151 ibid. pp. 53–54.
152 ibid. p. 53.
153 ibid. p. 54.
154 ibid. p. 52.
155 *QPD*, vol. CLXXXVI, 1945, p. 975.
156 Miss Abbott's Report to Annual Meeting, 29 Jul. 1948, Minutes of Annual General Meeting, ATNA Qld, 29 Jul. 1948.
157 Beatrice Roberts & A.L. Hart, 'What is the Trained Nurses' Guild?' *ANJ*, Dec. 1948, p. 262.
158 Minutes of Extraordinary General Meeting, ATNA Qld, 22 Oct. 1947.
159 Minutes of Annual Meeting, ATNA Qld, 22 Jul. 1949.
160 'Unity or Disunity in the Nursing Profession?' *ANJ*, Jan. 1949, p. 3.

Chapter 10

1 Minutes of Council Meeting, ATNA Qld, 10 Aug. & 3 Sep. 1947.
2 ibid. 8 Jan. 1946 & 8 Nov. 1949.
3 Gregory, *A Tradition of Care*, p. 75.
4 Minutes of Council Meeting, ATNA Qld, 10 Feb. 1948.
5 Miss Abbott's Report to Annual Meeting, Minutes of Annual General Meeting, ATNA Qld, 29 Jul. 1948.
6 Minutes of Council Meeting, ATNA Qld, 14 Sep. 1948, 12 Apr. & 27 May 1949.
7 Gregory, *A Tradition of Care*, p. 98.
8 Muriel K. Doherty, 'An Australian College of Nursing', *ANJ*, Jan. 1947, p. 6.
9 Minutes of Council Meeting, ATNA Qld, 14 May 1946.
10 ibid. 13 Aug. 1946.
11 Mary Dickenson & Glenda Law, 'Nurses in the National Health Scheme', *Australian Quarterly*, 46, 1, Mar. 1974, p. 36 & Gregory, *A Tradition of Care*, p. 104.
12 'History of Nursing Organizations in Australia', *ANJ*, Mar. 1949, p. 46.
13 Gregory, *A Tradition of Care*, p. 96.
14 'Australian Nursing Federation', *ANJ*, Feb.–Mar. 1946, p. 42.
15 Trembath & Hellier, *All Care and Responsibility*, pp. 126, 142–145.

16 Beatrice Roberts & A.L. Hart, 'What is the Trained Nurses' Guild?' *ANJ*, Dec. 1948, p. 262.
17 Minutes of Council Meeting, ATNA Qld, 3 Sep. 1947.
18 Dickenson, *An Unsentimental Union*, pp. 115–119.
19 Virginia Henderson, *Basic Principles of Nursing Care*, 2nd edn, International Council of Nurses, New York, 1969, p. 4.
20 Carol Fox, 'Antecedents of the 1986 Victorian Nurses' Strike', *Journal of Industrial Relations*, 32, 4, Dec. 1990, pp 465–487; Heather Gardner & Brigid McCoppin, 'The Politicisation of Australian Nurses: Victoria 1984–1986', *Politics*, 22, 1, May 1987, pp 19–34.
21 See for instance Sexton, *The New Nightingales*; the debate in the *Nursing Mirror* and *Nursing Times* in 1979, for example Anon., 'GNC: A reminder that the patient must come first', *Nursing Mirror*, 9 Aug. 1979, p. 6; Anthony Carr, 'Let strikers suffer the consequences', *Nursing Mirror*, 13 Sep. 1979, p. 12; Anthony Carr, 'Professional industrial action?', *Nursing Times*, 8 Feb. 1979, pp 224–225.
22 C.E. Grant, 'The A.T.N.A. and What It Stands For', *ANJ*, Apr. 1951, p. 57.
23 *QPD*, vol. CLXXXV, 1945, p. 916.

APPENDIX

Australasian Trained Nurses' Association, Queensland Branch, office-bearers, 1904 to 1950

Presidents

1904–1910	Dr Ernest Sandford Jackson (Patron from 1910 until his death in 1938)
1910–1912	Dr A.C.F. Halford
1912–1923	Dr John Barr McLean
1923–1934	Dr Alexander Hammett Marks (Patron from 1939)
1934–1941	Dr R.G. Quinn
1941–1943	Dr G.P. Dixon
1943–1948	Miss Eunice Muriel Paton
1948–1950	Miss Doris Bardsley

Vice-presidents

1904–1910, 1912–1937	Dr A.C.F. Halford
1904–1905	Miss Mary Elizabeth Weedon
1905–1910	Miss Lesa Caroline Marks
1910–1912	Dr George Herbert Hopkins
1910–1918	Mrs Marshall
1918–1921	Miss Fitzgerald
1921–1924	Mrs A. Dudley
1924–1926	Dr John Barr McLean
1933–1934	Miss Eunice Muriel Paten
1934–1939	Dr A.H. Marks
1937–1943	Miss Florence Chatfield (Patroness from 1945)
1939–1943	Miss Eunice Muriel Paten

1943–1950 Miss Christense Sorensen
1944–1945 Miss K.M. Caldwell
1945–1946 Miss Joan Stevenson Abbott
1946–1948 Miss Doris Bardsley
1948–1949 Miss C. Heeney
1949–1950 Miss Rosa Anna Micheli

Secretaries

1904–1912 Dr John Barr McLean
1904–1905 Miss Appleton
1905–1907 Miss Jane Bell
1907–1914 Miss Emily Louisa Hunter
1912–1935 Miss Florence Chatfield
1918–1921 Miss M. A. MacDonald
1921–1922 Miss Nelly M. Ingarfield
1922–1933 Miss Ellen Barron
1933–1946 Miss Doris Bardsley
1935–1937 Miss Joan Stevenson Abbott
1937–1942 Miss E. Scanlan
1943–1950 Miss Flora Cowan R. Moodie
1946–1949 Miss Rosa Anna Micheli
1949–1950 Miss C.E. Falconer

Treasurers

1904–1923 Dr Page
1924–1926 Dr Thomson Leckie
1926–1928 Dr Neville Graham Sutton
1928–1934 Dr R.G. Quinn
1934–1940 Dr Kenneth Wilson
1940–1943 Dr A.E. Paterson
1943–1945 Dr Kenneth Wilson
1945–1950 Miss W. Payne

Councillors

Unless specified all councillors are nurses representing general nurses. All councillors were addressed as 'Miss' unless otherwise specified.

* Doctors representing general nurses.
** Doctors representing midwifery nurses (obstetric nurses from 1945).
\# Nurses representing midwifery nurses.

From 1922 these categories changed to councillors representing general nurses and councillors representing midwifery nurses.
Councillor representing mental nurses.
Councillor representing child welfare nurses.

Joan Stevenson Abbott	1932–1935, 1943–1945, 1948–1950
Dr R.M. Allan**	1923–1926
E.H. Allen	1943–1950
Gertrude Jessie Andrews	1919–1924
Linda Gertrude Andrews	1937–1940
Appleton	1905–1909
Dr F. Arden*	1940–1941
C. Axelsen	1924–1925
I.M. Axelsen	1919–1920, 1925–1936
Doris Bardsley	1924–1933
Ellen Barron	1921–1922
Jane Bell	1904
L. Bell	1921–1940
Best	1906–1907
Alice Adelaide Billing	1930–1933
Bishop	1906–1910, 1915–1916, 1918–1921
Dr Eleanor Elizabeth Bourne*	1905–1907 and ** 1907–1911
Miss Effie Jane Bourne	1915–1916, 1918–1933
Violet McDonnell Bradford	1919–1928
Dr Brockway*	1904–1905
Brown#	1904–1907
R. Brown	1926–1928
J.W. Burgess ###	1945–1946
Dr Graham Butler**	1911–1923
Butterworth	1921–1922
Dr Byrne*	1908–1910
K.M. Caldwell	1932–1944, 1945–1946
Campbell	1911–1912
Capner#	1907–1913
Dr Carvosso*	1905–1906, 1908–1909
Florence Chatfield	1904–1912, 1935–1937
V. Clarke	1905–1906
Dr Clatworthy*	1907–1912
S.V. Coker	1936–1937
M. Cormack	1948–1950
Kathleen Amy Cowen	1932–1943
Dr D. Gifford Croll*	1924–1945
	1947–1950, medical member (adviser)
Crosse	1904–1908
E.M. Crowe	1944–1945

B.I. Cutting	1940–1941
U.N. Davidson	1923–1926
Dr Espie Dods*	1907–1931
Donaldson	1906–1910
Doyle#	1905–1906
Mrs Dudley	1918–1921
Jessie Frances Dunbar	1944–1948
T.J. Dunne	1922–1931
Durdin	1904
Dr P.A. Earnshaw*	1924–1926
E.M. Egger	1947–1948, # 1940–1947, 1948–1949
Ada England#	1926–1940
Everett	1910–1914, 1915–1916, 1918–1923
Sister Faith	1931–1939
C.E. Falconer	1944–1949
Faulkiner	1912–1914, 1918–1922
F. Fetherstonhaugh#	1913–1938
Fitzgerald	1904–1918
F. Fountain	1947–1949
E.M. Francis	1930–1942
Dr Gibson*	1904–1907
M. Glasgow	1946–1948
K. Gormley##	1928–1932
C.E.N. Grant	1944–1946
Florence Ethel Green	1931–1932
Dr Harding*	1909–1918
G.A. Harkness	1933–1944, 1945–1950
Julia Mary Hart	1926–1937
B. Hayes	1948–1949, ### 1949–1950
K. Heaven#	1938–1942
C.M. Heeney##	1932–1949
W.I. Hill	1949–1950
Holmes	1915–1916, 1918–1919
Dr Hopkins*	1906–1910, 1912–1921
Violet Ruby Hoskins	1937–1943, 1945–1947, * 1943–1945, 1947–1948
Nelly M. Ingarfield	1908–1919, 1920–1921, 1922–1928
Agnes Isambert	1912–1919
C.A. Johnson	1942–1947
H. Johnson	1940–1947, 1949–1950
R.J. Langford	1922–1926
Florence Louise Kilgour	1941–1948
Dr T. Leckie*	1922–1924
Dr Love**	1904–1907
M.A. MacDonald	1908–1918

Beatrice L. Macnish	1904–1908
Magee	1914–1918
Dr Charles Ferdinand Marks*	1904–1907
Dr Alexander Hammett Marks*	1922–1923
Miss Lesa Caroline Marks	1904–1905, 1910–1922
Mrs Marshall	1904–1910
E. McCorkindale#	1949–1950
Dr A.J. McDonnell*	1914–1923
R. McDougall	1949–1950
J. McHutchinson	1947–1949
Dr J.B. McLean*	1923–1924
McPherson	1904–1906
McStay#	1918–1922
Mee	1914–1918
Rosa Anna Micheli	1937–1945, ### 1945–1947
Flora Cowan R. Moodie#	1942–1943
Doris Mary Morley	1928–1932, 1946–1948
Munro	1909–1910
L. Munro#	1908–1910
Oakes	1910–1912
C. O'Connor	1945–1947
E. Ogilivie	1913–1930
Grace Pampling	1904–1921
Pate#	1911–1919
Eunice M. Paten	1919–1933, 1934–1939
W. Payne	1940–1945
Amy Perry	1909–1918
P. Price	1947–1948
Dr Aubrey David Dick Pye*	1932–1945
	1947–1950, medical member (adviser)
Dr R.G. Quinn	1926–1928
Ralston	1913–1914, 1918–1919
D. Ralston	1948–1950
Dr A.C. Roper*	1931–1932
E. Scanlan	1936–1937
Schmidt	1909–1913
Ivy Bartz Schultz	1948–1949
Lucy Scott#	1904–1905, 1906–1908
Sherlock#	1910–1911
R.M. Simpson	1928–1933
E. Sinclair	1947–1948
C. Smith	1904–1905
V. Smith	1949–1950
Christense Sorensen	1923–1943
Mrs A. Stewart	1907–1908

Dr Joyce Stobo	1931–1945 1947–1950, medical member (adviser)
E. Sully	1942–1944
Dr Sutton*	1904–1908
Dr N.G. Sutton*	1924–1926, 1928–1945, 1947–1950, medical member (adviser)
N.I. Thompson	1932–1935
Mrs Trundle	1904–1909
Dr Turner*	1904–1905
Dr Voss*	1906–1923
A.Waldie	1904–1906, 1908–1909
M.Waldie	1906–1907, 1908–1910
Waldie	1907–1908
Mary Elizabeth Weedon	1905–1906
Whipham	1908–1909
A.E. Wilcox	1933–1936
Williams	1910–1918, 1919–1923
Grace Margaret Wilson	1918–1919
Dr Kenneth Wilson**	1930–1938

The association with the Brisbane General Hospital is evident, especially in the early years of the ATNA in Queensland. Mary Weedon was Head Nurse (1885–1890) as was Lesa Marks (1893–1904). Matrons involved in the ATNA were Emily Hunter (1906–1914), Grace Wilson (1914), Effie Jane Bourne (1914–1928), Christense Sorensen (1928–1951) and Adelaide Billing (1952–1957). Joan Abbott, Doris Morley, W. Hill and Bartz Schultz held the position of Head of the School of Nursing. Many others such as Florence Chatfield and Eunice Paten trained at the hospital. Medical Superintendents of the Brisbane General Hospital were also actively involved in the ATNA. E. Sandford Jackson was Medical Superintendent from 1886 to 1898, as was J.B. McLean (1904–1931) and A.D.D. Pye (1933–1967). Others such as Eleanour Bourne, C.F. Marks, A.H. Marks, G.H. Hopkins and Neville Sutton held various positions as resident and visiting medical practitioners.

Sources: Minutes of Annual General Meetings and Annual Reports, ATNA Qld; *ANJ*; ATNA files, QIC. In these sources given names were included only on rare occasions. As most of the nurses trained or worked at the Brisbane General Hospital, details of some of their given names have been gained from H. Gregory & C. Brazil, *Bearers of the Tradition: Nurses of The Royal Brisbane Hospital 1888–1993*, Boolarong, Brisbane, 1993. Details of doctors came from J. Tyrer, *History of the Brisbane Hospital and its Affiliates*, Boolarong, Brisbane, 1993.

Select bibliography

This bibliography lists the major sources used. A full list of primary sources that were consulted can be found in Glenda Strachan, 'The History of the Australasian Trained Nurses' Association, Queensland Branch, 1904 to 1950', PhD thesis, University of Queensland, 1992. In the endnotes full references are provided to archival files, newspaper and contemporary journal articles, parliamentary debates and papers and legislation and industrial commission records.

Official and unpublished sources

Archive material

Queensland State Archives: Home Office files, 1886–1930.
Australian Archives, Australian Capital Territory; Attorney-General's Department, Department of Defence and Department of Health, New South Wales; Department of Health, Victoria; Department of Labour and National Service. Files covered the period 1938–1946.

Trade union records

RANF Queensland and Queensland Nurses' Union: ATNA minutes, annual reports and associated papers, 1904–1960.
RANF New South Wales: ATNA minutes, annual reports and associated papers, 1899–1910.
RANF Victoria: ATNA and RANF minutes, annual reports and associated papers, 1904–1970.

Archives of Business and Labour, Australian National University: E83—RANF files.

Nurses' records

Graduate Nurses' Association Archive, Royal Brisbane Hospital.

Industrial commission records

Commonwealth Arbitration Reports.
Commonwealth Public Service Arbitration Reports.
Australian Industrial Relations Commission Registry, File 145, The Trained Nurses' Guild.
Queensland Industrial Commission, decisions, transcripts and associated papers relating to nurses' and other cases.
Industrial Relations Commission, Victoria, Registered Nurses Case, 1986 & 1989.

Government publications

Census of the Commonwealth of Australia, April 1911.
Commonwealth Parliamentary Debates, 1941–1944.
Queensland Government Gazette.
Queensland Parliamentary Debates, Papers and Votes and Proceedings.
New South Wales Parliamentary Debates.
Victorian Government Gazette.
Victorian Parliamentary Debates and Papers.

Theses

Costar, Brian J. 'Labor, Politics and Unemployment: Queensland during the Great Depression'. PhD thesis, University of Queensland, 1981.
Gardner, Margaret Elaine. 'Women Workers, Trade Union Government and Strategies: The New South Wales Nurses' Association and Teachers' Federation'. PhD thesis, University of New South Wales, 1984.
Strachan, Glenda Jean. 'The Brisbane General Strike of 1912'. BA(Hons) thesis, University of Queensland, 1972.
Strachan, Glenda Jean. 'The History of the Australasian Trained Nurses' Association, Queensland Branch, 1904 to 1950', PhD thesis, University of Queensland, 1992.

Books

Abel-Smith, Brian. A *History of the Nursing Profession*, Heinemann, London, 1960.
Alford, Katrina. *Production or Reproduction? An economic history of women in Australia, 1788–1850*, Oxford University Press, Melbourne, 1984.

Alford, Katrina & McLean, Michelle. *Partners or Parasites of Men? Women's Economic Status in Australia, Britain and Canada, 1850–1900*, Working Paper in Economic History no. 66, Australian National University, Canberra, 1986.

Anderson, George. *Fixation of Wages in Australia*, Macmillan, Melbourne, 1929.

Anon. *Nursing in South Australia: First Hundred Years 1837–1937*, reprinted with supplements of 1939–1945 and 1989, Nurses' Memorial Foundation of SA Incorporated, Adelaide, 1989.

Australian Bureau of Statistics. *Labour Statistics Australia, 1993*, catalogue no. 6101.0, Commonwealth Government, Canberra, 1994.

Barker, Marianne. *Nightingales in the Mud: The Digger Sisters of the Great War 1914–1918*, Allen & Unwin, Sydney, 1989.

Bevege, Margaret, James, Margaret & Shute, Carmel, eds. *Worth Her Salt: Women at work in Australia*, Hale & Iremonger, Sydney, 1982.

Bolton, G.C. & Joske, Prue. *History of Royal Perth Hospital*, University of Western Australia, Perth, 1982.

Bolton, Geoffrey. *The Oxford History of Australia: Volume 5: 1942–1988: The Middle Way*, Oxford University Press, Melbourne, 1990.

Boreham, Paul, Pemberton, Alec & Wilson, Paul, eds. *The Professions in Australia: A Critical Appraisal*, University of Queensland Press, Brisbane, 1976.

Branca, Patricia. *Silent Sisterhood: Middle Class Women in the Victorian Home*, Croom Helm, London, 1975.

Bray, Mark & Rimmer, Malcolm. *Delivering the Goods: A History of the Transport Workers' Union in New South Wales 1888–1986*, Allen & Unwin, Sydney, 1987.

Buckley, Ken. *The Amalgamated Engineers in Australia, 1852–1920*, Australian National University, Canberra, 1970.

Buckley, Ken & Wheelwright, Ted. *No Paradise for Workers: Capitalism and the Common People in Australia 1788–1914*, Oxford University Press, Melbourne, 1988.

Bullough, Vern L. & Bullough, Bonnie. 'Nursing as a Profession' in Stewart, Phyllis L. & Cantor, Muriel G., eds. *Varieties of Work*, Sage, Beverly Hills, 1982.

——*The Emergence of Modern Nursing*, 2nd edn, Macmillan, Toronto, 1969.

Burgmann, Verity & Lee, Jenny, eds. *A Most Valuable Acquisition: A People's History of Australia since 1788*, McPhee Gribble, Melbourne, 1988.

——*Constructing a Culture: A People's History of Australia since 1788*, McPhee Gribble, Melbourne, 1988.

Butlin, S.J. *War Economy 1939–1942*, Australian War Memorial, Canberra, 1955.

Butlin, S.J. & Schedvin, C.B., *War Economy 1942–1945*, Australian War Memorial, Canberra, 1977.

Castle, Josephine. *Nursing at the Wollongong Hospital 1926–1982*, University of Wollongong Press, Wollongong, 1984.

Chambers, Coral. *Lessons for Ladies: A social history of girls' education in Australasia 1870–1900*, Hale & Iremonger, Sydney, 1986.

Clarke, Eddie. *Female Teachers in Queensland State Schools: A History 1860–1983*, Department of Education, Brisbane, 1985.

Committee of Inquiry into Nursing. *Nursing in Queensland*, Royal Australian Nursing Federation (Queensland Branch), Brisbane, 1971.

Commonwealth Bureau of Census and Statistics. *Labour Report 1947*, Commonwealth Bureau of Census and Statistics, Canberra, 1948.

Cope, Zachary. *Six Disciples of Florence Nightingale*, Pitman Medical, London, 1961.

Curson, Peter & McCracken, Kevin. *Plague in Sydney: The Anatomy of an Epidemic*, New South Wales University Press, Sydney, 1989.

Curthoys, Ann & Merritt, John. *Better Dead Than Red: Australia's First Cold War: 1945–1959: Volume 2*, Allen & Unwin, Sydney, 1986.

Darian-Smith, Kate. *On the Home Front: Melbourne in Wartime 1939–1945*, Oxford University Press, Melbourne, 1990.

Davidson, Alastair. *The Invisible State: The Formation of the Australian State 1788–1901*, Cambridge University Press, Cambridge, 1991.

Davies, Celia, ed. *Rewriting Nursing History*, Croom Helm, London, 1980.

Davis, John. *Florence Nightingale, or the Heroine of the East*, Arthur Hall, Virtue, London, 1856.

Davison, Graeme, McCarty, J.W. & McLeary, Ailsa, eds. *Australians 1888*, Fairfax, Syme & Weldon, Sydney, 1987.

Department of Labour and National Service. *Equal Pay: Some Aspects of Australian and Overseas Practice*, 3rd edn, Department of Labour and National Service, Melbourne, 1968.

Diamond, Marion. 'The Nightingale Nurse: A Case Study in Victorian Values' in Debenham, Helen & Slinn, Warwick, eds. *Australasian Victorian Studies Association Conference Papers 1982*, University of Canterbury, Christchurch, 1983.

Dickenson, Mary. *Democracy in Trade Unions: Studies in Membership Participation and Control*, University of Queensland Press, Brisbane, 1982.

——*An Unsentimental Union: The NSW Nurses Association 1931–1992*, Hale & Iremonger, Sydney, 1993.

Dickey, Brian. *No Charity There: A Short History of Social Welfare in Australia*, Nelson, Melbourne, 1980.

Dock, Lavinia L., ed. *A History of Nursing: From the Earliest Times to the Present Day with Special Reference to the Work of the Past Thirty Years*, vols 3 & 4, G.P. Putnam's Sons, New York, 1907–1912.

Dolan, Josephine A. *Goodnow's History of Nursing*, 11th edn, W.B. Saunders, Philadelphia, 1963.

Donahue, M. Patricia. *Nursing: The Finest Art: An Illustrated History*, C.V. Mosby, St Louis, 1985.

Ehrenreich, Barbara & English, Deirdre. *Witches, Midwives and Nurses: A History of Women Healers*, 2nd edn, Feminist Press, New York, 1973.

Ellem, Bradon. *In Women's Hands? A History of Clothing Trades Unionism in Australia*, New South Wales University Press, Sydney, 1989.

Etzioni, Amitai, ed. *The Semi-Professions and Their Organization: Teachers, Nurses, Social Workers*, Free Press, New York, 1969.

Fitzgerald, Ross. *A History of Queensland from 1915 to the 1980s*, University of Queensland Press, Brisbane, 1984.

Fitzgerald, Ross & Thornton, Harold. *Labor in Queensland from the 1880s to 1988*, University of Queensland Press, Brisbane, 1989.

Flanagan, Lynda. *One Strong Voice: The Story of the American Nurses' Association*, Lowell, Kansas City, 1976.

Flanders, Allan. *Management and Unions*, Faber & Faber, London, 1970.

Ford, Bill & Plowman, David, eds. *Australian Unions: An Industrial Relations Perspective*, 2nd edn, Macmillan, Melbourne, 1989.

Frank, Charles Marie. *Foundations of Nursing*, 2nd edn, W.B. Saunders, Philadelphia, 1959.

Gamarnikow, Eva, 'Sexual division of labour: the case of nursing' in Kuhn, Annette & Wolpe, AnnMarie. *Feminism and Materialism: Women and Modes of Production*, Routledge & Kegan Paul, London, 1978.

Game, Ann & Pringle, Rosemary. *Gender at Work*, George Allen & Unwin, Sydney, 1983.

Gammage, Bill & Spearritt, Peter, eds. *Australians: 1938*, Fairfax, Syme & Weldon, Sydney, 1987.

Gibbney, H.J. & Smith, Ann G., eds. *A Biographical Register 1788–1939*, vols 1 & 2, Australian National University, Canberra, 1987.

Goodman, Rupert. *Queensland Nurses: Boer War to Vietnam*, Boolarong, Brisbane, 1985.

——*Secondary Education in Queensland, 1860–1960*, Australian National University, Canberra, 1968.

Gregory, Helen. *A Tradition of Care: A History of Nursing at the Royal Brisbane Hospital*, Boolarong, Brisbane, 1988.

Gregory, Helen & Brazil, Cecelia. *Bearers of the Tradition: Nurses of the Royal Brisbane Hospital 1888–1993*, Boolarong, Brisbane, 1993.

Grieve, Norma & Burns, Ailsa, eds. *Australian Women: New Feminist Perspectives*, Oxford University Press, Melbourne, 1986.

Hagan, Jim. *The History of the A.C.T.U.*, Longman Cheshire, Melbourne, 1981.

Hare, F. *The Cold-bath Treatment of Typhoid Fever*, Macmillan, London, 1898.

Hasluck, Paul. *The Government and the People 1939–1941*, Australian War Memorial, Canberra, 1952.

——*The Government and the People 1942–1945*, Australian War Memorial, Canberra, 1970.

Henderson, Virginia. *Basic Principles of Nursing Care*, 2nd edn, International Council of Nurses, New York, 1969.

Hicks, Neville. *'This Sin and Scandal': Australia's Population Debate 1891–1911*, Australian National University, Canberra, 1978.

Hobbs, Victoria. *But Westward Look: Nursing in Western Australia 1829–1979*, University of Western Australia Press, Perth, 1980.

Hutson, J. *Six Wage Concepts*, Amalgamated Engineering Union, Sydney, 1971.

Hyslop, Anthea. *Sovereign Remedies: A history of Ballarat Base Hospital 1850s–1980s*, Allen & Unwin, Sydney, 1989.

Inglis, K.S. *Hospital and Community: A History of The Royal Melbourne Hospital*, Melbourne University Press, Melbourne, 1958.

International Council of Nurses. *Congress Papers*, International Council of Nurses, London, 1937.

Johnson, Terence J. *Professions and Power*, Macmillan, London, 1972.

Kingston, Beverley. *The Oxford History of Australia: Volume 3: 1860–1900: Glad, Confident Morning*, Oxford University Press, Melbourne, 1988.

——*My Wife, My Daughter, and Poor Mary Ann: Women and Work in Australia*, Nelson, Melbourne, 1975.

Krause, Elliott A. *The Sociology of Occupations*, Little, Brown and Company, Boston, 1971.

Kyle, Noeline. *Her Natural Destiny: The Education of Women in New South Wales*, New South Wales University Press, Sydney, 1986.

Lagemann, Ellen Condliffe, ed. *Nursing History: New Perspectives, New Possibilities*, Teachers College, New York, 1983.

Lawler, Jocalyn. *Behind the Screens: Nursing, Somology, and the Problem of the Body*, Churchill Livingstone, Melbourne, 1991.

Lawson, Ronald. *Brisbane in the 1890s: A Study of an Australian Urban Society*, University of Queensland Press, Brisbane, 1973.

Longhurst, Robert. *In the Footsteps of the Mercies: A History of Nursing at the Mater Misericordiae Public Hospitals, Brisbane*, Mater Misericordiae Public Hospitals, Brisbane, 1992.

Louis, L.J. *Trade Unions and the Depression: A Study of Victoria 1930–1932*, Australian National University, Canberra, 1968.

Lumby, Judy. *Nursing: Reflecting on an Evolving Practice*, Deakin University, Geelong, 1991.

MacDonald, Isabel. 'The Organisation of the Registered Nurse' in International Council of Nurses. *Congress Papers 1937*, International Council of Nurses, London, 1937.

MacDonnell, Freda. *Miss Nightingale's Young Ladies: The Story of Lucy Osburn and Sydney Hospital*, Angus and Robertson, Sydney, 1970.

Macintyre, Stuart. *The Oxford History of Australia: Volume 4: 1901–1942: The Succeeding Age*, Oxford University Press, Melbourne, 1986.

——*Winners and Losers: The pursuit of social justice in Australian history*, Allen & Unwin, Sydney, 1985.

Mackinolty, Judy, ed. *The Wasted Years? Australia's Great Depression*, George Allen & Unwin, Sydney, 1981.

Mackinolty, Judy & Radi, Heather, eds. *In pursuit of justice: Australian women and the law 1788–1979*, Hale & Iremonger, Sydney, 1979.

Maggs, Christopher, ed. *Nursing History: The State of the Art*, Croom Helm, London, 1987.

Maggs, Christopher. *The Origins of General Nursing*, Croom Helm, London, 1983.

Matthews, Jill Julius. *Good and Mad Women: The historical construction of femininity in twentieth century Australia*, George Allen & Unwin, Sydney, 1984.

McMurchy, Megan, Oliver, Margot & Thornley, Jeni. *For Love or Money: A pictorial history of women and work in Australia*, Penguin, Melbourne, 1983.

Mellish, J.M. *A Basic History of Nursing*, 2nd edn, Butterworths, Durban, 1990.

Melosh, Barbara. *'The Physician's Hand': Work Culture and Conflict in American Nursing*, Temple University, Philadelphia, 1982.

Millerson, Geoffrey. *The Qualifying Associations: A Study in Professionalization*, Routledge & Kegan Paul, London, 1964.

Minchin, Maureen K. *Revolutions and Rosewater: The Evolution of Nurse Registration in Victoria 1923–1973*, Hart Hamer, Melbourne, 1975.

Mitchell, Ann M. *The Hospital South of the Yarra: A history of Alfred Hospital Melbourne from foundation to the nineteen-forties*, Alfred Hospital, Melbourne, 1977.

Mitchell, Bruce. *Teachers, Education and Politics: A History of Organizations of Public School Teachers in New South Wales*, University of Queensland Press, Brisbane, 1975.

Murphy, Denis. *Ken Laidlaw: A White Collar Union Leader*, Australian Bank Employees Union, Brisbane, 1979.

Nairn, Bede & Searle, Geoffrey, eds. *Australian Dictionary of Biography*, vols 7–11, Melbourne University Press, Melbourne, 1979–1988.

National Women's Consultative Council. *Pay Equity for Women in Australia*, Australian Government Publishing Service, Canberra, 1990.

Neff, Wanda F. *Victorian Working Women: An Historical and Literary Study of Women in British Industries and Professions 1832–1850*, Frank Cass, London, 1966.

Nolan, Cynthia. *A Bride for St Thomas*, Constable, London, 1970.

Nutting, M. Adelaide & Dock, Lavinia L. *A History of Nursing: The Evolution of Nursing Systems from the Earliest Times to the Foundations of the First English and American Training Schools for Nurses*, vols 1 & 2, G.P. Putnam's Sons, New York, 1907–1912.

Offen, Karen, Pierson, Ruth Roach & Rendall, Jane, eds. *Writing Women's History: International Perspectives*, Indiana University, Bloomington, 1991.

Parker, Neville & Pearn, John, eds. *Ernest Sandford Jackson: The Life and Times of a Pioneer Australian Surgeon*, Australian Medical Association Queensland Branch, Brisbane, 1987.

Patmore, Greg. *Australian Labour History*, Longman Cheshire, Melbourne, 1991.

Patrick, Ross. *A History of Health & Medicine in Queensland 1824–1960*, University of Queensland Press, Brisbane, 1987.

——*The Royal Women's Hospital, Brisbane—The First Fifty Years*, Boolarong, Brisbane, 1988.

Pavey, Agnes E. *The Story of the Growth of Nursing as an Art, a Vocation, and a Profession*, 5th edn, Faber & Faber, London, 1959.

Punch, Peter. *Guidebook to Australian Industrial Law*, 4th edn, CCH, Sydney, 1984.

Reiger, Kerreen M. *The disenchantment of the home: Modernizing the Australian family 1880–1940*, Oxford University Press, Melbourne, 1985.

Reverby, Susan M. *Ordered to Care: The dilemma of American nursing, 1850–1945*, Cambridge University Press, Cambridge, 1987.

Rickard, John. *Class and Politics: New South Wales, Victoria and the Early Commonwealth, 1890–1910*, Australian National University Press, Canberra, 1976.

Roe, Jill, ed. *Social Policy in Australia: Some Perspectives 1901–1975*, Cassell, Sydney, 1976.

Rosser, Sue V. *Feminism within the Science and Health Care Professions: Overcoming Resistance*, Pergamon, Oxford, 1988.

Rowbotham, Judith. *Good Girls Make Good Wives: Guidance for Girls in Victorian Fiction*, Basil Blackwell, Oxford, 1989.

Ryan, Edna. *Two-thirds of a Man: Women & Arbitration in New South Wales 1902–08*, Hale & Iremonger, Sydney, 1984.

Ryan, Edna & Conlon, Anne. *Gentle Invaders: Australian Women at Work*, 2nd edn, Penguin, Melbourne, 1989.

Schultz, Bartz. *A Tapestry of Service: The Evolution of Nursing in Australia: Volume I: Foundation to Federation 1788–1900*, Churchill Livingstone, Melbourne, 1991.

Secondary Industries Division, Ministry of Post-War Reconstruction. *Australian Secondary Industry: The Demand for Female Labour: A Brief Study*, Central Drawing Office, Melbourne, 1947.

Sexton, Patricia Cayo. *The New Nightingales: Hospital Workers, Unions, New Women's Issues*, Enquiry, New York, 1981.

Seymer, Lucy Ridgely. *A General History of Nursing*, 4th edn, Faber & Faber, London, 1957.

Sheridan, Tom. *Division of Labour: Industrial Relations in the Chifley Years, 1945–1949*, Oxford University Press, Melbourne, 1989.

——*Mindful Militants: The Amalgamated Engineering Union in Australia 1920–1972*, Cambridge University Press, Cambridge, 1975.

Shryock, Richard H. *The History of Nursing: An Interpretation of the Social and Medical Factors Involved*, W.B. Saunders, Philadelphia, 1959.

Smith, F.B. *Florence Nightingale: Reputation and Power*, Croom Helm, London, 1982.

——*The People's Health, 1830–1910*, Croom Helm, London, 1979.

Spaull, Andrew & Sullivan, Martin. *A History of the Queensland Teachers' Union*, Allen & Unwin, Sydney, 1989.

Stacey, Margaret, Reid, Margaret, Heath, Christian & Dingwall, Robert, eds. *Health and the Division of Labour*, Croom Helm, London, 1977.

Starr, Paul. *The Social Transformation of American Medicine*, Basic Books, New York, 1982.

Summers, Anne. *Damned Whores and God's Police: The Colonization of Women in Australia*, Penguin, Melbourne, 1975.

Summers, H.J. *They Crossed the River: The Founding of the Mater Misericordiae Hospital, Brisbane, by the Sisters of Mercy*, University of Queensland Press, Brisbane, 1979.

Taperell, Kathleen, Fox, Carol & Roberts, Margaret. *Sexism in Public Service: The employment of women in Australian Government Administration*, Australian Government Publishing Service, Canberra, 1975.

Taylor, Sandra & Henry, Miriam, eds. *Battlers and Bluestockings: Women's Place in Australian Education*, Australian College of Education, Canberra, 1989.

Trembath, Richard & Hellier, Donna. *All Care and Responsibility: A History of Nursing in Victoria 1850–1934*, Florence Nightingale Committee, Melbourne, 1987.

Turner, Bryan S. *Medical Power and Social Knowledge*, Sage, London, 1987.

Twaddle, Andrew C. & Hessler, Richard M. *A Sociology of Health*, C.V. Mosby, Saint Louis, 1977.

Tyrer, John. *History of the Brisbane Hospital and its Affiliates*, Boolarong, Brisbane, 1993.

Vamplew, Wray, ed. *Australians: Historical Statistics*, Fairfax, Syme & Weldon, Sydney, 1987.

Vicinus, Martha. *Independent Women: Work and Community for Single Women 1850–1920*, Virago, London, 1985.

Vicinus, Martha, ed. *A Widening Sphere: Changing Roles of Victorian Women*, Methuen, London, 1977.

——*Suffer and Be Still: Women in the Victorian Age*, Methuen, London, 1972.

Walby, Sylvia. *Patriarchy at Work: Patriarchal and Capitalist Relations in Employment*, Polity, Oxford, 1986.

Walker, Allan S. *Medical Services of the R.A.N. and R.A.A.F.*, Australian War Memorial, Canberra, 1961.

——Middle East and Far East, Australian War Memorial, Canberra, 1953.
——*The Island Campaigns*, Australian War Memorial, Canberra, 1957.
Watson, J. Frederick. The History of the Sydney Hospital from 1811 to 1911, W.A. Gullick, Sydney, 1911.
White, Ruth. *Report to accompany the annotated bibliography on the role of the nurse in Australia*, University of New South Wales Tertiary Education Research Centre, Sydney, 1972.
Whitehouse, Gillian & Wiltshire, Kenneth. *The History of the Queensland Professional Officers' Association*, Royal Australian Institute of Public Administration, Brisbane, 1987.
Willis, Evan. *Medical Dominance: The division of labour in Australian health care*, George Allen & Unwin, Sydney, 1983.
Windschuttle, Elizabeth, ed. *Women, Class and History: Feminist Perspectives on Australia 1788–1978*, Fontana, Melbourne, 1980.
Woodham-Smith, Cecil. *Florence Nightingale 1820–1910*, McGraw-Hill, New York, 1951.
Wurth, Wallace C. *Control of Manpower in Australia: A General Review of the Administration of Man-Power Directorate, February, 1942–September, 1944*, Government Printer, Sydney, c.1944.

Journal articles

Aikens, Charlotte A. 'The Registration Movement: Its Past and Its Future', *The Trained Nurse and Hospital Review*, vol. 44, no. 1, Jan. 1910, pp. 1–11.
Allport, Carolyn. 'Left off the Agenda: Women, Reconstruction and New Order Housing', *Labour History*, no. 46, May 1984, pp. 1–20.
Allport, Karin. 'Equal pay for equal work? Of course. But how about equal pay for comparable work? Should housepainters make more than nurses?' *Across the Board*, vol. 17, no. 10, Oct. 1980, pp. 22–25.
Anon. 'Hours of Hospital Nurses', *Nursing Record & Hospital World*, 12 Sep. 1896, pp. 213–215.
Anon. 'Nursing Politics in New South Wales', *Nursing Record and Hospital World*, 16 Oct. 1897, pp. 313–315.
Anon. 'The Nurse—Laborer or Professional?' *The Modern Hospital*, vol. 8, no. 4, Apr. 1917, p. 269.
Anon. 'Training School for Nurses', *Australian Medical Journal*, 15 Nov. 1889, pp. 506–508.
Bacon, Asa S. 'Nurses and Factory Labor', *The Modern Hospital*, vol. 8, Apr. 1917, p. 299.
Baumgart, Alice & Kirkwood, R. 'Social reform versus education reform: university nursing education in Canada, 1919–1960', *Journal of Advanced Nursing*, vol. 15, no. 5, May 1990, pp. 510–516.
Baxter, Janeen. 'Gender and Class Analysis: The Position of Women in the Class Structure', *Australian and New Zealand Journal of Sociology*, vol. 24, no. 1, Mar. 1988, pp. 106–123.

Bennett, Laura. 'Equal pay and comparable worth and the Australian Conciliation and Arbitration Commission', *Journal of Industrial Relations*, vol. 30, no. 4, Dec. 1988, pp. 533–545.

——'Legal Intervention and the Female Workforce: The Australian Conciliation and Arbitration Court 1907–1921', *International Journal of the Sociology of Law*, vol. 12, no. 1, 1984, pp. 23–36.

——'The Construction of Skill: Craft Unions, Women Workers and the Conciliation and Arbitration Court', *Law in Context*, vol. 2, no. 1, 1984, pp. 118–132.

Black, Laurel. 'Social Democracy and Full Employment: The Australian White Paper, 1945', *Labour History*, no. 46, May 1984, pp. 34–51.

Broom, L. & Smith, J.H. 'Bridging Occupations', *British Journal of Sociology*, vol. 45, no. 4, Dec. 1963, pp. 321–334.

Brumberg, Joan Jacobs & Tomes, Nancy. 'Women in the Professions: A Research Agenda for American Historians', *Reviews in American History*, no. 10, Jun. 1982, pp. 275–296.

Bunting, Sheila & Campbell, Jacquelyn C. 'Feminism and nursing: Historical perspectives', *Advances in Nursing Science*, vol. 12, no. 4, Jul. 1990, pp. 11–24.

Bush, Mercia. 'Nursing as a Feminist Issue', *The Lamp*, Apr. 1981, pp. 25–29.

Church, Olga Maranjian. 'Historiography in Nursing Research', *Western Journal of Nursing Research*, vol. 9, no. 2, May 1987, pp. 275–279.

Clark, Mary Dormady. 'The Historical Basis for Nursing's Troubled Self-Image', *AAOHN Journal*, vol. 34, no. 4, Apr. 1986, pp. 168–170.

Colliere, Marie Francoise. 'Invisible care and invisible women as health-care providers', *International Journal of Nursing Studies*, vol. 23, no. 2, 1986, pp. 95–112.

Crew, Jennifer. 'Women's Wages in Britain and Australia during the First World War', *Labour History*, no. 57, Nov. 1989, pp. 27–43.

——'Women's Work and Wages—Britain and Australia Pre 1914', *Journal of Australian Studies*, no. 21, Nov. 1987, pp. 60–79.

Crisp, Helen. 'Women in Munitions', *Australian Quarterly*, vol. 13, no. 3, Sep. 1941, pp. 71–76.

Crowder, E. 'Historical Perspectives of Nursing's Professionalism', *Occupational Health Nursing*, vol. 33, no. 4, Apr. 1985, pp. 184–190.

Davies, Celia. 'Continuities in the development of hospital nursing in Britain', *Journal of Advanced Nursing*, vol. 2, 1977, pp. 479–493.

——'The Regulation of Nursing Work: An Historical Comparison of Britain and the U.S.A.', *Research in the Sociology of Health Care*, vol. 2, 1982, pp. 121–160.

——'Where next for nursing history?' *Nursing Times*, vol. 76, no. 21, 22 May 1980, pp. 920–922.

Deacon, Desley. 'Taylorism in the Home: The Medical Profession, the Infant Welfare Movement and the Deskilling of Women', *Australian and New Zealand Journal of Sociology*, vol. 21, no. 2, Jul. 1985, pp. 161–173.

Dickenson, Mary. 'The Nursing Profession as a Pressure Group', *Australian Journal of Social Issues*, vol. 11, no. 2, May 1976, pp. 88–98.

Dickenson, Mary & Law, Glenda. 'Nurses in the National Health Scheme', *Australian Quarterly*, vol. 46, no. 1, Mar. 1974, pp. 29–41.

Dickey, Brian. 'Health and the State in Australia, 1788–1977', *Journal of Australian Studies*, no. 2, Nov. 1977, pp. 50–63.

——'The Sick Poor in N.S.W., 1840–1880: Colonial Practice in an Amateur Age', *Journal of the Royal Australian Historical Society*, vol. 59, no. 1, Mar. 1973, pp. 16–30.

Dock, Lavinia L. 'Status of the Nurse in the Working World', *British Journal of Nursing*, 3 Jan. 1914, pp. 4–6.

Evans, E.P. 'Nursing in Australia', *International Nursing Review*, vol. 12, 1936, pp. 260–264.

Ewers, Dora. 'The History of Home Economics in New South Wales Schools', *Journal of the Home Economics Association of Australia*, vol. 1, no. 1, May 1969, pp. 14–29.

Fickeissen, Janet L. 'Lobbying for Registration Laws: Letters from the Past', *Journal of Nursing History*, vol. 1, no. 2, Apr. 1986, pp. 12–19.

Fox, Carol. 'Antecedents of the 1986 Victorian Nurses' Strike', *Journal of Industrial Relations*, vol. 32, no. 4, Dec. 1990, pp. 465–487.

Gardner, Heather & McCoppin, Brigid. 'The Politicisation of Australian Nurses: Victoria 1984–1986', *Politics*, vol. 22, no. 1, May 1987, pp. 19–34.

Geister, Janet M. 'Hearsay and Facts in Private Duty', *American Journal of Nursing*, vol. 26, no. 7, Jul. 1926, pp. 515–528.

Gray, David E. 'Attitudinal Militancy Amongst Australian Nurses', *Australian Journal of Social Issues*, vol. 19, no. 2, May 1984, pp. 125–133.

Hardy, Leslie & Rafferty, Anne Marie. 'Nursing and History', *Nursing Times*, vol. 78, no. 37, 15 Sep. 1982, pp. 1564–1565.

Hendricx, Betty. 'Social and Political Attitudes of Women Teachers In Queensland State Primary Schools 1875–1911', *Refractory Girl*, no. 4, Spring 1973, pp. 18–22.

Hewitt, Nancy A. 'Beyond the search for sisterhood: American women's history in the 1980s', *Social History*, vol. 10, no. 3, Oct. 1985, pp. 299–321.

Hunter, Rosemary. 'Women Workers and Federal Industrial Law: From *Harvester* to Comparable Worth', *Australian Journal of Labour Law*, vol. 1, no. 2, Sep. 1988, pp. 147–172.

Hunter, Thelma. 'Industrial Courts and Women's Wages in Australia', *Economic Record*, vol. 38, no. 84, Dec. 1962, pp. 438–451.

——'Some Factors Which Determine the Distribution of the Female Work Force', *Journal of Industrial Relations*, vol. 4, no. 2, Oct. 1962, pp. 108–119.

James, Janet Wilson. 'Writing and Rewriting Nursing History: A Review Essay', *Bulletin of the History of Medicine*, no. 58, Winter 1984, pp. 568–584.

Johnson, Penelope. 'Gender, Class and Work: The Council of Action for Equal Pay and the Equal Pay Campaign in Australia During World War II', *Labour History*, no. 50, May 1986, pp. 132–146.

Keneley, Monica. 'Handmaidens of Medicine: Working Conditions for Nurses in Late Nineteenth Century Victoria', *Journal of Australian Studies*, no. 22, May 1988, pp. 57–68.

Kennedy, Sally. 'Useful and Expendable: Women Teachers in Western Australia in the 1920s and 1930s', *Labour History*, no. 44, May 1983, pp. 18–26.

Lee, Jenny. 'A Redivision of Labour: Victoria's Wages Boards in Action, 1896–1903', *Historical Studies*, vol. 22, no. 88, Apr. 1987, pp. 352–372.

Lewis, Milton & MacLeod, Roy. 'Medical Politics and the Professionalisation of Medicine in New South Wales, 1850–1901', *Journal of Australian Studies*, no. 22, May 1988, pp. 69–82.

Lynagh, Joan E. & Fagin, Claire M. 'Nursing Comes of Age', *Image*, vol. 20, no. 4, Winter 1988, pp. 184–190.

Macarthy, P. G. 'Wages for Unskilled Work, and Margins for Skill, Australia, 1901–21', *Australian Economic History*, vol. 12, no. 2, Sep. 1972, pp. 142–160.

——'Wages in Australia, 1891 to 1914', *Australian Economic History Review*, vol. 10, no. 1, Mar. 1970, pp. 56–76.

MacDonald, Isabel. 'Nursing Progress in the Nineteenth Century', *The Nursing Record and Hospital World*, 29 Dec. 1900, pp. 512–518.

Matthews, Jill. 'Education for Femininity: Domestic Arts Education in South Australia', *Labour History*, no. 45, Nov. 1983, pp. 30–53.

——'Feminist History', *Labour History*, no. 50, May 1986, pp. 147–153.

Matthews, Mr Justice. 'A History of Industrial Law in Queensland with a Summary of the Provisions of the Various Statutes', *Journal of the Historical Society of Queensland*, vol. 4, 1949, pp. 150–181.

McCawley, Thomas William. 'Arbitration and Conciliation: Industrial Arbitration', *Queensland Industrial Gazette*, Aug. 1924, pp. 482–510.

——'Industrial Arbitration in Queensland', *International Labour Review*, vol. 5, Mar. 1922, pp. 385–409.

McGahey, Susan B. 'The Nursing Organisations in the Australasian Commonwealth', *The Nursing Record & Hospital World*, 21 Dec. 1901, pp. 494–497.

McGrath, E.C. 'The Future of Women In Industry', *Australian Quarterly*, vol. 15, no. 2, Jun. 1943, pp. 39–45.

McGuire, L. 'Surgical History of the Royal Brisbane Hospital', *Proceedings of the Division of Surgery Royal Brisbane Hospital*, 1985, pp. 6–15.

——'Surgical History of the Royal Brisbane Hospital—1931–1967', *Proceedings of the Division of Surgery Royal Brisbane Hospital*, 1987, pp. 5–14.

McManamny, Sally. 'Nurses' Work, Nurses' Worth', *Arena*, no. 77, 1986, pp. 119–128.

Meredith, Lesley. 'Anne Conlon Memorial Lecture 1986—Working Our Way to the Bottom: Women and Nursing', *Labour History*, no. 52, May 1987, pp. 96–102.

Nichol, W. 'Medicine and the Labour Movement in New South Wales, 1788–1850', *Labour History*, no. 49, Nov. 1985, pp. 19–37.

Oakley, Ann. 'What Price Professionalism? The Importance of Being a Nurse', *Nursing Times*, vol. 80, no. 50, 12 Dec. 1984, pp. 24–27.

Parsons, Margaret. 'The Profession in a Class by Itself', *Nursing Outlook*, vol. 34, no. 6, Nov.–Dec. 1986, pp. 270–275.

Power, Margaret. 'The Making of a Woman's Occupation', *Hecate*, vol. 1, no. 2, Jul. 1975, pp. 25–34.

——'The Wages of Sex', *Australian Quarterly*, vol. 46, no. 1, Mar. 1974, pp. 2–14.

——'Woman's Work Is Never Done—by Men: A Socio-Economic Model of Sex-Typing in Occupations', *Journal of Industrial Relations*, vol. 17, no. 3, Sep. 1975, pp. 225–239.

Reekie, Gail. 'Industrial Action by Women Workers in Western Australia during World War II', *Labour History*, no. 49, Nov. 1985, pp. 75–82.

——'Women's Responses to War Work in Western Australia 1942–1946', *Studies in Western Australian History*, no. 7, Dec. 1983, pp. 46–67.

Reverby, Susan. 'A Caring Dilemma: Womanhood and Nursing in Historical Perspective', *Nursing Research*, vol. 36, no. 1, Jan.–Feb. 1987, pp. 5–11.

Ryan, Edna. 'Equal pay, comparable worth and the central wage fixing system', *Australian Feminist Studies*, no. 6, Autumn 1988, pp. 7–15.

Sheridan, Tom. 'Planners and the Australian Labour Market 1945–1949', *Labour History*, no. 53, Nov. 1987, pp. 99–113.

Spearritt, Katie. 'The Market for Marriage in Colonial Queensland', *Hecate*, vol. 16, no. 1/2, 1990, pp. 23–42.

Strachan, Glenda. ' "A good nurse cannot be bought with money": The Development of the Professional and Industrial Roles of the Nursing Organization in Queensland, Australia, 1904–1950', *Nursing History Review*, no. 3, 1995, pp. 235–256.

——'Sacred Office, Trade or Profession? The Dilemma of Nurses' Involvement in Industrial Activities in Queensland, 1900 to 1950', *Labour History*, no. 61, Nov. 1991, pp. 147–163.

Sykes, E.I. 'The Queensland System of Industrial Relations', *Journal of Industrial Relations*, vol. 2, no. 1, Apr. 1960, pp. 62–65.

Thomson, D.C. 'Commonwealth Arbitration Powers and the Hospital's Wage Structure', *Hospital Administration*, vol. 6, Jul. 1958, pp. 29, 47–50.

Turner, Bryan S. 'The Vocabulary of Complaints: Nursing, Professionalism and Job Context', *Australian and New Zealand Journal of Sociology*, vol. 22, no. 3, Nov. 1986, pp. 368–386.

Wagner, David. 'The Proletarianization of Nursing in the United States, 1932–1946', *International Journal of Health Services*, vol. 10, no. 2, 1980, pp. 271–290.

Whelan, Dominica. 'Women and the Arbitration System', *Journal of Australian Political Economy*, no. 4, Mar. 1979, pp. 54–60.

Williamson, Noeline. 'The Employment of Female Teachers in the Small Bush Schools of New South Wales, 1880–1890: A Case of Stay Bushed or Stay Home'. *Labour History*, 43, Nov. 1982, pp. 1–12.

——'The Feminization of Teaching in New South Wales: A Historical Perspective', *Australian Journal of Education*, vol. 27, no. 1, 1983, pp. 33–44.

Willis, Evan. 'Sister Elizabeth Kenny and the Evolution of the Occupational Division of Labour in Health Care', *Australian and New Zealand Journal of Sociology*, vol. 15, no. 3, Nov. 1979, pp. 30–38.

INDEX